KEY TOPICS IN

ACCIDENT AND EME

MEDICINE

SECOND EDITION

The KEY TOPICS Series

Advisors:

T.M. Craft *Department of Anaesthesia and Intensive Care, Royal United Hospital, Bath, UK*
C.S. Garrard *Intensive Therapy Unit, John Radcliffe Hospital, Oxford, UK*
P.M. Upton *Department of Anaesthesia, Royal Cornwall Hospital, Treliske, Truro, UK*

Anaesthesia, Third Edition, Clinical aspects
Obstetrics and Gynaecology, Second Edition
Accident and Emergency Medicine, Second Edition
Paediatrics, Second Edition
Orthopaedic Surgery
Otolaryngology, Second Edition
Ophthalmology
Psychiatry
General Surgery
Renal Medicine
Trauma
Chronic Pain
Oral and Maxillofacial Surgery
Oncology
Cardiovascular Medicine
Neurology
Neonatology
Gastroenterology
Thoracic Surgery
Respiratory Medicine
Orthopaedic Trauma Surgery
Critical Care

Forthcoming titles include:
Acute Poisoning
Opthalmology, Second Edition
Urology
Evidence Based Medicine

KEY TOPICS IN

ACCIDENT AND EMERGENCY MEDICINE

SECOND EDITION

Rupert Evans
Consultant in Emergency Medicine,
University Hospital of Wales, Cardiff, UK

Derek Burke
Consultant in Accident and Emergency Medicine,
The Children's Hospital NHS Trust, Sheffield, UK

BIOS

First published 1994 (ISBN 1 872748 67 8)
Second Edition 2001 (ISBN 1 85996 132 0)

A CIP catalogue record for this book is available from the British Library.

ISBN 1 85996 132 0

BIOS Scientific Publishers Ltd
9 Newtec Place, Magdalen Road, Oxford OX4 1RE, UK
Tel. +44 (0)1865 726286. Fax +44 (0)1865 246823
World Wide Web home page: http://www.bios.co.uk/

Important Note from the Publisher
The information contained within this book was obtained by BIOS Scientific Publishers Ltd from sources believed by us to be reliable. However, while every effort has been made to ensure its accuracy, no responsibility for loss or injury whatsoever occasioned to any person acting or refraining from action as a result of information contained herein can be accepted by the authors or publishers.

The reader should remember that medicine is a constantly evolving science and while the authors and publishers have ensured that all dosages, applications and practices are based on current indications, there may be specific practices which differ between communities. You should always follow the guidelines laid down by the manufacturers of specific products and the relevant authorities in the country in which you are practising.

Production Editor: Andrea Bosher.
Typeset by Jayvee Computer Services, Trivandrum, India
Printed by The Cromwell Press, Trowbridge, UK

CONTENTS

ABBREVIATIONS

A&E	Accident and Emergency
AIS	Abbreviated Injury Score
ARDS	acute/adult respiratory distress syndrome
ATFL	anterior talo-fibular ligament
BAEM	British Association for Accident and Emergency Medicine
BHR	bronchial hyper-responsiveness
BLS	basic life support
CBF	cerebral blood flow
CCDC	Consultant in Communicable Disease Control
CFL	calcaneo-fibular ligament
COHb	baseline carboxyhaemoglobin
COPD	chronic obstructive pulmonary disease
CPPD	calcium pyro phosphate dihydrate
CPK	creatine phosphokinase
CPP	cerebral perfusion pressure
CPHM	Consultant in Public Health Medicine
CSA	Casualty Surgeons Association
CPAP	continuous positive airways pressure
DBP	diastolic blood pressure
DVT	deep vein thrombosis
ECG	echocardiogram
EMD	electro-mechanical dissociation
EMLA	eutectic mixture of local anaesthetics
EMRS	Emergency Medicine Research Society
ESR	erythrocyte sedimentation rate
FEV_1	forced expiratory volume
FFAEM	Faculty of Accident and Emergency Medicine
GABA	gamma-aminobutyric acid
GCS	Glasgow Coma Scale
GHB	gamma-hydroxybutyrate
HUS	haemolytic-uraemic syndrome
ICP	intracranial pressure
IFEM	International Federation of Emergency Medicine
ILCOR	International Liaison Committee on Resuscitation
IOFB	intraocular foreign bodies
IPCS	International Programme on Chemical Safety
ISS	Injury Severity Score
IUCD	intra-uterine contraceptive device
MABP	mean arterial blood pressure
MIBK	methyl isobutyl ketone
NAI	non-accidental injury
NIBP	non-invasive automated blood pressure
NIPPV	non-invasive intermittent positive pressure ventilation

OPG	orthopantomographs
ORS	oral rehydration solution
PEA	pulseless electrical activity
PEEP	positive end-expiratory pressure
PEF	peak expiratory flow
PTFL	posterior talo-fibular ligament
PTSD	post-traumatic stress disorder
RAPD	relative afferent papillary response
RTS	Revised Trauma Score
SAC	Specialist Advisory Committee
SHOT	serious hazards of transfusion
SIDS	sudden infant death syndrome
T-RTS	Triage Revised Trauma Score
TRISS	Trauma Score Injury Severity Score
TS	Trauma Score
UTI	urinary tract infection

Names of Medical Substances

In accordance with directive 92/27/EEC, this book adheres to the following guidelines on naming of medicinal substances (rINN, Recommended International Non-proprietary Name; BAN, British Approved Name).

List 1 – Both names to appear

UK Name	**rINN**
[1]adrenaline	epinephrine
amethocaine	tetracaine
bendrofluazide	bendroflumethiazide
benzhexol	trihexyphenidyl
chlorpheniramine	chlorphenamine
dicyclomine	dicycloverine
dothiepin	dosulepin
eformoterol	formoterol
flurandrenolone	fludroxycortide
frusemide	furosemide
hydroxyurea	hydroxycarbamide
lignocaine	lidocaine
methotrimeprazine	levomepromazine
methylene blue	methylthioninium chloride
mitozantrone	mitoxantrone
mustine	chlormethine
nicoumalone	acenocoumarol
[1]noradrenaline	norepinephrine
oxypentifylline	pentoxyifylline
procaine penicillin	procaine benzylpenicillin
salcatonin	calcitonin (salmon)
thymoxamine	moxisylyte
thyroxine sodium	levothyroxine sodium
trimeprazine	alimemazine

List 2 – rINN to appear exclusively

Former BAN	**rINN/new BAN**
amoxycillin	amoxicillin
amphetamine	amfetamine
amylobarbitone	amobarbital
amylobarbitone sodium	amobarbital sodium
beclomethasone	beclometasone
benorylate	benorilate
busulphan	busulfan
butobarbitone	butobarbital
carticaine	articane
cephalexin	cefalexin
cephamandole nafate	cefamandole nafate
cephazolin	cefazolin
cephradine	cefradine
chloral betaine	cloral betaine
chlorbutol	chlorobutanol
chlormethiazole	clomethiazole
chlorathalidone	chlortalidone
cholecalciferol	colecalciferol
cholestyramine	colestyramine
clomiphene	clomifene
colistin sulphomethate sodium	colistimethate sodium
corticotrophin	corticotropin
cysteamine	mercaptamine
danthron	dantron
desoxymethasone	desoximetasone
dexamphetamine	dexamfetamine
dibromopropamidine	dibrompropamidine
dienoestrol	dienestrol
dimethicone(s)	dimeticone
dimethyl sulphoxide	dimethyl sulfoxide
doxycycline hydrochloride (hemihydrate hemiethanolate)	doxycycline hyclate
ethancrynic acid	etacrynic acid
ethamsylate	etamsylate
ethinyloestradiol	ethinylestradiol
ethynodiol	etynodiol
flumethasone	flumetasone
flupenthixol	flupentixol
gestronol	gestonorone
guaiphenesin	guaifenesin

[1] In common with the BP, precedence will continue to be given to the terms adrenaline and noradrenaline.

hexachlorophane	hexachlorophene
hexamine hippurate	methenamine hippurate
hydroxyprogesterone hexanoate	hydroxyprogesterone caproate
indomethacin	indometacin
lysuride	lisuride
methyl cysteine	mecysteine
methylphenobarbitone	methylphenobarbital
oestradiol	estradiol
oestriol	estriol
oestrone	estrone
oxethazaine	oxetacaine
pentaerythritol tetranitrate	pentaerithrityl tetranitrate
phenobarbitone	phenobarbital
pipothiazine	pipotiazine
polyhexanide	polihexanide
potassium cloazepate	dipotassium clorazepate
pramoxine	pramocaine
prothionamide	protionamide
quinalbarbitone	secobarbital
riboflavine	riboflavin
sodium calciumedetate	sodium calcium edetate
sodium cromoglycate	sodium cromoglicate
sodium ironedetate	sodium feredetate
sodium picosulphate	sodium picosulfate
sorbitan monostearate	sorbitan stearate
stilboestrol	diethylstilbestrol
sulphacetamide	sulfacetamide
sulphadiazine	sulfadiazine
sulphadimidine	sulfadimidine
sulphaguanadine	sulfaguanadine
sulphamethoxazole	sulfamethoxazole
sulphasalazine	sulfasalazine
sulphathiazole	sulfathiazole
sulphinpyrazone	sulfinpyrazone
tetracosactrin	tetracosactide
thiabendazole	tiabendazole
thioguanine	tioguanine
thiopentone	thiopental
urofollitrophin	urofollitropin

PREFACE

Accident and Emergency Medicine has become a more prominent specialty in view of the ever increasing numbers of patients admitted as emergencies. There is a need for the Accident and Emergency specialist to have a wide knowledge to deal with emergencies as they enter the department.

The Fellowship Examination and the Higher Specialist Training programme in Accident and Emergency Medicine suggest a core curriculum.

Key Topics in Accident and Emergency Medicine contains certain essential information regarding the emergency management of the wide variety of conditions. It is intended to provide the reader with short articles covering a wide variety of topics which are particularly relevant to the Higher Specialist Trainee in their continuing professional development.

The book is written by active Emergency Medicine clinicians specifically for those involved in the specialty, including nurses and paramedics.

Rupert Evans, Derek Burke

ACKNOWLEDGEMENTS

The authors wish to acknowledge Dr Elizabeth Jones, Dr Liam Penny, Dr Rhys M Jones and Mr Mark Poulden.

ABDOMINAL PAIN

Conditions presenting with abdominal pain to the A&E department comprise those requiring immediate resuscitation, those requiring referral to an in-patient team for further assessment and treatment, and those that may safely be discharged. Although a diagnosis will not always be made, a full history, physical examination and a few simple investigations will usually suffice to manage the majority of cases.

Examination

Shock presents with some or all of the classical signs of tachycardia, hypotension, peripheral shut down and altered conscious level. In children and young healthy adults compensatory mechanisms will often make the signs of early shock less obvious. Similarly in the elderly the classical signs of shock may be less obvious or masked by the effects of certain drugs, e.g. β blockers. Cardiogenic shock secondary to myocardial infarction should be considered in all patients with shock and abdominal pain before aggressive fluid resuscitation is commenced.

Clinical features suggesting a surgical cause for abdominal pain include, abdominal tenderness, guarding, rebound, rigidity and absent bowel sounds. The abdomen, groins and genitalia should be carefully palpated for aortic aneurysm, hernias and testicular torsion. The presence of any of these is an indication for referral for a surgical opinion.

Investigations

Few investigations are helpful in the assessment of abdominal pain in the A&E department. Urine testing and where appropriate pregnancy testing should be considered as part of the routine clinical examination. The following are the commonest tests employed:

- urinalysis is mandatory in all cases looking for evidence of urinary tract infection (particularly important in children) and diabetic ketoacidosis;
- a pregnancy test is mandatory in all females of childbearing potential. A negative serum β HCG test virtually rules out a viable ectopic pregnancy. A negative urinary β HCG does not. Therefore if the diagnosis of ectopic pregnancy is considered and a urinary β HCG result is negative, a serum test should be taken to confirm the finding;
- serum amylase is measured to look for evidence of pancreatitis. A negative result does not exclude the diagnosis;
- despite its widespread use, white cell count is of little or no help in the diagnosis or management of abdominal pain;
- erect chest X-ray will demonstrate free gas under the diaphragm in a proportion of cases of perforated abdominal viscera; a normal film does not exclude the diagnosis. A chest film may also reveal intra-thoracic causes for abdominal pain, e.g. pneumonia.

- supine abdominal films. The majority of X-ray departments do not routinely perform supine abdominal views for the acute abdomen;
- ultrasound. This may be useful for excluding gynaecological or hepatobilary causes of abdominal pain.

Management

The shocked patient is resuscitated with high flow oxygen and intravenous fluids. A surgical opinion should be sought early as many of these cases will require urgent laparotomy.

Patients who are stable and have signs of surgical pathology should be referred for a surgical opinion. Once the decision is taken that the diagnosis is surgical, time should not be wasted on requesting further investigations to pin down the diagnosis. Non-surgical causes of abdominal pain should always be considered and sought. Non-surgical causes of abdominal pain.

- Gastro-intestinal:
  (a) diverticulitis;
  (b) gastroenteritis;
  (c) inflammatory bowel disease;
  (d) mesenteric adenitis;
  (e) pancreatitis.
- Hepatobiliary:
  (a) biliary colic;
  (b) cholecystitis;
  (c) hepatitis.
- Urinary tract:
  (a) acute urinary retention;
  (b) epididymo-orchitis;
  (c) pyelonephritis;
  (d) renal colic;
  (e) ureteric colic;
  (f) urinary tract infection.
- Obstetric/Gynaecological:
  (a) abruptio placentae;
  (b) endometriosis;
  (c) labour;
  (d) mittleschmerz;
  (e) ruptured ovarian cyst;
  (f) salpingitis;
  (g) torsion of ovarian tumour or appendage.
- Medical:
  (a) diabetic ketoacidosis;
  (b) drug withdrawal;
  (c) myocardial infarction;
  (d) pericarditis;

(e) pleurisy;
(f) pneumonia;
(g) pulmonary embolism;
(h) shingles;
(i) upper respiratory tract infection;
(j) uraemia.

Further reading

Ellis BW. *Hamilton Bailey's Emergency Surgery*. London: Butterworth-Heinemann, 1995.
Lumley JSP. *Hamilton Bailey's Demonstration of Physical Signs in Clinical Surgery*. London: Arnold, 1997.

Related topics of interest

Abdominal trauma (p. 4); Gynaecology (p. 168); Myocardial infarction (p. 246); Obstetric emergencies (p. 250); Urological conditions (p. 1334)

ABDOMINAL TRAUMA

Unrecognized abdominal injury is a frequent cause of preventable death after trauma. *A high index of suspicion* is required as signs are often subtle, or masked by other injuries, alcohol, or drugs. As many as 20% of patients with acute haemoperitoneum have benign abdominal findings when first examined in the Accident and Emergency department. Early evaluation by a surgeon is essential.

Examination

A positive examination is the most reliable clinical sign of abdominal trauma. However, a negative physical examination may hide significant intra-abdominal injury.

1. ***Inspect.*** Include the lower chest, abdomen, flank, back and perineum.

2. ***Palpate*** for signs of pain, muscle guarding and rebound tenderness.

3. ***Percuss*** to elicit subtle rebound tenderness and peritoneal irritation.

4. ***Auscultate*** for bowel sounds and bruits.

5. ***Rectal examination.*** This is performed for evidence of blood, sphincter tone, prostate position (high-riding prostate indicates urethral damage) and bony fragments.

6. ***Vaginal examination.*** This is performed in women for blood and bony fragments.

7. ***Penile examination.*** Evidence of blood at the urethral meatus strongly suggests a urethral tear. Inspect the scrotum and perineum for evidence of bruising.

8. ***Gluteal examination.*** Penetrating injuries in this are associated with a 50% incidence of significant intra-abdominal injury.

Management

After the *ABC and initial resuscitation* the following are performed:

1. ***Blood sampling*** for blood group and crossmatching, together with samples for full blood count, including haematocrit, amylase, urea and electrolytes, glucose, alcohol, and human chorionic gonadotrophin (HCG).

2. ***A nasogastric tube*** is inserted to remove gastric contents, relieve gastric distension and to detect the presence of blood in the aspirate. The tube is passed orally in those with a suspicion of basal skull fracture to prevent passage through the cribriform plate into the brain.

3. ***A bladder catheter*** will help decompress the bladder, assess for haematuria and allow monitoring of urine output. Caution in the following patients:

- Inability to void;
- Unstable pelvic fracture;
- A high-riding prostate;
- Blood at the urethral meatus;
- Scrotal haematoma.

as these are indicative of urethral trauma and signify the need for a urological opinion.

4. In addition to chest and pelvic X-rays a lateral cervical spine and abdominal film may be helpful. Sub-diaphragmatic air or extraluminal air in the retroperitoneum are signs of hollow viscus injury while loss of psoas shadow may suggest retroperitoneal blood.

5. Diagnostic peritoneal lavage. In adults the DPL is considered *98% sensitive* for intraperitoneal bleeding. The procedure should be performed by the surgeon caring for the patient. Either an *open or closed technique* is acceptable.

The only absolute *contraindication* is an existing indication for laparotomy. Relative contraindications include previous abdominal surgery, morbid obesity, advanced cirrhosis, and pre-existing coagulopathy. The open technique is preferred in patients with advanced pregnancy.

A positive test is indicated by the following:

- Free aspiration of blood;
- Gastrointestinal contents;
- Vegetable fibres or bile;
- $\geq$ 100 000 RBC/mm^3;
- $\geq$ 500 WBC/mm^3;
- Gram's stain with bacteria present.

False negatives are found in 2% of cases and are usually related to injuries of the pancreas, duodenum, diaphragm, small bowel or bladder.

False positive results are caused by pelvic fracture, inadequate local haemostasis or accidental injury to intraperitoneal organs.

Complications include local haemorrhage, peritonitis, trauma to the abdominal and retroperitoneal structures and wound infection.

6. Ultrasound scan. Ultrasound provides a rapid non-invasive means of diagnosing intra-abdominal injury. It is useful in detecting free intraperitoneal fluid in experienced hands and is often the investigation of choice in children. The ultrasound scan should be performed in the resuscitation room. Can also detect splenic and hepatic haematoma, but is operator dependent.

7. CT scan. The CT scan provides information regarding specific organ damage and its extent. Can also visualize the retroperitoneal and pelvic organs. Hollow viscus injury is not readily detected. The CT should only be performed in the stable patient.

Indications for laparotomy

1. ***Hypotension*** with evidence of abdominal injury
   - Gunshot wounds.
   - Stab wounds.
   - Blunt trauma with gross blood on diagnostic peritoneal lavage.
2. ***Peritonitis*** – early or subsequent.
3. ***Recurrent hypotension*** despite adequate resuscitation.
4. ***Extraluminal air.***
5. ***Injured diaphragm.***
6. ***Intraperitoneal perforation*** of urinary bladder on cystography.
7. ***CT evidence*** of injury to the pancreas, gastrointestinal tract, and specific injuries to the liver, spleen, or kidney.
8. ***Positive contrast study*** of upper and lower gastrointestinal tracts.

Further reading

Committee on Trauma. *Advanced Trauma Life Support.* American College of Surgeons, 1993.

Robertson C and Redmond AD. *The Management of Major Trauma.* Oxford Handbooks in Emergency Medicine, Oxford, 1991.

Related topics of interest

Genitourinary trauma (p. 164); Head Injury (p. 173); Maxillofacial Injury (p. 226); Thoracic trauma (p. 321)

ACCIDENT AND EMERGENCY LANDMARKS

1967 The first Consultant in A&E Medicine, Mr Maurice Ellis, is appointed at the Leeds General Infirmary.

1967 Establishment of the Casualty Surgeons Association (CSA) on 12th October.

1967 First Committee meeting of the Casualty Surgeons Association held at the British Medical Association on 12th October and attended by Mr M Ellis (Chairman), Mr E Abson, Mr D Caro, Mr J Collins, Mr J Hindle, Mr J James, Mr McCarthy, Mr J Pascall and Mr I Stillman.

1968 First Annual General Meeting of the Casualty Surgeons Association held at the Walsall General Hospital on 23rd March at which Mr M Ellis was elected as President, Mr D Caro was elected as Vice-President, Mr E Abson was elected as Honorary Secretary and Mr J Hindle was elected as Honorary Treasurer.

1972 Appointment of 30 further Consultants in Accident and Emergency Medicine made by the Department of Health following pressure from existing Consultants in the specialty.

1972 The first Consultant-led Department opens.

1975 Establishment of the Specialist Advisory Committee (SAC) in Accident and Emergency Medicine to establish a recognized training programme.

1977 First Senior Registrars appointments.

1983 Establishment of the FRCSEd in Accident and Emergency Medicine and Surgery.

1983 Establishment of the Emergency Medicine Research Society (EMRS).

1985 Adoption of Journals 'British Journal of Accident and Emergency Medicine' and 'Archives of Emergency Medicine'.

1986 First International Conference on Emergency Medicine with Mr G Bodiwala, Mr S Lord, Mr W Rutherford, Mr I Stewart, Dr J Thurston, Dr D Williams and Mr D Wilson forming the Organizing Committee.

1988 The joint statement by the Royal College of Paediatrics and Child Health, Casualty Surgeons Association and the British Association of Paediatric Surgeons declares there should be a children's specialist A&E centre in every large conurbation.

1989 Establishment of the Future Strategies Group to consider the establishment of an Intercollegiate Faculty and Examination in Accident and Emergency Medicine. Members: Dr H Baderman, Mr G Bodiwala, Major General N Kirby, Dr K Little, Mr S Miles, Dr C Robertson, Dr J Thurston, Dr D Williams (Chairman), Mr D Wilson and Mr D Yates.

1990 First Professorial appointment in Accident and Emergency Medicine to Professor D W Yates is appointed at Hope Hospital, Salford.

1990 Change in the name of the Association to the British Association for Accident and Emergency Medicine (BAEM) reflecting the changing emphasis of the specialty.

1991 Establishment of Association's official scientific Journal 'Archives of Emergency Medicine'.

1991 Establishment of an Intercollegiate Board in Accident and Emergency Medicine. Members: Mr I Anderson (RCP & S Glas), Dr H Baderman (A&E), Dr P Baskett (RCAnaes), Dr E Beck (RCP London), Major General N Kirby (A&E), Dr K Little (RCSEd/SAC A&E), Dr P O'Connor (RCP Ireland), Professor N O'Higgins (RCS Ireland), Dr C Robertson (RCPEd), Dr D Williams (A&E/Chairman) and Professor D Yates (RCSEng).

1991 Establishment of the International Federation of Emergency Medicine (IFEM).

1992 Silver Jubilee of the British Association for Accident and Emergency Medicine (formerly the Casualty Surgeons Association).

1992 Formation of a Steering Group to establish the Intercollegiate Faculty of Accident and Emergency Medicine. Members: Mr G Bodiwala (BAEM), Professor N Browse (RCSEng), Mr A Dean (RCSEd), Mr T Hide (RCP & S Glas), Major General N Kirby (BAEM), Dr K Little (SAC A&E), Mr S Miles (BAEM), Dr J Nimmo (RCPEd), Dr D Pyke (RCP London), Dr J Stoddart (RCAnaes), Dr D Williams (BAEM/Chairman) and Professor D Yates (BAEM).

1993 Formation of the Intercollegiate Faculty of Accident and Emergency Medicine. Inauguration Ceremony held on Tuesday 2nd November at the Royal College of Surgeons of England.

1993 First General Meeting of the Faculty of Accident and Emergency Medicine held on Tuesday 14th December 1993 at the Royal College of Physicians of London. First Officers of the Faculty: President: Dr D J Williams, Vice-President: Major General N G Kirby, Dean: Professor D W Yates, Treasurer: Mr G G Bodiwala and Registrar: Dr J G B Thurston.

1994 Fifth International Conference on Emergency Medicine with Mr G Bodiwala, Major General N Kirby, Mr C Perez-Avila, Mr I Stewart, Dr J Thurston, Dr D Williams and Professor D Yates forming the Organizing Committee.

1996 First specialty examination of the Faculty of Accident and Emergency Medicine (FFAEM) held in Glasgow in October.

1997 The Faculty of Accident and Emergency Medicine is granted its own coat of arms. The Faculty is aspiring to Royal College status within a decade.

1997 There are nearly 400 Consultants and 300 trainees in the specialty.

1998 Establishment of the Joint Committee on Higher Training in Accident and Emergency Medicine at the Royal College of Surgeons of England under the auspices of the Faculty of Accident and Emergency Medicine.

1998 The British Association for Accident and Emergency Medicine celebrates its 1000th member.

1998 Publication of the Association's revised document entitled 'The Way Ahead 1998'.

1999 Establishment of the Government's Accident and Emergency Modernization Programme led by Mr M Lambert.

ACUTE LIMB ISCHAEMIA

Acute limb ischaemia will result in irreversible tissue necrosis within 6 hours and requires urgent surgical revascularization. Patients with irreversible ischaemia will require an urgent amputation unless the patient is not fit for a surgical procedure.

Aetiology

Acute limb ischaemia is caused by the following:

- Acute thrombotic occlusion of a pre-existing stenotic lesion (60%). Factors predisposing to acute thrombosis include dehydration, hypotension, unusual posture or activity, malignancy, hyperviscosity syndromes and thrombophilia (including protein C, S and anti-thrombin III deficiency; activated protein C resistance, factor V Leiden; and antiphospholipid syndrome).
- Embolus (30%). 80% of peripheral emboli arise from the left atrial appendage in association with atrial fibrillation. Other sources include the left ventricle, heart valves, prosthetic grafts, aneurysms, paradoxical embolism and atrial myxoma.
- Iatrogenic injury.
- Trauma.
- Popliteal aneurysm.
- Aortic dissection.

Clinical features

Symptoms and signs of acute limb ischaemia include:

- Pain.
- Pallor.
- Pulseless.
- Perishing cold.
- Paraesthesia – leading to anaesthesia (unable to feel touch, foot or hand).
- Paralysis – unable to wiggle toes or fingers.

Apart from paralysis and anaesthesia the symptoms and signs of acute ischaemia are non-specific. Anaesthesia and paralysis are the key to diagnosing complete ischaemia that requires emergency surgical treatment.

Pain on squeezing the calf indicates muscle infarction and impending irreversible ischaemia.

Acute arterial occlusion is associated with a 'marble' white limb and is associated with spasm in the distal arterial tree. As the spasm relaxes the skin becomes mottled and blue/purple with a reticular pattern and blanches with pressure. At this stage the limb is still salvageable. Later the mottling becomes darker and does not blanch. This is more likely to be irreversible.

Differentiation of embolus and acute arterial thrombosis (thrombosis in situ)

Clinical features	*Embolus*	*Thrombosis*
Severity	Complete (no collaterals)	Incomplete (collaterals)
Onset	Seconds or minutes	Hours or days
Limb affected	Leg 3:1 arm	Leg 10:1 arm
Multiple sites	Up to 15%	Rare
Embolic source	Present (usually atrial fibrillation)	Absent
Previous claudication	Absent	Present
Palpation of artery	Soft, tender	Hard, calcified
Bruits	Absent	Present
Contralateral leg pulses	Present	Absent
Diagnosis	Clinical	Angiography
Treatment	Embolectomy, warfarin	Medical, bypass, thrombolysis

Management

This is a surgical emergency. It is important to obtain the opinion of a vascular surgeon in order to preserve the limb. If there are no contraindications (acute aortic dissection, multiple trauma etc) give an intravenous bolus of Heparin to limit thrombus propagation and protect the collateral circulation.

If ischaemia is complete the patient must be taken directly to theatre and not to angiography as this will delay treatment. If ischaemia is incomplete pre-operative angiography may help the decision-making process regarding treatment.

1. Acute embolus. Brachial Artery – This is not usually limb threatening and in elderly patients non-operative treatment is acceptable. Younger patients may require embolectomy.

Lower Limb Embolus – This is usually limb threatening and requires immediate surgical revascularization. Emboli usually lodge at the common femoral bifurcation.

Femoral embolus is associated with profound ischaemia to the level of the upper thigh. A femoral pulse does not exclude a diagnosis. Embolectomy may be performed under local, regional or general anaesthesia.

The in-patient mortality is reported between 10–20% but is secondary to other illnesses such as heart failure or cerebrovascular accident.

2. Saddle embolus. Acute embolic occlusion of the aortic bifurcation present as follows:

- Femoral pulses present.
- Marble white or mottled to the waist.
- Paraplegia (secondary to ischaemia of the cauda equina).

Immediate bilateral embolectomy restores lower limb perfusion but many patients still perish from the reperfusion injury, or secondary disease.

3. ***Popliteal aneurysm.*** This aneurysm may cause ischaemia by thrombus formation, or acting as a source of embolus. Thrombolysis is often the best treatment. Once the circulation is restored bypass should be performed to exclude the aneurysm.

4. ***Atheroembolism.*** The patient characteristically presents with the blue toe (finger) syndrome which may mimic Raynaud's phenomenon. It must be promptly identified as it may deteriorate rapidly and require amputation.

5. ***Trauma.*** This may be secondary to limb fractures and dislocations (supracondylar fracture in children, tibial fracture in adult), blunt trauma and penetrating injuries. Other causes include arterial cannulation (coronary angioplasty, aortic balloon pump) exsanguinating tourniquet. Presence of distal pulses does not exclude arterial injury. Pulse oximetry, Doppler and measuring ankle brachial pressure index may be helpful, but in cases of doubt proceed to angiogrphy.

6. ***Intra-arterial drug administration.*** This leads to spasm and microvascular thrombosis. The leg is mottled and digital gangrene is common, but pedal pulses are usually palpable. Treatment is supportive and the patient will require heparinization. Look for rhabdomyolysis and evidence of compartment syndrome.

Post-ischaemic syndromes

The following complications may occur after an acute ischaemic event:

- Re-perfusion injury. This is as a result of release of oxygen free radicals. Acidosis and hyperkalaemia may occur due to leakage from the damaged cells, causing cardiac arrhythmias and myoglobinaemia. Acute respiratory distress syndrome may also develop.
- Compartment syndrome.
- Chronic pain syndromes.

Further reading

Callum K, Bradbury A. Acute limb ischaemia. *British Medical Journal*, 2000; **320:** 764–7.

ACUTE MONOARTHRITIS

Acute inflammatory monoarthritis is a common clinical problem. Trauma is the commonest cause of acute joint pain and swelling in patients attending an A&E Department. Around 5–10% of patients will present with non-traumatic conditions.

An acute non-traumatic monoarthritis may be caused by a number of conditions. Septic arthritis must be excluded. Poor outcomes, include death or joint destruction. Patients with an acute inflammatory arthritis need immediate access to a specialist rheumatology service with inpatient facilities.

Differential diagnosis of acute non-traumatic monoarthritis

A number of different conditions can present as an acute monoarthritis.

Major diagnoses of monoarthritis

Disease	*Cause*
Infection	Bacterial Gonococcal Non-gonococcal Tuberculous Fungal Viral
Crystal induced arthritis	Monosodium urate (gout) Calcium pyrophosphate dihydrate – (Pseudo gout)
Reactive arthritis	Bacterial Viral
Trauma and mechanical problems	
Malignancy	
Systemic disease	

History

Obtain a thorough history. In particular, obtain the following features:

- History of severe pain/night pain which suggests a more sinister pathology.
- Systemic symptoms including fever, sweats, malaise, weight loss.
- Previous episodes/family history.
- Gastrointestinal symptoms.
- Upper respiratory tract, genitourinary symptoms.
- Sexual history.
- Foreign travel.
- Intravenous drug abuse.

- Conjunctivitis, urethritis, diarrhoea (reactive arthritis).
- Alcohol excess.
- Drug therapy, e.g. diuretics/sulphonamides.
- Back pain.
- Psoriasis.
- Inflammatory bowel disease.
- Mouth ulcers/skin rashes (psoriasis, erythema nodosum, lupus pernio, vasculitis), alopecia.

Examination

A thorough examination should include looking at the following:

1. General

- Temperature, pulse and blood pressure.
- Mouth.
- Eyes.
- Skin.
- Hands (splinter haemorrhages, nail fold infarcts, purpuric lesions).
- Feet.

2. Joint examination

The following signs and symptoms are typical:

- Joint line tenderness.
- Restricted, painful joint movement.
- Erythema.
- Local increase in skin temperature.
- Joint and soft tissue swelling.
- Loss of joint function.
- Periarticular muscle wasting.
- Cellulitis and local lymphadenopathy.

Investigations

1. Arthrocentesis. This is considered mandatory if possible and recommended by the Royal College of Physicians report of a joint working group of the British Society for Rheumatology. Use a non-touch technique to aspirate synovial fluid and should be undertaken or supervised by an experienced clinician. It should be performed at the first opportunity and the fluid immediately examined. Its appearance should be recorded. Send for microscopy (including polarizing microscopy) Gram stain, culture and sensitivities and cytology. If the patient's synovial cell count is greater than 60 000 cells/mm^3 with a predominance of polymorphs will confirm the diagnosis of septic arthritis.

2. Full blood count.

3. Erythrocyte sedimentation rate (ESR), plasma viscosity or C reactive protein.

4. Uric acid.

5. ***Blood cultures.***

6. ***Plain joint radiographs.***

7. ***Cervical and urethral swabs*** in cases of suspected gonococcal/reactive arthritis.

8. ***Swabs of skin lesions/throat swab*** if appropriate.

9. ***Anti-streptolysin titre*** in cases of suspected streptococcal infection.

Gonococcal septic arthritis

Infective agent is *Neisseria gonorrhoea.* Mainly affects young adults. Three times more common in women. May be preceded by migratory tendonitis or arthritis. A 'septic' rash with a small number of scattered pustules is frequently seen. Usually affects large joints – knee, wrist and ankle. The organism may be isolated from the genital tract in 50–80% of cases. Blood cultures may be positive early when the skin lesions are present but is less likely to be positive once the monoarthritis has developed. Synovial fluid positive in 30% of cases. Polymerase chain reaction test may be useful in culture negative suspected cases. Refer to Genito-Urinary Medicine for follow-up and exclude co-existing infection and arrange contact tracing. Treatment with Ciprofloxacin usually responds rapidly.

Non-gonococcal septic arthritis

Septic arthritis is an acute infection of the joint. A review of septic arthritis in one English health district over 10 years found 75 cases. Tends to occur in children, the elderly, immunocompromised, patients with joint disease (e.g. rheumatoid arthritis), after invasive joint procedures such as needle aspiration, arthroscopy and patients with prosthetic joints, or intravenous drug abusers. Organisms may enter the joint by local spread, e.g. from penetrating wounds or secondary to local osteomyelitis where the metaphysis of the affected bone is intracapsular or by haematogenous spread. 80% of cases are monoarticular. Large joints are most frequently infected.

1. ***Causative organisms***

Staphylococcus aureus (40–50%) is the commonest infecting organism in all age groups. In children under the age of 5 years *Haemophilus influenzae* is commonly implicated.

Other organisms implicated in septic arthritis include:

- *Staphylococcus epidermis* 10–15%.
- Gram-negative bacteria 15–20%.
- Non-group A, B haemolytic streptococci 15%.
- Anaerobic bacteria <5%.
- *Streptococcus pneumoniae* <5%.
- *Haemophilus influenzae* <5%.

Clinical features

1. ***Children.*** Septic arthritis is commonest in the under-5 age group. The source of the infection is usually a skin lesion or respiratory tract infection. It most frequently affects the large joints of the body. In older children a single joint is usually involved, in the neonatal period multiple joints may be involved. The child will be toxic, unwell with a fever and tachycardia. The joint is swollen, hot, red and exquisitely painful to even the smallest of movement. These signs may not be as florid in the early stages in the younger child or baby.

2. ***Adults.*** In the elderly the clinical signs and symptoms may not be as florid as in the child. They may present initially with confusion and fever. Pain at the site of infection may be minimal.

Radiology

The early X-rays will usually be normal, although widening of the joint space may indicate an effusion. In neonates osteomyelitis of the adjacent bone may be visible. In the late stages the X-rays will show bone destruction with periosteal new bone formation and loss of joint space. Such changes may not occur if the condition is diagnosed early and treated promptly. Ultrasound examination will reveal an effusion and may be used to guide a needle for aspiration.

Management

If there is the possibility of septic arthritis, then treat aggressively with intravenous antibiotics after taking synovial fluid and blood cultures. The choice of antibiotics depends on the finding in the gram film, subsequent culture results and on the general condition of the patient.

If 'blind' therapy is needed, intravenous flucloxacillin (1 g four times a day) and benzylpenicillin (600–1200 g four times a day) are appropriate for adults. An alternative for initial treatment in adults is Cefotaxime 2 mg three times daily.

Children need a cephalosporin because of the potential infection with a β lactamase-producing organism. Proven septic arthritis is treated with antibiotics for at least 6 weeks.

The choice of antibiotic should reflect the clinical scenario and consider seeking expert microbiological advice.

Refer patient to orthopaedic team who will consider arthroscopy and formal joint irrigation.

Gout

It is an underdiagnosed condition which presents as recurrent acute inflammation due to release of microcrystals of monosodium urate. The prevalence of gout is 6/1000 men and increases with age. Peak age in men is between 40 and 50 and women over 60. Any joint may be involved. However, the first metatarsophalangeal joint is the most common (90%) – the classical podagra. Initial episode is monoarticular in 90% of cases and involves the first metatarsophalangeal joint in 50% of cases.

Hyperuricaemia is a common but not essential feature and it is important to appreciate that the serum urate concentration may be normal in an acute attack.

The following criteria were described by Bennett and Wood in 1968:

- A clear history of at least two attacks of painful joint swelling with complete resolution within two weeks.
- A clear history or clinical diagnosis of podagra.
- The presence of a tophus.
- A rapid response to Colchicine within 48 hours.

Two of these criteria are required for the clinical diagnosis, but a definitive diagnosis can be made if crystals of sodium monourate are found in synovial fluid or the tissues.

Predisposing factors include:

- Family history.
- Obesity.
- High purine diet.
- Hypertension.
- Hyperlipidaemia.
- Excess alcohol intake.
- Renal impairment.
- Drugs. Increase production of uric acid – for example, cytotoxic drugs. Reduce uric acid excretion, for example, thiazide and loop diuretics.

In most cases of gout decreased urinary excretion of urate is the most common metabolic abnormality. Confirmation of the diagnosis is by joint aspiration and the presence of negative birefringent needle-shaped crystals (under polarized light microscopy).

Treatment – An acute attack may take up to seven days to settle. A non-steroidal anti-inflammatory drug is the treatment of choice and should be given in full dosage unless there is a history of peptic ulcer, renal impairment or cardiac failure. Colchicine is an alternative but is poorly tolerated by elderly patients. Intra-articular steroids and systemic steroids may be useful in older patients with impaired renal function. Long-term prophylaxis with Allopurinol should not be started until one month after an acute attack has subsided because it can worsen or prolong the attack.

Pseudo-gout (calcium pyrophosphate dihydrate – CPPD)

Characterized by crystal deposition of calcium pyrophosphate dihydrate. Incidence increases with age and more common in females. Is the most common cause of monoarthritis in the elderly. The knee is most commonly affected.

The following metabolic conditions are associated with CPPD:

- Haemochromatosis.
- Hyperparathyroidism.
- Hypomagnesaemia.
- Hypophosphatasia.
- Wilson's disease.
- Gout.
- Ochronosis.

Confirmation of the diagnosis is by aspiration of synovial fluid which reveals rhomboid or rod-like crystals which are weakly positively birefringent on polarized light microscopy. Plain radiographs may reveal calcification of fibro cartilage and hyaline cartilage.

Treatment – Treat symptomatically with non-steroidals and consider joint aspiration. Advise resting the joint and consider local steroid injection.

Reactive arthritis

May be precipitated by a wide variety of infections which include:

1. Bacteria

- Salmonella.
- Shigella.
- Yersinia.
- Campylobacter.
- Borrelia.
- Chlamydia.
- Streptococcal.

2. Viruses

- Rubella.
- Hepatitis B.
- Epstein–Barr.
- Cytomegalovirus.
- HTLV-1.
- HIV.
- Paramyxovirus (mumps).

The acute monoarthritis should be treated with non-steroidal anti-inflammatories. Antibiotic treatment should be given where appropriate.

Reiter's syndrome has the classic triad of reactive arthritis, urethritis and uveitis secondary to enteric urogenital infection. Mostly occurs in young adults and associated with the HLA B27 antigen.

Lyme disease is caused by the spirochete, *Borrelia burgdorferi*, which is transmitted by the tic *Ixodes ricinus*, commonly from the deer. Arthritis occurs in 60% of cases and often involves the knee as a monoarthritis. The pathognomonic rash, erythema chronicum migrans is diagnostic. Other complications include cardiac, neurological and rheumatological symptoms. For patients with an acute arthritis consider a course of Amoxycillin or Azithromycin. However, patients with systemic manifestations require specialist treatment.

Malignancy

An acute monoarthritis in a child should always raise the suspicion of leukaemia. The knee is the most commonly involved joint from secondaries of the breast, lung, gastrointestinal tract and malignant melanoma. Paraneoplastic syndromes can present with arthritis, e.g. hypertrophic osteoarthropathy, usually secondary to lung cancer.

Systemic disease

Many systemic illnesses present with an acute monoarthritis. These include:

- Connective tissue disorders.
- Vasculitis.
- Inflammatory bowel disease.
- Sarcoidosis.
- Rheumatoid arthritis.

Further reading

Esterhui JL Jnr, Gelb I. Adult septic arthritis. *Orthopaedic Clinics of North America*, 1991; **22**(3): 503–14.

Report of a Joint Working Group of the British Society for Rheumatology and the Research Unit of the Royal College of Physicians. Guidelines and a proposed audit protocol for the initial management of an acute hot joint. *Journal of the Royal College of Physicians of London*, 1992; **26:** 83–5.

Shaw DA, Casser JR. Acute septic arthritis in infancy and childhood. *Clinical Orthopaedics and Related Research*, 1990; **257:** 212–5.

Till SH, Snaith ML. Assessment, investigation and management of acute monoarthritis. *Journal of Accident and Emergency Medicine*, 1999; **16:** 355–61.

Related topics of interest

Febrile convulsion (p. 153); Limping child (p. 204)

ACUTE PANCREATITIS

Acute pancreatitis is an acute inflammatory process of the pancreas that can involve peripancreatic tissue or remote organs. Acute pancreatitis is classified as mild or severe. Severe disease is characterized by organ failure, or local complications such as necrosis, pseudocysts or fistulae. Pancreatitis should be considered in the differential diagnosis of all patients with abdominal pain and the serum amylase checked. The incidence of acute pancreatitis is approximately 5 cases per 100 000 of the population per annum. Most episodes are mild and self-limiting. A total of 20% of patients develop a severe attack and the overall mortality is 5–10%.

Acute pancreatitis typically presents with a continuous, boring upper abdominal pain, which often radiates to the back (50%). Other features include:

- Nausea and vomiting.
- Mild pyrexia.
- Shock/respiratory failure/renal failure in severe cases.
- Abdominal examination may reveal upper abdominal distension and tenderness. Reduced bowel sounds may be present as a consequence of the small bowel ileus. Signs of peritoneal irritation are often absent on initial presentation.
- Respiratory failure – Hyperventilation, basal pleural effusions, atelectasis, adult respiratory distress syndrome.
- Hypocalcaemia is common (due to saponification of fat); tetany (due to loss of ionized calcium) is rare.
- Local complications – pancreatic necrosis, with or without infection, pseudocyst and pancreatic fistulae.
- Retroperitoneal haemorrhage which manifests as periumbilical bruising (Cullen's sign) or loin bruising (Grey–Turner's sign) discolouration – both rare and develop after several days.

Laboratory diagnosis

Serum amylase typically rises within 2–12 hours of the onset of symptoms and levels over 1000 IU/l are strongly suggestive of acute pancreatitis. Serum amylase has a low specificity (<70%) when the upper limit of normal is used. Other conditions cause rises in serum amylase (perforated viscus, ischaemic bowel etc).

Serum lipase has a greater sensitivity and specificity (90–95%).

Urinary dipstick trypsinogen 2 has a negative predictive value of 99%.

Aetiology

Identifying the cause of acute pancreatitis is important – The risk of recurrence may be predicted and eliminating the cause may prevent further attacks.

Conditions associated with acute pancreatitis include:

- Gall stones – 45%.
- Alcohol – 35%.
- Idiopathic – 10–15%.
- Drugs – Azathioprine, oestrogens, corticosteroids etc.
- Trauma.

- Hypercalcaemia.
- Viral infection – Coxsackie B, mumps, HIV etc.
- Ischaemia or embolism.
- Vasculitis.
- Hypothermia.
- Hyperlipidaemia.
- Post-ERCP.
- Pancreatic tumours.
- Pregnancy.
- Venoms – scorpion bite, certain spiders.
- Familial pancreatitis.

Pathophysiology

The trigger for acute pancreatitis is a burst of free radical activity in the pancreatic acinar cells. Pancreatic secretions are diverted into the pancreatic interstitium, leading to autodigestion of pancreatic tissue as well as systemic effects from circulating enzymes which are drained away via the venous system. The inflammatory process attracts neutrophils, which further exacerbates the process by releasing proteases with their tissue destructive capabilities. The systemic inflammatory response is characterized by vasodilatation and capillary leakage. In severe cases this results in hypovolaemia, hypotension and hypoxaemia which may result in multisystem organ failure. Once initiated the pathophysiological process cannot be inhibited or reversed.

Severity

It is important to assess the severity of an episode of pancreatitis so patients can receive optimal treatment.

The most commonly used severity score is that developed by *Ranson*. This predicts severity within the first 48 hours of admission. All patients with more than three of Ranson's criteria should probably be admitted to either an HDU or ICU.

The *APACHE II* score has also been used to assess the severity of pancreatitis. This can be used at any stage of the disease and a score of >8 suggests a patient should be admitted to either an HDU or ICU.

C reactive protein levels are high in pancreatitis and associated with a more severe disease. Late rises in C reactive protein levels after initial fall may indicate the development of pancreatic sepsis or further exacerbation of the disease.

Investigations

- SaO_2.
- Serum amylase.
- FBC.
- U&E, calcium, LFTs, glucose.
- Coagulation screen.
- ABG.
- Chest X-ray.
- ECG.

Ranson's criteria

On admission	*Value*
Age	> 55 years
White cell count	> 16 000 mm^3
Lactate dehydrogenase	> 350 IU/l
Aspartate transaminase	> 250 U/l
Glucose	> 11 mmol/l
Within 48 hours	
Fall in haematocrit	> 10%
Urea rise	> 1.8 mmol/l
Calcium	< 2 mmol/l
Base deficit	> 4
Estimated fluid sequestration	> 6 l
PaO_2	< 8 kPa
Number of risk factors	Mortality (%)
0–2	< 1
3–4	+/– 15
5–6	+/– 40
>6	+/– 100

Imaging

1. Ultrasound. This is not particularly useful as the pancreas can be difficult to visualize because of the associated ileus. However, it may identify the presence of gall stones.

2. CT. This investigation provides a better method of viewing the pancreas and is accurate both in providing the diagnosis and in recognizing complications (pancreatic necrosis, pseudocysts and intra-abdominal fluid collections) and grading the severity of the pancreatitis.

Indications for CT scanning

- Ranson score >3 or APACHE II >8.
- Patients not improving after 72 hours of supportive therapy.
- Patients who deteriorate after initial improvement.

CT grading of acute pancreatitis

Grade	*CT findings*
A	Normal pancreas
B	Pancreatic enlargement focal or diffuse
C	Pancreatic enlargement with mild peri-pancreatic inflammation
D	Enlarged pancreas associated with single fluid collection
E	Enlarged pancreas with fluid collections in at least two areas

The grading is important as patients with grade ABCD have a <2% chance of developing a pancreatic abscess whilst those with grade E have a 57% chance.

Dynamic CT pancreatography is helpful in diagnosing pancreatic necrosis. Necrosis is the forerunner of pancreatic infection and is otherwise difficult to diagnose. CT-guided aspiration of necrotic areas may also be performed.

Management

1. Supportive management

- Oxygen therapy.
- Respiratory failure secondary to pleural effusions or ARDS is treated as appropriate.
- Full haemodynamic monitoring should be established.
- Aggressive fluid replacement.
- Hypotension and decreased cardiac output if not responsive to fluid replacement may require inotropes and vasopressors.
- Pain relief by intravenous opiates or thoracic epidural.
- Nil by mouth – nasogastric aspiration.
- Prophylactic antibiotics are not routinely given. They may be considered for those predicted to develop severe pancreatitis or those with signs of pancreatic infection.
- Hyperglycaemia is common and treated appropriately.
- Treat other electrolyte abnormalities, particularly hypocalcaemia and hypomagnesaemia.
- Specific modulators of disease activity such as somatostatin, aprontinin, gabexate, octreotide, PAF inhibitors are currently under evaluation.
- Renal compromise should be treated with volume replacement. Aim to maintain an adequate urine output (30 ml/hr). Treat renal failure as appropriate.

2. Surgery. Eight per cent of patients with gall stones develop pancreatitis and of these around 10% will die. After an episode of pancreatitis there is a >50% chance of a further episode occurring within six months.

It is a reasonable approach to perform ERCP and stone extraction in all patients with severe pancreatitis that do not improve rapidly. If improvement occurs cholecystectomy can then be performed electively.

Other indications for surgery include:

- Acute abdomen where the diagnosis of pancreatitis is unclear.
- Infected pancreatic necrosis.
- Pancreatic abscess (although this may be aspirated under CT).

3. Peritoneal lavage. As yet there is no consensus regarding the role of peritoneal lavage in pancreatitis.

Further reading

Coad NR. The management of acute severe pancreatitis. *British Journal of Intensive Care*, 1999; **March/April:** 38–44.

Mergener K, Baillie J. Acute pancreatitis. *British Medical Journal*, 1998; **316:** 44–48.

ADDER BITES

The adder (*Vipera berus* or European adder) is found widely throughout Western Europe. It is the only indigenous poisonous snake in the UK. Adder envenomations cause significant morbidity, although rarely result in death. There have only been reported 14 deaths in the UK since 1876, the last in 1975. More than 100 people bitten are treated in hospital each year.

The snake measures some 50–60 cm in length at maturity and is distinguishable by a black/brown dorsal zig-zag patterning and a V-shaped marking on the head.

The adder is most commonly located on dry, sandy heaths, sand dunes, rocky hillsides, moorlands and woodland edges.

The adder will tend to bite when provoked during summer months. Only approximately 50% of bites will result in envenomation.

Snake venom

Snake venoms contain 200+ components, mostly proteins which include:

- Enzymes – procoagulants serine proteases and arginine esterhydrolases that activate the blood clotting cascade resulting in disseminated intravascular coagulation.
- Proteases – result in tissue damage.
- Phospholipases A_2 – damage membranes and block neuromuscular transmission.
- Zinc metalloproteinase haemorrhagins – damage vascular endothelium.
- Non-enzymatic polypeptide toxins – e.g. post-synaptic neurotoxins that bind competitively with acetylcholine.

Other components include bradykinin-potentiating compounds, angiotensin-converting enzyme inhibitors and sanafotoxins.

Toxicity

Immediate pain at the site is common. Puncture marks are frequently visible and usually comprise two marks about a centimetre apart. Localized swelling is usually apparent within two hours and is a certain indicator of envenomation.

Early features include abdominal pain, vomiting, diarrhoea, sweating and pallor. Hypotension may be transient, persistent and may be fatal. Swelling may spread involving the whole extremity. Bruising may develop after one to two days. Local lymph nodes may become painful and enlarge. Angioneurotic oedema, urticaria and bronchospasm have been reported.

Severe effects

- Hypertension may occur. Non-specific ECG changes (T-wave inversion and ST depression and heart block) and arrhythmias and evidence of myocardial infarction.
- Coagulopathy is rare, though spontaneous haemorrhage in the lungs, gastro-intestinal and urinary tracts has been reported.
- Neutrophil leucocytosis, haemolysis and thrombocytopaenia.

- Creatine phosphokinase elevation.
- Pyrexia.
- Drowsiness, coma and convulsions.
- Pulmonary oedema.
- Acute pancreatitis.
- Cerebral oedema.
- Adult respiratory distress syndrome (ARDS).
- Acute renal failure.
- Death occurs 6–60 hours after envenomation.

Treatment

1. ***First aid treatment.*** Reassure the victim and transfer to hospital with the affected extremity immobilized. Do not cut or suck out the wound, as this may introduce infection and aggravate bleeding. Do not use tourniquets.

Do not advise patients to bring live specimens to hospital because of the risk of further bites. Additionally the adder is protected under the Wildlife and Countryside Act 1981 which makes it illegal to kill or injure wild specimens unless the snake was posing an immediate and foreseeable serious threat to pets and livestock and only if the slaughter was undertaken by an authorized person.

2. ***Hospital treatment***

- All cases require observation for a minimum of two hours, even if a puncture site is not visible.
- Clean the bite site.
- Immobilize or splint the extremity.
- Give anti-tetanus prophylaxis as appropriate.
- Asymptomatic patient after two hours may be discharged.
- Patients with clinical effects require admission for a minimum of 12 hours with cardiac monitoring.
- Record routine observations including pulse, blood pressure and respiratory rate hourly.
- Monitor ECG, urea and electrolytes, full blood count, clotting screen and creatine phosphokinase (CPK).
- Give anti-emetics for persistent vomiting.
- Shock and angioneurotic oedema should be treated initially with adrenaline and antihistamines.
- Fluid administration for hypotension.
- Appropriate analgesia for pain.
- In severe cases consider anti-venom treatment.
- Wound management.

Zagreb anti-venom

1. ***Indications***

- Persistent (>2 hours) fall in blood pressure (systolic to <70 mmHg or a decrease of more than 50 mmHg from normal or admission value) with or without signs of shock.

- Any other evidence of systemic envenomation e.g. pulmonary oedema, spontaneous bleeding, haematuria, coagulopathy, pulmonary oedema or haemorrhage, ECG abnormality, marked neutrophil leucocytosis (>20 × 10^9/l), or raised creatinine phosphokinase.
- Severe local envenomation within 2 hours of the bite (even in the absence of systemic signs) i.e. swelling beyond the next major joint from bite site. Any cases involving significant swelling of forearm or leg should also receive anti-venom.

2. ***Dose of antivenom.*** For adder bites use European Viper-venom serum (Zagreb).

- 1 × 10 ml ampoule diluted into 2–3 volumes of isotonic saline administered by slow intravenous injection at a rate not exceeding 2 ml/minute, or by intravenous infusion.
- The dose may be repeated after 1–2 hours if severe signs of envenomation persist, or if blood coagulability is not restored within 6 hours.
- Caution should be taken in patients with previous hypersensitivity to equine antisera.
- Additionally atopic individuals and those with allergic histories may get increased risk of anti-venom reactions. Nonetheless, such reactions are rare. Consider premedication of high risk patients with subcutaneous adrenaline, antihistamine and steroids.
- Treat allergic reactions conventionally with epinephrine (adrenaline) etc.
- Serum sickness may develop (one to two weeks after antivenom) and is characterized by fever, urticaria, arthralgia and albuminuria. Treatment may include oral steroids and antihistamines.
- Skin and conjunctival 'hypersensitivity' tests do not predict early (anaphylactoid) or late (serum-sickness type) antivenom reactions.
- The dose of antivenom given to children is the same as the adult dose.

Response to antivenom

There may be marked symptomatic improvement soon after treatment and blood pressure and consciousness may be restored. Spontaneous systemic bleeding usually stops within 15–30 minutes and blood coagulation restored within 6 hours (provided a neutralizing dose is given) systemic envenomation may recur hours or days after initial response. Observe patients in hospital for at least 3 days.

Antivenom reactions

- Early (anaphylactic/anaphylactoid) reactions develop within 30 minutes. The case of the boy with asthma who died from anaphylactic shock after Pasteur antivenom in England in 1957 has been widely publicized and resulted in unreasonable adverse rejection of the antivenom.

  Most reactions are not IgE mediated hyposensitivity reactions but complement activation.

  Treatment – As acute anaphylaxis.

- Pyrogenic reactions are caused by endotoxin contamination and result in fever, rigors, febrile convulsions in children, vasodilatation and fall in blood pressure.

Treatment – Cool the patient and give antipyretics.

- Late reaction (serum sickness) may develop 5–24 days later. Clinical features include fever, itching, urticaria, arthralgia, lymphadenopathy, periarticular swelling, mononeuritis multiplex and albuminuria.

  Treatment – Oral antihistamines and oral Prednisolone.

Contact telephone numbers

Professor DA Warrell, Centre for Tropical Medicine, University of Oxford, John Radcliffe Hospital. Telephone: 01865 221332/220968/220279; Fax: 01865 220984; E-mail: david.warrell@ndm.ox.ac.uk

AIRWAY

In the standard ABC sequence of resuscitation airway management has the highest priority. This is because hypoxia due to airway obstruction can cause brain damage within a few minutes and will rapidly lead to cardiac arrest.

Causes of airway obstruction

- Decreased conscious level.
- Anatomical disruption of the airway (e.g. trauma).
- Obstruction of the lumen:
  (a) foreign body;
  (b) blood;
  (c) vomitus.
- Intrinsic compression:
  (a) haematoma;
  (b) tumour;
  (c) infection (croup, epiglottitis);
  (d) Oedema (burn, allergy, angioneurotic oedema).
- Extrinsic compression:
  (a) haematoma;
  (b) retropharyngeal abscess.

Difference between the airway in children and adults

Although the airways of adults and children have the same anatomical components, there are differences due to the relative sizes of the structures, which are important when managing airway problems in children:

- the occiput is large with a relatively short neck resulting in flexion of the neck;
- the face is relatively small;
- the tongue is large and obstructs the airway with ease;
- the floor of the mouth is soft allowing digital compression to occur;
- the trachea is short and relatively straight making intubation of the right main bronchus easier than in adults.

Assessment of the airway

In the conscious patient the most striking feature of airway obstruction is the presence of abnormal sounds. Inspiratory Stridor and hoarseness are associated with upper airway obstruction. The presence of gurgling sounds suggests the presence of fluid in the upper airway. Wheezing is characteristic of lower airway obstruction.

In-patients with partial airways obstruction signs of respiratory distress and hypoxia should be sought. These include increased respiratory rate (or in severe cases decreased respiratory rate or ineffective ventilation), use of accessory muscles, cyanosis and decreased conscious level. In addition children may exhibit nasal flaring, recession (supraclavicular, intercostal, or subcostal), see-sawing of the sternum or tracheal tug.

In the unconscious patient the presence of respiratory effort should be checked by looking for movement of the chest, listening for breath sounds at the mouth and feeling for the warmth of exhaled air. The airway is inspected for the presence of foreign bodies. In children blind sweeps of the mouth are contraindicated because of the risk of damage to the soft tissues.

If the patient is not breathing the airway must be opened up to ensure a clear and unobstructed passage from the mouth to the lungs. If this does not restore spontaneous respiration, then the patient should be ventilated. When attempting to secure the airway, the simplest and least invasive manoeuvre or technique should be used which is consistent with maintaining the airway. More complex manoeuvres or techniques generally require more skill and have more complications. Suction and oxygen must be immediately available.

Basic airway management

The simplest airway manoeuvre is the head tilt and chin lift. In the majority of cases of airway obstruction this will ensure a clear airway. If a head tilt and chin lift fail to open the airway, or if cervical spine injury is suspected a jaw thrust may be used. If inspection of the airway reveals a foreign body, this is removed manually or by suction (but see note above about blind sweeps of the airway in children).

If the above manoeuvres fail to open the airway, or if a single-handed operator cannot maintain the airway and carry out other manoeuvres such as ventilation whilst maintaining the airway, an airway adjunct may be used. The oropharyngeal airway is the commonest such adjunct. Conscious or semi-conscious patients better tolerate the nasopharyngeal airway.

Advanced airway management

If the airway cannot be secured using a basic technique then a more advanced technique can be used. The most common of the advanced techniques is orotracheal intubation. Alternative techniques to orotracheal intubation are the nasotracheal route or the use of the laryngeal airway mask.

Surgical airway

If use of the above techniques fails to secure the airway, a surgical airway is indicated. Two techniques are described: needle cricothyroidotomy and surgical cricothyroidotomy.

The simplest technique is the needle cricothyroidotomy. A 14G cannula is inserted into the cricoid membrane and is connected via a 'Y' connector to wall oxygen at 15 litres/minute (or 1 litre/minute per year of life in children). The open port of the 'Y' connector is occluded for 1 second in 4. This technique buys time while expert help is sought. The technique allows oxygenation to be continued but does not provide adequate ventilation. The progressive onset of hypercarbia limits the duration of this technique to about 40 minutes.

An alternative to needle cricothyroidotomy is surgical cricothyroidotomy. In this technique a small incision is made in the cricoid membrane and a 4–6 mm endotracheal or tracheostomy tube is inserted into the trachea. This technique is contraindicated in children under the age of 12 years.

Formal tracheostomy is not generally considered to be a technique suitable for use in an emergency situation.

Ventilation

A proportion of patients will breath spontaneously once a patent airway has been secured. Patients who do not begin to breathe spontaneously should be ventilated. This can be achieved by one of four methods:

- mouth to mouth ventilation (exhaled air contains about 16% oxygen);
- mouth to mask (with supplemental oxygen a concentration of up to 50% oxygen can be delivered);
- self-inflating bag with oxygen reservoir (with full flow oxygen a concentration of oxygen of 85–90% can be delivered);
- anaesthetic circuit (up to 100% oxygen concentration).

Choking

The diagnosis of choking is usually obvious in the acute case. The patient presents with acute onset of stridor associated with coughing and gagging. In children the clinical picture is usually less obvious. A diagnosis of choking should be considered in any child with signs of airway obstruction or acute collapse.

During the routine assessment of the airway in the collapsed patient difficulty in establishing a patent airway despite adequate positioning should suggest the possibility of choking.

1. Management. The airway is opened and inspected; obvious foreign bodies are removed. If the patient has stopped breathing five rescue breaths should be attempted. If air cannot be introduced into the lungs the patient should be given five back blows followed by five chest thrusts. The airway is reassessed and further rescue breaths attempted. If the airway has still not been cleared a further five back blows are given followed by five abdominal thrusts. This cycle of back blows and chest thrusts followed by reassessment of the airway and further rescue breaths followed by back blows and abdominal thrusts is continued until the foreign body is expelled. In infants abdominal thrusts are contraindicated because of the risk to intra-abdominal organs. The sequence to be followed is five back blows followed by five chest thrusts, reassess the airway, attempt five rescue breaths and repeat the five back blows followed by five chest thrusts as necessary.

Further reading

Advanced life Support Group. *Advanced Cardiac Life Support.* London: Arnold, 1997.
Advanced life Support Group. *Advanced Paediatric Life Support.* London: BMJ Publishing Group, 1999.

Related topics of interest

Coma (p. 97); Head injury (p. 173); Inhalational injuries (p. 192); Major injuries – initial management (p. 215); Maxillofacial injury (p. 226); Sedation (p. 286)

ANALGESIA

Elizabeth Jones

Definition of pain – An unpleasant sensory or emotional experience associated with actual or potential tissue damage.

The aim of analgesia prescribing should be the abolishment of pain within the A&E Department once it has been identified (i.e. often before X-ray) and commencement of pain relief procedures for subsequent patient management in other departments. Regular analgesic prescribing is much preferred to a PRN approach.

Pain assessment

- Necessary for selection of the correct drug, route and dose. Re-assessment and review of requirements essential.
- Scoring systems – Physiological (BP, HR, RR).
  Patient reporting (Visual Analogue Scale, McGill pain questionnaire).

Approaches available

1. Non-pharmacological

Emotional: A warm, friendly and non-threatening environment.
Comprehensive explanations.

Physical: Splinting of fractures, cold treatment.

2. Pharmacological

Local: LA techniques.

Mild pain

1. Paracetamol (p.o., p.r.). A useful analgesic and anti-pyretic especially in the elderly because of the relatively few side effects at correct doses. However, it is very dangerous in overdose as it causes delayed onset liver failure.

2. Non steroidal anti-inflammatory drugs. Additional anti-inflammatory properties make these appropriate for many conditions presenting to A&E, although full anti-inflammatory effect may take up to 3 weeks.

Gastric and renal side effects mean that they should be avoided in patients with known peptic ulcer disease and used with caution in patients with renal impairment. They should be used with caution if patients have a history of asthma or allergy to aspirin.

Diclofenac is used with good effect for renal colic. Paracetamol and an NSAID in combination should be considered as it provides greater analgesia than the simple additive effect, one would expect.

Moderate pain

1. Morphine (p.o., i.m., i.v.). Morphine is the standard opiate for severe pain and the drug with which all others are compared. When given intravenously the peak action occurs within two to three minutes with a half-life of two to four hours.

In addition to analgesia it increases venous capacitance and hence is beneficial in pulmonary oedema and myocardial infarction.

Side-effects include:

- Nausea.
- Vomiting.
- Constipation.
- Drowsiness.
- Respiratory depression.
- Hypotension.
- Pupillary constriction.

The correct dose is that which gives good analgesia without significant side effects and is determined by titrating in small increments and waiting to assess the effect.

Resuscitation equipment should be readily available. (Naloxone is a potent opiate antagonist. It has a rapid but short-lived effect thus it may be necessary to repeat the dose or set up an intravenous infusion.) Oral preparations are available but are limited by a high first-pass metabolism that may result in an inadequate analgesic effect.

2. Diamorphine. Usually given intravenously for e.g. myocardial infarction and pulmonary oedema. Possibly causes less nausea and hypotension. Smaller doses and need for reconstitution may explain less common usage.

A 'morphine-sparing' effect of paracetamol and NSAIDs has been shown and these 'simple' analgesics should be considered as well as strong opiates in patients in severe pain.

3. Pethidine (i.m., i.v.). A short-lasting analgesic that causes less respiratory depression than morphine. Effects on smooth muscle (ureteric and biliary spasm) have in the past limited the use of morphine for acute abdominal pain, when pethidine has been advocated, but it is important to note that even at high doses pethidine is a less effective analgesic.

Combined preparations

The addition of codeine 60 mg produces additional pain relief but may be accompanied by dizziness and a degree of sedation. Doses less than this may add little to the analgesic effect.

1. Co-codamol. Paracetamol 500 mg + codeine 8 mg (or 30 mg).

2. Co-dydramol. Paracetamol 500 mg + dihydrocodeine 10 mg.

3. Co-proxamol. Paracetamol 325 mg + dextropropoxyphene 32.5 mg.

Preparations on sale to the public often contain paracetamol and codeine or codeine-like drugs on their own, or with aspirin, therefore consideration of the patients 'home pharmacy' is important when prescribing combination analgesics.

Route

This will depend on many factors including the particular drug, gastric function (e.g. nausea and vomiting) and urgency of analgesia required.

1. Oral. Convenient and acceptable to patients. Not indicated if vomiting is a symptom. Problems with oral morphine include unpredictable or delayed absorption because of delayed gastric emptying associated with trauma. Similarly a large bolus may be delivered once gastric motility returns. Other problems arise from the variable high first-pass metabolism of opiates which result in unpredictable bioavailability.

2. Per rectum. Useful alternative to oral especially in pyrexia and vomiting (paracetamol); as alternative to i.m. in renal colic (diclofenac).

3. Intravenous. Rapid onset of analgesic effects of e.g. morphine, but also of side effects. Intermittent doses inevitably lead to troughs of pain. This can be reduced by continuous i.v. infusions or patient-controlled analgesia systems more commonly found on the wards.

4. Intranasal. A major advance for use in Emergency Departments, particularly in children.

Others

1. Inhalation agents. e.g. Entonox (50% nitrous oxide and 50% oxygen). Self-administered to cover short-duration procedures. Low water solubility results in a rapid onset (two to three minutes) and rapid recovery. It produces a degree of sedation which may potentiate the sedative effect of other drugs. Nitrous oxide diffuses into air filled spaces therefore absolute contraindications include:

- Pneumothorax.
- Recent head injury.
- Abdominal injury.
- Decompression sickness.
- Otitis media.

2. Local anaesthetic agents. Topical, local, regional, epidural and spinal techniques.

3. General anaesthesia.

Analgesia in children

Despite the widespread acceptance of the ability of children of all ages (including the fetus) to experience pain, underprescribing of analgesics in children is still widespread. Part of the problem is that pain assessment parameters and scoring systems vary, depending on the age of the child. Children may themselves by reluctant to ask for analgesia, especially if the route is painful e.g. i.m.

Assessment of pain

- Extent of the injury.
- Behavioural signs of pain: crying, grimacing, restlessness, loss of interest in play.
- Physiological signs: sweating, heart rate, respiratory rate.
- Assessment by parents and experienced nurses.
- Formal pain scores: CRIES (neonates); Objective pain scale, CHEOPS (infant and toddler); Wong and Baker Faces scale, Linear analogue scales (3–7 years); analogue scales and Adjectival self report ($\geq$7 years).

Non-drug approaches

1. Emotional

- Child-friendly environment with parental involvement.
- Distraction techniques: blowing bubbles, toys, videos, music.
- Careful explanation in appropriate language to child and parent.
- Hypnosis.

2. Physical

Splinting of fractures.

Drugs and doses

Doses calculated per kg body weight. A guide to the weight of a child aged 1–10 years is obtained by the formula:

$$\text{Weight in kgs} = (\text{age in years} + 4) \times 2.$$

Be wary of over dosage in obese children.

Mild pain

1. Paracetamol. Children over 1 year

- Oral: No loading dose.
  Regular dose 20 mg per kg 6 hourly.
- P.r.: Loading dose up to 40 mg per kg.
  Regular dose 20 mg per kg 6 hourly.
- Max: 90 mg per kg per day.

Infants and neonates: Same regime except doses every 8 hours to give a max daily dose 60 mg per kg.

Review these doses after 48 hours and taper doses after 72 hours.
Reduce doses if: hepatic impairment, hypovolaemia, dehydration.

2. NSAIDs. Useful as they have an opioid-sparing effect. NSAIDs should not be used in renal failure, hepatic failure, aspirin sensitivity or coagulopathy.

3. Ibuprofen. Oral 20 mg per kg per day in 4 divided doses.
Can be used in children 6 months upwards.

4. Diclofenac. Oral or p.r. 3 mg per kg per day in 3 divided doses.
Can be used in children over 1 year.

Moderate pain

1. Codeine phosphate. P.o. or p.r. 1 mg per kg per dose 4–6 hourly.
Max daily dose 6 mg per kg.
Useful when bridging the gap between intravenous and oral analgesia especially in neonates or ex-premature babies and those children who cannot be given NSAIDs.

Severe pain

1. Morphine

- Oral: Dose 1 month–1 year 0.5 mg per kg per day in 6 divided doses.
  Despite high 1st pass metabolism this is useful when opioid analgesia is required, oral fluids are being tolerated and mild or moderate analgesics are insufficient.
- i.v.: Children over 1 year 200 mcg per kg per dose.
  Given after dilution in 10 ml of sterile water.
  Slowly give an initial dose of 2 ml followed by further increments of 1 ml according to pain scores at 5 minute intervals.
  Younger children may be given opiates provided great care is taken in calculating the dose and the same principles of dilution and incremental delivery are applied:

6–12 months	100 mcg per kg per dose.
3–6 months	50 mcg per kg per dose.
1–3 months	25 mcg per kg per dose.

Respiratory rates, oxygen saturations and level of sedation must be monitored.
Intranasal diamorphine avoids first-pass metabolism.Research has shown this to be at least as effective as i.m. morphine and a popular route of administration by parents and nurses.

2. Anti-emetics. These are not normally required in young children. If one is required: cyclizine i.v. (1 mg per kg, 8 hourly, max daily dose 3 mg per kg per day) is useful, but must be diluted to reduce pain on injection.

Others

1. Entonox. Useful for a wide range of procedures in A&E which require potent analgesia for a short period of time e.g. infiltration of LA, suture insertion or removal and dressing changes. It works best in co-operative children over 5 years.

2. Local anaesthesia. Topical preparations: these are very useful for anaesthetising the skin prior to intravenous cannulation or venepuncture. They need 45–60 minutes to work. However, application in the A&E department will facilitate procedures on the ward.

3. Local infiltration. Pre-emptive oral analgesia, careful explanations, fine needles, warmed lignocaine all reduce pain on infiltration.

- Lignocaine: Max dose 3 mg per kg, 4 hourly.
- Bupivacaine: Max dose 2 mg per kg, 8 hourly.
- Note: Ideal weight should be used in obese children.

Further reading

British Association for Accident and Emergency Medicine. *Guidelines for Analgesia in Children in the Accident & Emergency Department*, 1997.

ANAPHYLAXIS

Anaphylaxis is the syndrome elicited in a hypersensitive individual on subsequent exposure to the sensitizing antigen. Reactions range from mild pruritus and urticaria to anaphylactic shock and death.

'Anaphylactoid' reactions are similar, but are not IgE mediated and not related to prior sensitization. They require identical treatment.

Antibiotics (especially penicillin) and radiographic contrast agents are the most common causes of serious anaphylactic events, with rates of about 1 per 2300 new attendances at an Accident & Emergency Department. Fatal anaphylactic reactions are estimated at 1 per million population per year, but this is probably under-reported because of diagnostic uncertainty, e.g. confusion with asthma.

Other precipitants include insect stings, foods, plants, chemicals, latex and exercise.

Anaphylaxis may progress slowly or rapidly. Its onset may be delayed for up to 6 hours. Five per cent of patients have a biphasic response with the recurrence occurring 1–72 hours after the acute event.

Aetiology

Anaphylaxis may arise in three ways:

- Exposure to a foreign protein results in the generation of an IgE-antibody response. During re-exposure, antigen results in degranulation of mast cells and perhaps basophils, releasing chemical mediators such as histamine, prostaglandins, leukotrienes, and platelet-activating factor.
- Immune complexes or other agents activate the complement cascade, resulting in the formation of anaphylatoxins that trigger the release of mast cells and basophils directly.
- Certain agents such as hyperosmolar solutions and radio-contrast mediums can stimulate the release of mediators directly by an as yet unknown mechanism.

Clinical features

Diagnosis of anaphylaxis relies on the association of the typical clinico-pathologic features in association with exposure to a foreign substance.

Diagnosis is clinical and includes the following features:

1. ***Airway.*** Angioedema, tongue swelling, laryngeal oedema progressing to airway obstruction.

2. ***Breathing.*** Bronchospasm and pulmonary oedema.

3. ***Circulation.*** Hypotension and cardiovascular collapse.

4. ***General.*** Faintness, syncope, feeling of impending doom.

5. ***Cutaneous.*** Pruritis, erythema, urticaria.

6. ***Gastrointestinal.*** Nausea and vomiting, abdominal pain and diarrhoea.

The onset of symptoms and signs vary from immediate to hours with the majority occurring within one hour and the timing of onset depends on the sensitivity of the person, the route, quantity and rate of delivery of the antigen. A biphasic reaction may occur.

1. General symptoms. Faintness, syncope, seizures, confusion or a feeling of impending doom.

2. Cutaneous. Pruritus, flushing, erythema, urticaria and in severe cases angio-edema. Mucous membranes can also be involved.

3. Respiratory symptoms. Breathlessness, wheeze, chest tightness. In severe cases upper airway obstruction due to oedema of the larynx and epiglottis (angio-edema) may result.

4. Cardiovascular collapse. Secondary to peripheral vasodilatation, increased vascular permeability and intravascular volume depletion. Arrhythmias and ischaemia may result.

5. Gastrointestinal symptoms. Nausea, vomiting, abdominal cramps and diarrhoea.

The differential diagnosis includes those associated with:

- Loss of consciousness (e.g. syncope, epilepsy, myocardial infarction and arrhythmias).
- Acute respiratory conditions (asthma, epiglottis, foreign body obstruction and pulmonary embolism).
- Disorders with cutaneous or respiratory manifestations (mastocytosis, carcinoid, hereditary angioedema and reactions to drugs).

Treatment

- The recommendations for management were published by the Resuscitation Council (UK) in 1999 and are summarized in the algorithms below for adults and children.
- Cardiopulmonary resuscitation must be performed as per Advanced Life Support guidelines if the need arises.
- All victims should recline in a position of comfort.
- Oxygen should be administered at high flow rate (10–15 litres per minute).
- Epinephrine (Adrenaline) should be administered intramuscularly to all patients with clinical signs of airway swelling, breathing difficulty or hypotension.

  The dose of Epinephrine (adrenaline) for adults is 0.5 ml of 1:1000 solution (500 μg). This may be repeated after approximately 5 minutes if there is no clinical improvement or the patient has deteriorated.

  The EpiPen or Anapen and the EpiPen Jr and Anapen Jr inject 300 μg or 150 μg, respectively.

  Intravenous (adrenaline) in a dilution of at least 1:10000 (never 1:1000) is hazardous and must be reserved for patients with profound shock that is immediately life-threatening and for special indications, e.g. during anaesthesia. The injection must be given as slowly as seems reasonable whilst monitoring the heart rate and ECG.

- Severe reactions are manifest by inspiratory stridor, wheeze, cyanosis, pronounced tachycardia and decreased capillary refill.
- An antihistamine (Chlorpheniramine) should be administered. Administer by slow intravenous injection to avoid drug-induced hypotension.
- Hydrocortisone should be administered after severe attacks to help avert late sequelae. This is particularly important for asthmatics if they have been treated with corticosteroids previously. Administer by slow intravenous injection to avoid inducing further hypotension.
- If severe hypotension does not respond rapidly to drug therapy intravenous fluids should be infused. A bolus infusion of 1–2 litres may be needed for an adult. Children should receive a 20 ml/kg bolus.
- All patients should be warned of the possibility of recurrence of symptoms and in some circumstances should be observed for 8–24 hours. This particularly applies to the following:

  (a) Severe reactions with slow onset.
  (b) Reactions in severe asthmatics or with a severe asthmatic component.
  (c) Reactions with the possibility of the continuing absorption of allergen.
  (d) Patients with a previous history of biphasic reactions.

- An inhaled β_2 agonist such as Salbutamol is a useful treatment for bronchospasm.
- It is essential to inform the patient of the suspected allergen to avoid future reactions. This may necessitate referral to a specialist allergy clinic. All patients should also wear a Medicalert-type bracelet.

Anaphylaxis reactions for children: Treatment by first medical responder

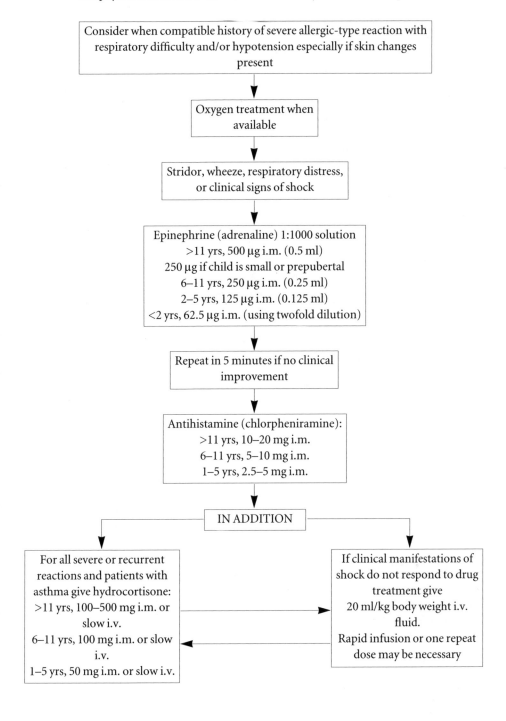

Consider when compatible history of severe allergic-type reaction with respiratory difficulty and/or hypotension especially if skin changes present

↓

Oxygen treatment when available

↓

Stridor, wheeze, respiratory distress, or clinical signs of shock

↓

Epinephrine (adrenaline) 1:1000 solution
>11 yrs, 500 μg i.m. (0.5 ml)
250 μg if child is small or prepubertal
6–11 yrs, 250 μg i.m. (0.25 ml)
2–5 yrs, 125 μg i.m. (0.125 ml)
<2 yrs, 62.5 μg i.m. (using twofold dilution)

↓

Repeat in 5 minutes if no clinical improvement

↓

Antihistamine (chlorpheniramine):
>11 yrs, 10–20 mg i.m.
6–11 yrs, 5–10 mg i.m.
1–5 yrs, 2.5–5 mg i.m.

↓

IN ADDITION

For all severe or recurrent reactions and patients with asthma give hydrocortisone:
>11 yrs, 100–500 mg i.m. or slow i.v.
6–11 yrs, 100 mg i.m. or slow i.v.
1–5 yrs, 50 mg i.m. or slow i.v.

If clinical manifestations of shock do not respond to drug treatment give 20 ml/kg body weight i.v. fluid.
Rapid infusion or one repeat dose may be necessary

Anaphylaxis reactions for adults: Treatment by first medical responder

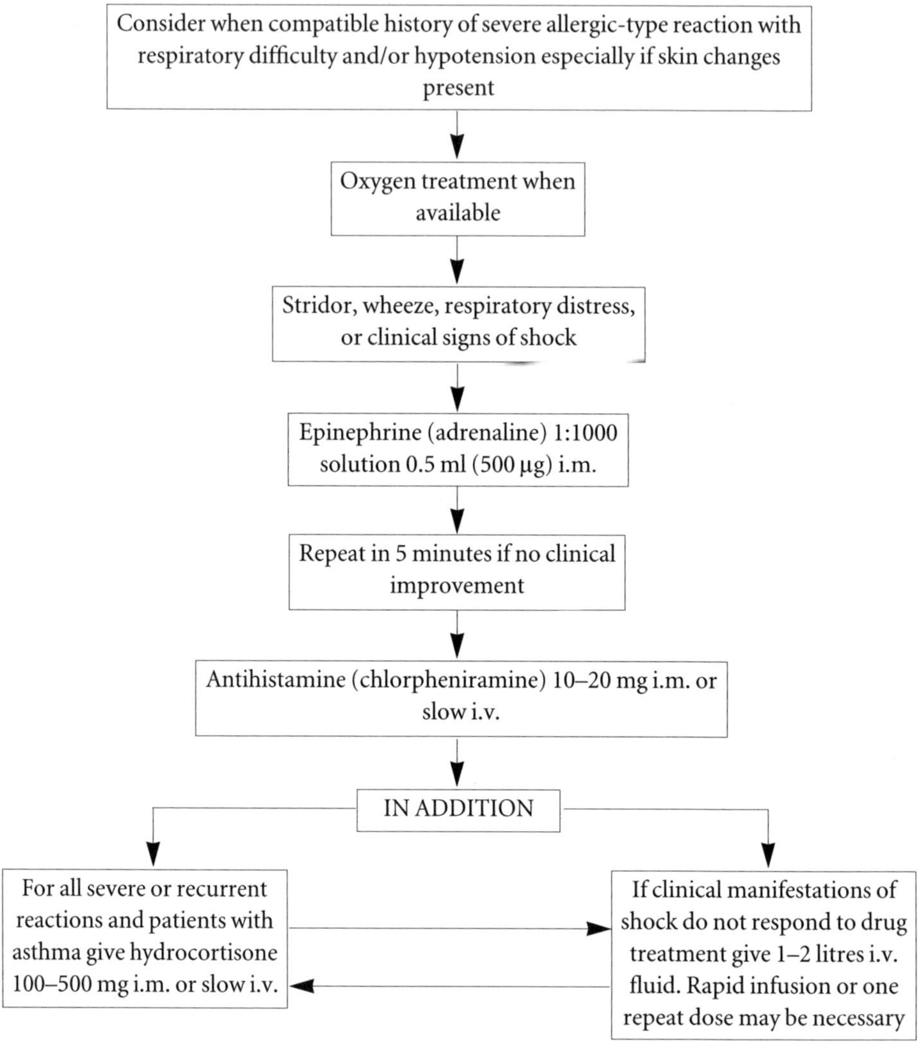
Consider when compatible history of severe allergic-type reaction with respiratory difficulty and/or hypotension especially if skin changes present
Oxygen treatment when available
Stridor, wheeze, respiratory distress, or clinical signs of shock
Epinephrine (adrenaline) 1:1000 solution 0.5 ml (500 µg) i.m.
Repeat in 5 minutes if no clinical improvement
Antihistamine (chlorpheniramine) 10–20 mg i.m. or slow i.v.
IN ADDITION
For all severe or recurrent reactions and patients with asthma give hydrocortisone 100–500 mg i.m. or slow i.v.
If clinical manifestations of shock do not respond to drug treatment give 1–2 litres i.v. fluid. Rapid infusion or one repeat dose may be necessary

Further reading

Bochner BS, Lightenstein LM. Anaphylaxis. *The New England Journal of Medicine*, 1991; **324:** 1785–90.

Brueton MJ *et al.* Management of anaphylaxis. *Hospital Update*, 1991; **5:** 386–98.

Handley AJ. Resuscitation Council (UK). *Advanced Life Support Manual*, 1992.

Project Team of the Resuscitation Council (UK). Emergency medical treatment of anaphylactic reactions. *Journal of Accident and Emergency Medicine*, 1999; **16:** 243–7.

Related topic of interest

Shock (p. 291)

ANKLE SPRAIN

Ankle injuries commonly present to the A&E department estimated at a rate of 1 per 10000 people per day. The dominant ankle is more likely to be involved. Ankle injuries can cause significant morbidity. These include functional instability, mechanical instability, chronic pain, stiffness and recurrent swelling.

A sprain is defined as the acute rupture of a ligament (often mistakenly called a strain, a strain is an acute tear in a muscle).

Classification of sprains

1. Grade 1 injuries. It involves partial tearing of the fibres with little associated functional loss and no joint instability. This is the most common type of sprain. Pain and localized swelling are the characteristic features.

2. Grade 2 injuries. Extensive tearing of the ligament with some joint instability evident on radiographic stress views although the joint cannot be fully opened up. Like the grade 1 injury, pain and localized swelling are characteristic. This type of sprain is uncommon. The instability usually only becomes evident days or weeks after the injury when the patient returns because the sprain is not getting better.

3. Grade 3 injuries. Complete rupture of the ligament with joint instability both clinically and radiographically. On stress views the joint can be opened up completely. The injury is painless or has minimal pain because the ligament is completely torn. This type of sprain is rare in ankle injuries.

Lateral ligament

Most ankle sprains occur due to inversion injuries (85%).

The lateral complex comprises of the following three ligamentous structures:

- the anterior talo-fibular ligament (ATFL).
- the calcaneo-fibular ligament (CFL).
- the posterior talo-fibular ligament (PTFL).

These ligaments oppose inversion forces on the joint. Inversion injuries lead first to tearing and then to the rupture of the anterior talo-fibular (65% as an isolated injury), then calcano-fibular and finally posterior talo-fibular ligaments. Complete disruption of all three leads to joint instability. In some patients the subtalar complex may also be injured. The CFL is rarely injured in isolation.

Medial ligament

Medial ligament injury (15% of injuries) is rare and usually involves malleolar fractures.

The medial or deltoid ligament opposes eversion forces on the joint. Eversion injuries first lead to tearing and the rupture of the deltoid ligament. Severe forces can lead to a Maissoneuve fracture possibly associated with ankle joint diastasis (see below). Eversion injuries are more likely to result in chronic pain or chronic instability.

History/examination

Establish the mechanism of injury. Enquire regarding previous ankle injuries. Ask about the presence of immediate or delayed pain, swelling and ability or inability to bear weight. Observe for oedema, ecchymosis or deformity. Palpate for tenderness, crepitus or deformity. Assess active and passive range of movement as well as weight-bearing ability.

Examine the following:

- Proximal fibula.
- Lateral malleolus and ligament.
- Medial malleolus and ligament.
- 5th metatarsal base.
- Calcaneum.
- Achilles tendon.

The entire length of the fibula should be examined up to and including the head. This is to ensure that the uncommon *Maissoneuve fracture* is not missed. The Maissoneuve fracture is caused by an eversion injury and involves the tearing of the deltoid ligament in association with a proximal fibula fracture. This fracture may cause instability of the ankle joint if the deltoid ligament is completely ruptured and diastasis of the inferior tibiofibular ligament is ruptured in addition.

Stress testing for ligament instability is difficult particularly in an acute setting. The following tests are performed:

1. ***Talar tilt test:***
   - The foot is placed in 20–30° of plantar flexion and slight adduction and gentle inversion stress are applied to the calcaneal midfoot.
   - If both the anterior talofibular and the calcaneofibular ligaments are ruptured, the examiner will detect talar tilt or movement of the talus in the mortise.
2. ***Anterior drawer test:***
   - The foot is placed in 10–15° of plantar flexion and gentle forward traction is placed on the heel.
   - With anterior talofibular ligament rupture, the deltoid ligament becomes the centre of rotation and a dimple may be seen just anterior to the lateral malleolus and forward motion of the talus detected by the examiner.
   - For this test, 3 mm of movement may be significant; 1 cm of movement is certainly significant.
3. ***Perform and document a neurovascular exam.***
   - Check dorsalis pedis and posterior tibial pulses, capillary refill and sensation.

The Ottawa ankle rules

The Ottawa ankle rules were developed as a clinical decision support tool to minimize exposure to radiation without increasing missed fracture rate. Originally validated in adults their use has now been validated in children over two years of age.

Ankle X-rays comprise approximately 10% of A&E X-rays. Only about 15% of these demonstrate a fracture.

The decision as to whether to X-ray an ankle to exclude a fracture is a balance between the small, but not zero, risk associated with exposing patients to unnecessary diagnostic radiation and the risk of missing significant injuries.

The rules are applied to adults (less than 55 years old) or children (over 2 years) who present with an acute ankle or midfoot injury. The lateral malleolar zone extends up from the tip of the lateral malleolus to include the lower 6 cm of the posterior border of the fibula. The medial malleolar zone extends from the tip of the medial malleolus to include the lower 6 cm of the posterior border of the tibia. The midfoot zone includes the navicular medially and the base of the fifth metatarsal laterally.

Weight-bearing is defined as the ability to take four steps.

Indications for an ankle X-ray

The patient complains of pain in the malleolar zone *and* any of the following:

- bone tenderness at the lateral malleolar zone, or
- bone tenderness at the medial malleolar zone, or
- inability to weight-bear both immediately after the injury *and* in the A&E department.

Indications for a foot X-ray

The patient complains of pain in the midfoot zone *and* any of the following:

- bone tenderness at the lateral midfoot zone, or
- bone tenderness at the medial midfoot zone, or
- inability to weight-bear both immediately after the injury *and* in the A&E department.

Use of these rules has been found to reduce the number of X-ray requests by up to 33% without a significant increase in missed fractures.

X-rays

Standard AP and lateral views of the ankle suffice to make diagnosis in most cases. There is no indication for stress views in the acute situation because of the pain associated with the injury. Complete ligamentous rupture is rare. If there is a clinical suspicion of a Maissoneuve fracture (tenderness along the upper fibula) then full views of the tibia and fibula are required. A mortise view (45° oblique film with the ankle in dorsiflexion) is occasionally necessary.

Treatment

The aim of treatment in the short term is to relieve pain and reduce swelling and in the long term to reduce the duration of morbidity.

The acronym **RICE** describes the standard treatment:

- Rest: in the first day or two after the injury the ankle will be too painful to move. Short-term rest eases discomfort and does not increase morbidity.
- Ice: for the first 48 hours local application of ice (frozen peas, or an ice pack, wrapped in a towel to prevent cold injury) intermittently (for 20 minutes at 4 hourly intervals) causes vasoconstriction which reduces capillary leak and therefore swelling. There is no benefit to be derived from using ice after the first 48 hours.
- Compression: adequate compression increases tissue hydrostatic pressure and reduces capillary leakage and swelling. Ordinary tubigrip does not produce sufficient compression to affect tissue hydrostatic pressure significantly.
- Elevation: swelling as well as contributing to the pain of a sprain also reduces mobility in the joint. Elevation of the affected part reduces swelling. Elevate the leg above the waist when not exercising including during sleep.

Analgesia, NSAIDs and/or paracetamol provides symptomatic relief of pain. Non-weight-bearing exercises should be commenced as soon after the injury as possible.

Mobilization

Patients must be encouraged to mobilize as soon as possible and normally.

Grade 2 injuries may require a more formal compression dressing such as a stirrup strap or air stirrup splint. More severe cases may require further assessment by the physiotherapist or may require further investigation as other injuries may occasionally be associated.

Surgical repair in a severe grade 3 injury may be considered in active sports persons.

There is no indication for the routine use of plaster of Paris immobilization in the management of ankle sprains. Such immobilization leads to stiffness in the joint and may lead to loss of proprioceptive reflexes.

Outcome

Gradual progression to full weight-bearing can usually take place within a week in most instances. Return to full activity, including sports may take up to 6 weeks. Some patients present with failure to progress to full recovery several weeks after injury. These will usually have either grade 2 or 3 tears which can be seen on stress views or problems associated with loss of proprioceptive reflexes which may respond to physiotherapy.

Differential diagnosis

Differential diagnosis includes the following:

- Achilles tendon rupture.
- Peroneal tendon subluxation.
- Septic joint.
- Osteomyelitis.

Further reading

Libetta C, Burke DP, Brennan PO, Yassa JG. Validation of the Ottawa ankle rules in children. *Journal of Accident and Emergency Medicine*, 1999; **16:** 342–4.

Liu SH, Nguyen TM. Ankle sprains and other soft tissue injuries. *Current Opinion in Rheumatology*, 1999; **11:** 132–7.

Stiell IG, Greenberg GH, McKnight RD, Nair RC, McDowell I, Worthington JR. A study to develop clinical decision rules for the use of radiography in acute ankle injuries. *Annals of Emergency Medicine*, 1992; **21:** 384–90.

Stiell IG, Greenberg GH, McKnight RD, Nair RC, McDowell I, Reardon M, Stewart JP, Maloney J. Decision rules for the use of radiography in acute ankle injuries. Refinement and prospective validation. *JAMA*, 1993; **269:** 1127–32.

Related topics of interest

Calf pain – musculoskeletal causes (p. 178); Overuse injury (p. 263)

ANTERIOR KNEE PAIN

Anterior knee pain is common. There are a range of distinct clinical conditions causing anterior knee pain. History and examination usually allow a diagnosis to be made clinically.

Osgood–Schlatter disease

This is a traction apophysitis of the epiphysis at the insertion of the patellar tendon into the tibial tuberosity. The peak incidence occurs between the ages of 10–14 years. The patient is usually an active boy who complains of localized pain in the anterior aspect of the knee. Examination reveals a prominent tibial tuberosity with localized tenderness. This is a self-limiting condition. Acute exacerbations are treated with rest and NSAIDs. There is no need to advise long-term restriction of activity if the discomfort is tolerable, merely short periods of rest during acute exacerbations. Reassurance should be given that the condition will settle spontaneously as the epiphysis fuses. In severe cases the knee can be immobilized in plaster for several weeks to enforce rest.

Sinding–Larsen–Johansson syndrome

This is a traction apophysitis of the inferior pole of the patella. Similar in presentation to Osgood–Schlatter the tenderness is localized to the inferior border of the patella. Management and prognosis is as for Osgood–Schlatter disease.

Chondromalacia patellae

This condition occurs in teenagers and young adults. Girls are more often affected than boys. The presentation is anterior knee pain, particularly when exercising and characteristically when climbing upstairs. The patient often complains of a sensation that the knee gives way. The knee is generally tender, particularly over the patella.

Treatment is symptomatic with rest and NSAIDs. If the symptoms are severe enough to restrict activity quadriceps wasting may occur. If this is present physiotherapy is advised. The majority of cases settle spontaneously, the more recalcitrant cases may require arthroscopic lateral retinacular release.

Osteochondritis dessicans

This condition also occurs in teenagers and young adults. A fragment of bone and articular cartilage separates from the femoral condyle (usually medial) forming a loose body within the knee joint. The patient presents with anterior knee pain and possibly an effusion in the acute phase. There may be a history of the knee giving way or locking.

Plain X-ray of the knee including an intracondylar (tunnel) view may reveal either the bone fragment or the defect in the condyle. The patient should be referred to the orthopaedic clinic for consideration of fixation or removal of the fragment.

Patella dislocation

This condition most commonly affects young women. Although there is rarely a history of significant trauma to the knee, the patient will have usually been taking part in sport or vigorous exercise. The diagnosis is clear on examination. The patella can be seen to be dislocated laterally. The patient is often apprehensive and unwilling to let the knee be examined.

There is rarely any need to use force to reduce the patella. The heel of the affected leg is place on a rolled up towel and the patient encouraged to relax. As the knee gently relaxes into hyperextension the patella often reduces spontaneously. The knee is placed in a splint and the patient referred to the orthopaedic clinic. On occasions the patient will present with a history of a dislocated patella which has been reduced (or has spontaneously reduced) before arrival at hospital. Examination will usually reveal tenderness over the medial retinacular fibres and a haemarthrosis. Patients with recurrent dislocation of the patella may require surgical correction of the patellar malalignment.

Quadriceps/patellar ligament rupture

Rupture of the patellar tendon is most common in the under 40s, rupture of the quadriceps is most common in the over 40s. The patient complains of sudden onset of severe pain in the front of the knee following forceful contraction of the knee or a fall onto the flexed knee. There is swelling of the knee and a defect in the tendon may be palpable. The patient cannot raise the straight leg against gravity or resistance.

The treatment is surgical repair. This injury is often missed because of failure to examine for straight leg raising ability in the injured knee.

Bursitis

A variety of bursae may be found around the knee. Some communicate with the knee joint itself. Inflammation due to local trauma causes pain and swelling of the bursa.

The treatment is rest and analgesia. In chronic cases the bursa may be surgically excised. In some instances the degree of inflammation will lead to concerns that the bursa is infected. Some advocate aspiration and microscopy to exclude infection.

Further reading

Bourne MH, Hazel WA Jnr, Scott SG, Sim FH. Anterior knee pain. *Mayo Clinic Proceedings*, 1988; **63**(5): 482–91.

Jacobson KE, Flandry FC. Diagnosis of anterior knee pain. *Clinics in Sports Medicine*, 1989; **8**(2): 179–95.

ANTIBIOTICS

Antibiotics are one of the most commonly prescribed group of drugs both in the hospital and community setting. Concern over the emergence of resistance to the common first-line antibiotics and increasingly second- and third-line choices has led to a growing demand for rational use of these drugs.

Rational use depends on the decision that an antibiotic is required in the first instance then a decision as to which drug to use, appropriate dose and the route of administration.

Within Accident and Emergency departments policies on the use of antibiotics vary. Some departments advocate the liberal use of antibiotics both for treatment and prophylaxis. Others are more conservative.

When choosing an antibiotic three groups of considerations should be taken into account before a decision is made as to which drug it to be used, host factors, pathogen factors and factors related to the specific antibiotic.

Host factors

- Infection type, site and severity.
- Age.
- Allergies.
- Ethnic origin.
- Compliance.
- State of immune system.
- Previous or concurrent antibiotic treatment.
- Hepatic function.
- Renal function.
- Ability to tolerate oral route.
- Prosthetic implants (e.g. heart valves).
- Whether breastfeeding.
- Whether pregnant.
- Whether taking the oral contraceptive pill.

Pathogen factors

- Organism involved (or in the absence of culture results the likely organism involved).
- Antibiotic sensitivities (either from culture and sensitivity reports or known local pattern of sensitivity).

Antibiotic factors

- Local policy.
- Route of administration.
- Side effects.
- Contraindications.
- Cost.

Side effects of treatment

1. Anaphylaxis. Although uncommon this is a potentially life-threatening complication. Any previous history suggestive of allergy to a class of antibiotics (urticarial rash, bronchospasm, angioedema or circulatory collapse) should lead to the use of another class of drug. Many patients claim to be allergic to antibiotics, especially the penicillins. Closer questioning will often reveal that the history of allergy is spurious, e.g. diarrhoea or failure of therapy. In the uncommon instance when a patient claims to be allergic to several classes of antibiotic, specific tests can be carried out by a specialist in allergy to confirm or refute the claim.

2. Super infection. Broadspectrum antibiotics are more likely to lead to the selection of resistant organisms and lead to overgrowth of these organisms (superinfection). This can manifest itself in several ways: fungal infections (e.g. candida), pseudomembranous colitis, vaginitis, pruritis ani.

3. Drug-specific effects. Disulfiram-like reaction with alcohol associated with Metronidazole use. Tetracycline staining of developing teeth. Ototoxicity of aminogylcosides.

4. Others. Diarrhoea and/or vomiting are common side effects of many antibiotics. Skin rashes may occur in up to 10% of cases.

Resistance to antibiotics and other antimicrobial agents (HSC 1999/049)

The House of Lords Science and Technology Select Committee published its report in April 1998 'Resistance to Antibiotics and other Antimicrobial agents'. In this report they highlighted concern at the emergence and spread of antimicrobial resistance and its impact on the treatment of infection. They said:

'this enquiry has been an alarming experience, which leaves us convinced that resistance to antibiotics and other anti-infective agents constitutes a major threat to public health and ought to be recognized as such more widely than it is at present'.

In March 1999 the Government responded with the publication of Health Service Circular 1999/049. This set out actions for the NHS:

The goal is for the NHS to:

- minimize morbidity and mortality due to antimicrobial resistant infection, including hospital acquired infection;
- contribute to the control of antibiotic resistant organisms;
- to this end, facilitate more efficient and effective use of NHS resources.

This will be achieved through:

- strengthening prevention and control of communicable disease, including infection control;
- optimizing antimicrobial prescribing;
- improving surveillance of communicable disease and infection caused by antimicrobial resistant organisms, and monitoring antimicrobial usage to provide the information base for action.

These actions are currently being implemented.

Further reading

British Medical Association & Royal Pharmaceutical Society. *British National Formulary*, September 1999.
Department of Health. Health Service Circular 1999/049: *Resistance to Antibiotics and Other Antimicrobial Agents*, March 1999.
House of Lords Select Committee on Science and Technology. Report: *Resistance to Antibiotics and Other Antimicrobial Agents.* The Stationery Office. April 1998.

Related topics of interest

Anaphylaxis (p. 38); Bites and envemonations (p. 65); Meningococcal disease (p. 237); Tetanus (p. 317)

ANTIDOTES

Modern resuscitation techniques and supportive care are the mainstay of management of a seriously poisoned patient. In view of this some antidotes have been rendered unnecessary because patients will make a full recovery provided vital functions are maintained. However, in certain circumstances, antidotes may be lifesaving or may shorten the duration of toxicity or diminish its severity, increasing the chances of recovery and reducing side effects.

The International Programme on Chemical Safety (IPCS) on antidotes have recommended antidotes with their indications. The IPCS definition of an antidote is as follows, 'A therapeutic substance administered to counteract the adverse effects of a specified xenobiotic'.

IPCS list of antidotes and other useful agents in the treatment of human poisoning

The antidotes presented are considered useful in the treatment of acute human poisoning and their availability in terms of *urgency of use* in treatment is classified as follows:

A. Required to be immediately available (within 30 minutes).
B. Required to be available within 2 hours.
C. Required to be available within 6 hours.

Their *effectiveness in practice* is classified as follows:

1. Effectiveness well documented e.g. reduced lethality in animal experiments and reduction of lethality or severe complications in human cases.
2. Widely used, but not yet universally accepted as effective due to lack of research data, and requiring further investigation concerning effectiveness or indications for use.
3. Questionable usefulness.

List of Antidotes

Antidotes	*Indications*
A1	
Atropine	Organophosphorus Compounds and Carbamates
Beta-blockers (β-1 and β-2, preferably short acting)	Beta-adrenergic agonists
Calcium gluconate or other soluble calcium salts	HF, fluorides, oxalates
Dicobalt edetate	Cyanide
Digoxin-specific fab antibody fragments	Digoxin/Digitoxin, other digitalis glycosides
Ethanol	Methanol, ethylene glucol
Glucagon	Beta-blockers
Glucose (Hypertonic)	Insulin

[*Continued*]

Antidotes	*Indications*
Hydroxocobalamin	Cyanide
Isoprenaline (Isoproterenol)	Beta-blockers
4-Methylpyrazole	Ethylene glycol
Methylthioninium chloride	Methaemoglobinaemia
Naloxone	Opiates
Oxygen	Cyanide, carbon monoxide, hydrogen sulfide
Phentolamine	Alpha-adrenergic agonists
Physostigmine	Central anti-cholinergic syndrome from atropine and derivatives
Prenalterol	Beta-blockers
Protamine sulphate	Heparin
Sodium nitrite	Cyanide
Sodium nitroprusside	Ergotism
Sodium thiosulfate	Cyanide
A2	
Amyl nitrite	Cyanide
Dantrolene	Drug-induced hyperthermia
Diazepam	Organophosphorus compounds
4-Dimethylaminophenol (4-DMAP)	Cyanide
Pyridoxine	Isoniazide, Hydrazines
B1	
Acetylcysteine	Paracetamol (Acetaminophen)
Desferri-oxamine	Iron
Flumazenil	Benzodiazepines
Folinic acid	Folinic acid antagonists
Methionine	Paracetamol (Acetaminophen)
Neostigmine	Neuromuscular block (curare type), peripheral anticholinergic effects
B2	
4-Dimethylaminophenol (4-DMAP)	Cyanide
Obidoxime	Organophosphorus compounds
Potassium ferric hexacyanoferrate (Prussian blue C177520)	Thallium
Pralidoxime	Organophosphorus compounds
Silibinin	Amanitines
Succimer (DMSA)	Mercury (organic, inorganic)
Unithiol (DMPS)	Cobalt, gold, lead, mercury (inorganic), nickel

B3	
Benzylpenicillin	Amanitines
Dimercaprol	Arsenic
C1	
Penicillamine	Copper (Wilson's disease)
Phytomenadione (vitamin K_1)	Coumarin derivatives
C2	
Edetate calcium disodium	Lead
Oxygen-hyperbaric	Carbon monoxide
Trientine (Triethylene tetramine)	Copper (Wilson's disease)
C3	
N-Acetylpenicillamine	Mercury (inorganic & vapour)
Pentetic acid (DTPA)	Cobalt
Succimer (DMSA)	Antimony, arsenic, bismuth, cadmium, cobalt, copper, gold, lead, platinum, silver

Agents used to prevent absorption of poisons to enhance elimination, or to treat symptomatically the effects on body functions

Agents	*Indications – Uses*	*Status*
Ipecacuanha	Emetics	A2
Magnesium citrate, sulfate, hydroxide, mannitol, sorbitol, lactulose, sodium sulfate, phosphate, bicarbonate, polyethylene glycol electrolyte lavage solution	Cathartics and solutions used for whole gut lavage	B3 B3 B3 B3 B2
Sodium bicarbonate	Agents to alkalinize urine or blood	A1
Activated charcoal (for adsorbable poisons)	Agents to prevent absorption of toxic substances by the GI tract	A1
Starch (for iodine ingestion)		A3
Calcium gluconae gel (for hydrofluoric acid)	Agents to prevent skin absorption or damage	A1
Polyethylene glycol (Macrogol 400) (for phenol)		A1
Dimethicone (for soaps, shampoos)	Anti-foaming agents	

Other therapeutic agents useful for the treatment of poisoning

Agents	*Indications – symptoms arising from poisoning*
Benztropine	Dystonia
Chlorpormazine	Psychotic states with severe agitation
Corticosteroids	Acute allergic reactions, laryngeal oedema, (systemic/topical/bronchoconstriction, mucosal oedema inhaled)
Diazepam	Convulsions, excitation, anxiety, muscular hypertonia
Diphenydramine	Dystonia
Dobutamine	Myocardial depression
Dopamine	Myocardial depression, vascular relaxation
Epinephrine (adrenaline)	Anaphylactic shock, cardiac arrest, myocardial depression
Frusemide	Fluid retention, left ventricular failure
Glucose	Hypoglycaemia
Haloperidol	Hallucinations and other psychotic states
Heparin	Hypercoagulability states
Magnesium sulphate	Cardiac arrhythmias
Mannitol	Cerebral oedema, fluid retention
Oxygen	Hypoxia
Pancuronium	Muscular rigidity, convulsions, mechanical ventilation
Promethazine	Allergic reactions
Salbutamol	Bronchoconstriction (systemic/inhaled)
Sodium bicarbonate	Metabolic acidosis, cardiac disturbances (in cyclic antidepressant overdose)

ASTHMA

Asthma affects over 5% of the population in industrialized countries and there is evidence that the prevalence and severity are rising. The diagnosis and treatment is relatively straightforward yet asthma is still underdiagnosed and undertreated with resultant avoidable deaths. The mortality from asthma is approximately 2000 per year in the UK.

Asthma is defined as widespread narrowing of the airways which changes in severity over periods of time due to bronchial hyper-responsiveness (BHR). Symptoms include intermittent wheeze, chest tightness, cough and shortness of breath.

Pathologically it manifests as widespread airway narrowing with bronchial smooth muscle contraction, mucosal oedema and inflammatory cell infiltration. Reversibility of airway's obstruction is characteristic and BHR is defined as a 20% fall in the 1 second forced expiratory volume in response to a provoking dose of histamine or methacholine of less than 8 μmol.

A number of stimuli may activate the inflammatory response and include – inhaled allergens, infection, exercise, anxiety, cold, and drugs.

Acute asthma

Patients with severe or life-threatening attacks may not be distressed and may not have all these abnormalities. The presence of any should alert the doctor.

1. ***Features of acute severe asthma include:***

- Cannot complete sentences in one breath.
- Respiratory rate ≥ 25 breaths per minute.
- Pulse ≥ 110 beats per minute.
- Peak expiratory flow (PEF) ≤ 50% of predicted or best.

2. ***Life-threatening features include:***

- PEF <33% of predicted or best.
- Silent chest, cyanosis, or feeble respiratory effort.
- Bradycardia or hypotension.
- Exhaustion, confusion, or coma.
- Normal or high $PaCO_2$.
- Severe hypoxia: PaO_2 < 8 kPa (60 mmHg) irrespective of treatment with oxygen.
- Low pH (or high H^+).

3. ***Monitoring***

- Peak expiratory flow rate – repeat measurement of PEF 15–30 minutes after starting treatment.
- Pulse oximetry – maintain SaO_2 > 92%.
- Arterial blood gases – repeat blood gas measurements if:
  (a) initial PaO_2 < 8 kPa (60 mmHg);
  (b) $PaCO_2$ was normal or raised;
  (c) patient deteriorates.

4. ***Management.*** Acute severe asthma is life-threatening and requires urgent and aggressive management based on clinical assessment and repeated objective measurement of respiratory function.

5. ***The aims of management are to:***

- Prevent death.
- Restore the patient's clinical condition and lung function to their best possible levels as soon as possible.
- Maintain optimal function and prevent early relapse.

6. ***Treatment consists of:***

- High flow oxygen in all cases.
- Bronchodilators – salbutamol 5 mg or terbutaline 10 mg via oxygen-driven nebulizer.
- Steroids – prednisolone tablets 30–60 mg or hydrocortisone 200 mg i.v., or both.
- No sedative of any kind.

Mild asthma

1. ***PEF greater than 75% of predicted:***

- Treat with oxygen and inhaled bronchodilators.
- Observe for 60 minutes and discharge if patient stable and PEF > 75%.
- Ensure patient has supply of drugs, correct inhaler technique and written instructions. Arrange GP follow up and inform of need to return if symptoms worsen.

Moderate asthma

1. ***PEF 50–75%:***

- Treat with oxygen and nebulized bronchodilator.
- Observe for 60 minutes, and discharge if PEF stable and >60%.
- Drugs to include prednisolone 30–40 mg for 7 days, regular inhaler steroid and bronchodilator.
- Follow up by GP and chest clinic, crisis plan and PEF monitoring.

Severe asthma

1. ***PEF 33–50%:***

- Measure arterial blood gases and monitor closely.
- Admit.

Life-threatening asthma

1. ***PEF <33%:***

- Seek senior help.
- Add ipatropium 0.5 mg to the nebulized beta-agonist.

- Give i.v. aminophylline 250 mg over 20 minutes or salbutamol or terbutaline 250 μg over 10 minutes. Do not give bolus aminophylline to patients already taking oral theophylline.
- Chest radiography to exclude pneumothorax.
- Admit to ICU.

2. Indications for ventilation

- Deteriorating PEF, worsening or persisting hypoxia or hypercapnia.
- Exhaustion, feeble respirations, confusion or drowsiness.
- Coma or respiratory arrest.

Further reading

British Thoracic Society and others. *Guidelines for the management of asthma: a summary. British Medical Journal*, 1993; **306:** 776–82.

Related topics of interest

Airway (p. 28); Anaphylaxis (p. 38)

BABY CHECK

Baby Check is a scoring system to quantify whether a baby of less than 6 months is acutely ill. It is not a substitute for clinical judgement and is not applicable to conditions such as injury, convulsions, abscess and chronic conditions that clearly warrant admission.

One version is to be used by parents and the other for doctors. A combination of 7 symptoms and 12 signs are checked and these provide the user with individual scores derived from the regression coefficients. The total score provides the user with a risk assessment of severity of illness.

Parents

The score provides the parent with a guide to decide whether medical advice should be sought:

1. ***Score 0 to 7***. The baby is only a little unwell, and medical attention should not be necessary.

2. ***Score 8 to 12.*** The baby is unwell, but is unlikely to be seriously ill. Seek advice from your doctor, health visitor or midwife, as necessary.

3. ***Score 13 to 19.*** The baby is ill. Contact your doctor and arrange for your baby to be seen.

4. ***Score 20 or more.*** The baby may be seriously ill and should be seen by a doctor straight away.

A randomized controlled trial in 13 general practices in Glasgow showed that distributing Baby Check to an unselected group of mothers did not affect use of health services for infants up to 6 months of age.

Hospital

A study showed that the Baby Check was of some value in predicting those babies 'needing hospital admission' with a score over 20 resulting in a 100% admission rate. It also revealed that conditions such as apnoeic episodes, feeding problems, trauma and rashes often gave low scores despite the obvious need for admission. Conditions such as bacterial pneumonia, meningitis and intussusception all scored over 20.

1. Have these symptoms been present in the last 24 hours?

	SCORE
• Has the baby vomited at least half the feed after each of the last three feeds?	4
• Has the baby had any bile-stained vomiting?	13
• Has the baby taken less fluids than usual in the last 24 hours? If so score for the total amount of fluids taken as follows:	
*Taken slightly less than usual (more than 2/3 normal)	3
*Taken about half usual amount (1/3–2/3 normal)	4
*Taken very little (less than 1/3 normal)	9

*Breastfeeding mothers should estimate the amount taken.
*Fluids that have been vomited should still be scored.

- Has the baby passed less urine than usual? 3
- Has there been any frank blood (not streaks) mixed with the baby's stools? 11
- Has the baby been drowsy when awake? If so, score as follows:
  - *occasionally drowsy 3
  - *drowsy most of the time 5

  *Do not score irritability or increased sleeping.
- Has the baby had an unusual cry (sounds unusual to mother)? 2

2. *Now examine the baby awake*

- Is the baby more floppy than you would expect? 4
- Talk to the baby. Is the baby watching you less than you expect? 4
- Is the baby wheezing (not snuffles or upper respiratory noises) on expiration? 3
- Is the baby responding less than you would expect to what is going on around? 5

3. *Now examine the baby naked for the following checks*

- Is there any indrawing (recession) of the lower ribs, sternum or upper abdomen? If so, score as follows:
  - *just visible with each breath? 4
  - *obvious and deep indrawing with each breath? 15
- Is the baby abnormally pale or has the baby looked very pale in the last 24 hours? 3
- Does the baby have blue fingernails or toenails? 3
- Squeeze the big toe to make it white. Release and observe colour for 3 seconds. Score if the toe is not pink within 3 seconds, or it was completely white to start with. 3
- Has the baby got an inguinal hernia? 13
- Has the baby an obvious generalized truncal rash or a sore and weeping rash covering an area greater than 5 × 5 cm? 4
- Is the baby's rectal temperature 38.3°C or more? 4
- Has the baby cried (more than just a grizzle) during this assessment? 3

Further reading

Morley CJ *et al.* Baby Check: a scoring system to grade the severity of acute systemic illness in babies under 6 months old. *Archives of Disease in Childhood*, 1991; **66:** 100–5.

Thomas H *et al.* Randomised controlled trial of effect of Baby Check on use of health services in first 6 months of life. *British Medical Journal*, 1999; **318:** 1740–4.

Thornton AJ *et al.* Field trials of the Baby Check score card in hospital. *Archives of Disease in Childhood*, 1991; **66:** 115–20.

Related topic of interest

Trauma scoring and injury scaling (p. 329)

BACK PAIN

Back pain is common. Eighty percent of the population experience the symptom at some time in their life. In the majority of cases it is self-limiting. Significant pathology is present in approximately 3% of all cases, but in the under 20s accounts for 10% of causes and in the over 55s 20%. Back pain may be classified as traumatic or non-traumatic.

Traumatic

If the mechanism of injury suggests the possibility of significant trauma then the patient is managed as a major trauma case. Full spinal immobilization is maintained until spinal injury is excluded on clinical and radiological grounds

Where the mechanism of injury suggests that significant trauma is unlikely (e.g. minor injury, bending, straining or sneezing) the patient is fully assessed to exclude nerve root irritation, acute disc prolapse and in the case of the elderly, pathological fracture due to osteoporosis.

1. Examination. In addition to assessing the ability to straight leg raise, the patient is assessed for motor (using the MRC scale) and sensory function and reflexes in the distribution of the following nerve roots:

- L2 nerve root
  (a) Motor: Hip flexion (L3, L4).
  (b) Sensory: Front of thigh proximally.
  (c) Reflex: None.
- L3 nerve root
  (a) Motor: Knee extension (L3, L4).
  (b) Sensory: Front of thigh.
  (c) Reflex: Knee jerk (L3, L4).
- L4 nerve root
  (a) Motor: Knee extension (L3, L4); Foot inversion; Ankle dorsiflexion (L4, L5).
  (b) Sensory: Medial calf.
  (c) Reflex: Knee jerk (L3, L4).
- L5 nerve root
  (a) Motor: big toe dorsiflexion; Ankle dorsiflexion (L4, L5).
  (b) Sensory: Lateral calf; medial foot.
  (c) Reflex: None.
- S1 nerve root
  (a) Motor: Foot and toe plantar flexion; foot eversion (S1, L5).
  (b) Sensory: Lateral foot.
  (c) Reflex: Ankle jerk.

2. Medical Research Council scale for assessing motor strength

- M5: Normal power.
- M4: Active movement against gravity and resistance.
- M3: Active movement against gravity.
- M2: Active movement but not against gravity.
- M1: Flicker or trace of contractions.
- M0: No contraction.

3. Straight leg raise (SLR). The degree of SLR is measured with the patient lying flat on his back. The ability to raise the legs up perpendicular to the body is recorded as 90° SLR. The SLR is assessed for each leg independently.

4. Signs indicating cauda equina compression (central disc prolapse)

- Difficulty evacuating the bowels or bladder.
- Weakness in both legs.
- Saddle area anaesthesia (S2–S5 dermatomes).
- Reduced or absent tone in the anal sphincter (assessed by rectal examination).

5. Management. Patients with signs of cauda equina compression should be referred to the orthopaedic team. Cauda equina compression constitutes an orthopaedic emergency. Early decompression is required to preserve bladder function. Patients with severe pain not responsive to standard analgesics or non-steroidal anti-inflammatory drugs, or who are immobilized by the pain may require admission.

Non-traumatic

In many cases of back pain no history of trauma is elicited. Once serious pathology has been excluded, the majority of such cases settle with simple analgesia or non-steroidal anti-inflammatory drugs and gentle mobilizations. The important conditions causing back pain in this group of patients vary with age and include:

1. Age less than 30

- Ankylosing spondylitis.
- Discitis.
- Eosinophilic granuloma.
- Osteomyelitis.
- Rheumatoid arthritis.
- Scheuermann's disease.

2. Age over 30

- Aortic aneurysm.
- Bone metastases:
  - (a) breast;
  - (b) kidney;
  - (c) lung;
  - (d) prostate;
  - (e) thyroid.
- Myeloma.
- Retroperitoneal disease.

3. *Age over 60 (in addition to above)*

- Osteoarthritis.
- Osteoporosis.
- Spinal stenosis.

4. *Features suggesting a significant underlying cause for back pain*

- Constant pain unrelated to activity (particularly night pain).
- Onset of neurological symptoms (including urinary symptoms).
- ESR >25 mm/hour.

Further reading

American Academy of Orthopaedic Surgeons. *Low Back Pain: a Scientific and Clinical Overview.* American Academy of Orthopaedic Surgeons, 1996.

Related topic of interest

Spine and spinal cord trauma (p. 307)

BITES AND ENVENOMATIONS

Bites are a common cause of presentation to the A&E department in the UK, the majority are minor. Some may however lead to significant morbidity due to tissue damage and infection and on occasion may cause death. Snake bites in the UK are uncommon and rarely fatal. Wasp and bee stings are common but rarely cause significant sequelae, but death due to anaphylaxis may occur, particularly in the 0.5% of the population who are hypersensitive to the venom. Wasp and bee stings kill more individuals in the UK each year than snake bites.

Non-venomous bites

These can be classified into two groups:

1. ***Crush injuries*** (dogs, human and herbivores). The tremendous crushing force of such bites leads to tissue destruction (both soft tissue and bone), devitalization and contamination leading in many cases to infection.

2. ***Penetrating injuries*** (cats and rodents). These may lead to the inoculation of wounds and underlying joints and tendon sheaths with pathogenic organisms. The apparently trivial appearance of the surface wound fails to reflect the degree of penetration.

Microbiology

Human bites present the highest risk of infection. Saliva contains many pathogenic organisms including staphylococci, streptococci, anaerobes and proteus. Dog and cat saliva may also contain *Pasteurella multocida.* Monkey bites may transmit the Herpes simplex virus.

Localized soft tissue infection is the commonest complication, but osteomyelitis, septic arthritis and tendon sheath infection may also occur.

As with all contaminated wounds the risk of tetanus should be considered and tetanus status checked and acted on accordingly.

Hepatitis B and rabies can also be transmitted by bites. The possibility of transmission of HIV should be considered after human bites.

Investigation

- Consider an X-ray looking for underlying bone or joint involvement or for a foreign body if a part of a tooth has been broken off.
- Routine wound culture is not required.
- If the possibility of Hepatitis B or HIV transmission is considered local protocols should be followed.

Management

The management of a bite follows the same principles of management as for any wound. The wound is thoroughly cleaned and debrided. The cleaned wound is explored looking for foreign body and bone, joint or tendon involvement. Antibiotics are no substitute for poor wound management. The decision as to whether the bite should be closed and antibiotics used rests on an assessment of whether the wound is at high or low risk of infection.

High-risk wounds

These include human bites, bites involving the hands, wrists and feet, bites in the elderly, immunocompromised, diabetics and those with peripheral vascular disease. These should generally be left to heal by secondary intention or undergo delayed primary suture at 2–3 days if there is no evidence of infection.

Low-risk wounds

Minor wounds of the head and face that do not meet any of the above criteria for high-risk wounds may be considered low risk (except in infants). These may be sutured immediately to achieve a good cosmetic result.

Antibiotic prophylaxis

All but the most superficial of bites require antibiotic prophylaxis.

A combination of Penicillin V and Flucloxacillin is adequate for the majority of bites, although some would advocate Augmentin (co-amoxiclav) as routine prophylaxis for bites. For those who are penicillin-sensitive Erythromycin may be used.

Rabies

For those who have been bitten in an area where rabies is endemic rabies postinoculation prophylaxis should be considered and discussed with a local expert in infectious diseases.

Venomous stings

Bees and wasp stings are the commonest cause of venomous sting in the UK. Other causes include the lesser weever fish sting, stingray and several species of jelly fish.

Bee and wasp stings

The majority of the population (99.5%) are unsensitized to bee and wasp stings. Several hundred stings being required to induced a life-threatening reaction. In those few individuals who are hypersensitive a single sting may be enough to cause death. The commonest manifestation is localized pain and swelling. Treatment is based upon the symptoms. The sting is removed (it should not be squeezed as this will increase the release of venom). If anaphylaxis ensues it is treated accordingly. Individuals with a history of severe reactions may carry a pre-loaded adrenaline syringe.

Weever fish stings

The lesser weever fish (*Echiichthys vipera*) and greater weever fish (*Trachinus draco*) both possess approximately six venomous spines in the dorsal fin and a single spine in each main gill cover. The venom (an ichthyocanthotoxin) contains several thermolabile proteins including 5-hydroxytryptamine, a kinin or kinin-like substance, adrenaline, noradrenaline, histamine, possibly serotonin as well as several enzymes.

Immediately after envenomation the patient develops intense pain at the site of puncture. The pain can increase in severity and last for up to 24 hours. The limb may feel numb with associated erythema and oedema which may extend proximally from the wound. Inflammation of the wound may continue for up to 14 days.

Systemic symptoms include agitation, pallor, anxiety and headaches, nausea, vomiting, sweating and syncope.

Management should be to immerse the wound in hot water (approximately 40°C or as hot as can be tolerated) for about 20 minutes. This dramatically eases the pain as the toxin is thermolabile. Analgesia as appropriate. Local wound toilet, debridement and tetanus are provided as necessary.

Antihistamines may relieve the local inflammatory response. Occasionally an allergic reaction may occur.

Jelly fish stings

The stinging part of a jelly fish is known as a nematocyst. Within the nematocyst is a hollow tube containing the venom. Immediate first aid involves removing any nematocysts which have not released their venom. This should be done by rinsing with sea water or applying vinegar or 5% acetic acid. Rubbing the area or application of fresh water will stimulate the release of more venom. The venom is heat labile and immersion of the affected part in hot saline (not fresh water) gives symptomatic relief from the intense pain.

Stingray

Local symptoms and signs include intense pain, oedema around the wound, erythema and petechiae.

Systemic symptoms and signs include nausea and vomiting, muscle cramps, diaphoresis, syncope, headache, muscle fasciculations, and cardiac arrhythmias. Treatment aims to reverse local and systemic effects of the venom, alleviate pain, and prevent infection. Antitetanus prophylaxis is important. Treatment for anaphylaxis may be necessary.

Further reading

Harborne DJ. Emergency treatment of adder bites: case reports and literature review. *Archives of Emergency Medicine*, 1993; **10:** 239–43.

Rest JG, Goldstein EJ. Management of human and animal bite wounds. *Emergency Medicine Clinics of North America*, 1985; **3:** 117–26.

Warrell DA, Fenner PJ. Venomous bites and stings. *British Medical Bulletin*, 1993; **49:** 423–39.

Related topics of interest

Adder bites (p. 24); Antibiotics (p. 50); Tetanus (p. 317)

BRITISH ASSOCIATION FOR ACCIDENT AND EMERGENCY MEDICINE EMERGENCY MANAGEMENT OF RADIATION CASUALTIES

Reproduced with the permission of BAEM

Principles of management

There are two types of radiation casualties, irradiated and contaminated. Normally radiation casualties will be taken to designated National Arrangements for Incidents (involving) Radio-activity (NAIR) hospitals, although they may present to the nearest Accident and Emergency Unit. Some patients may be suffering from serious life threatening injuries. Patients who are contaminated may have external and internal contamination. As long as reasonable precautions are taken the patients should present no significant risk to staff. Contact the nominated NAIR staff who will measure the level of contamination and provide appropriate advice. Irradiated patients present no risk to staff.

First priority must be given to life saving procedures. Standard ALS and ATLS procedures should be employed. The emphasis throughout management should be to remove contamination whilst limiting its spread. Augmented universal precautions will greatly reduce the risk of spread of contamination. Normal casualty handling will go a long way to achieving this.

Correct management will require preparation in advance: A local plan should be written to implement the following guidance.

Facilities

- An area should be marked out where ambulances and crews can be monitored after arrival and decontamination if necessary.
- A separate entrance and treatment area (designated or 'dirty') in which the patients can be isolated/decontaminated should be marked out. This area should be equipped with shower/irrigation facilities (ideally with a holding tank for effluent). Flushing down a main drain may be acceptable. The local council, water company and the National River Authority should be informed.

  If this is not available, an adjacent area should be set aside for staff and patients decontamination and waste storage. Flooring and walls to 2 metres should be constructed from chemically resistant plastic.
- Disposable paper sheets with plastic backing should be placed on the floor and along all transit areas, and then taped together. Portable equipment should be removed and non-disposable items covered with polythene sheeting. The necessary equipment should be taken into the 'dirty' area rather than using standard treatment areas.
- Where practical air handling equipment should be switched off. A separate unit may be advisable.

Staffing

- Call the A&E Consultant. A senior member of the Accident and Emergency and Medical staff must be identified as the Incident Manager. He/she will stay out of the immediate clinical area and monitor the overall conduct of the incidents in the A&E Department. Another senior clinician will be required as the team leader in the contaminated area. Strong leadership is essential to maintain team cohesiveness, minimize anxiety, and ensure meticulous control of cross contamination.
- A controller should be nominated to record details of all personnel in contact with the contaminated area. The number of personnel involved must be kept to a minimum. All patients and staff must be checked for contamination before leaving the designated area.
- All staff who may come into contact with radio-active materials should be issued with overalls, long plastic aprons, caps, boots/overshoes and two pairs of gloves. The inner gloves should be taped to the sleeves and the outer gloves discarded when contaminated. Overalls should be of the Tyvek Type F. standard. Respiratory protection for both staff and patients can be ensured by the use of appropriate masks (3M Type 4255 (Alternatives include 3M 8835/4257)) . The 4800 General Purpose Safety Goggles (Grade I) should be used.
- Patients and staff must not eat, drink or smoke within the designated area.

Techniques for emergency decontamination

The patient should be delivered double blanketted by the ambulance service. Cotton blankets are extremely effective at absorbing external contamination. The levels of contamination should be monitored either directly or indirectly by taking moist cotton swabs from exposed areas and storing them in labelled containers. If it is likely that patients have inhaled particles, high nasal swabs (dry swab stored in labelled holder without a transport medium) should be taken as early as possible and the time recorded. The earlier the swab is taken the greater the accuracy of estimation of dose to guide subsequent treatment. Any urine, vomit, faeces, debrided tissue, wound washings, etc. should be placed in labelled containers. Analysis will provide essential data for the estimation of radiation dose and clinical management.

Undress the patient carefully to reduce the spread of contamination. If the patient is transported in a bag, remove the bag by turning the contaminated inner surface inwards. *Roll blankets inwards. Roll clothes outwards.* Carefully remove headwear, gloves, footwear and clothes by gently cutting with scissors and folding the cut material outwards and under to provide a clean surface. Cover wounds prior to surface decontamination.

For limbs wash contaminated skin with soap under running water. Avoid splashing. Over-generous use of water can spread contamination. Clean nails with a brush for four to five minutes. For trunk areas the ideal would be localized decontamination with the repeated use of large moist swabs. If monitoring confirms residual contamination, repeat the procedure twice more if necessary with soap and water. If contamination still remains, use acid 3.2–5% potassium permanganate solution for 4–5 minutes and remove the brown staining by application of 5% sodium bisulphite – this gives visual confirmation of coverage and removal. Rinse thoroughly. If contamination remains the whole procedure may be repeated as long as the skin remains undamaged. If contaminants are not easily removed, advice must be sought. Cling-film/Opsite may be useful for alpha emiting material particles, as sweating forces particles outwards. As an alternative dry vacuuming or 'Vax' type vaccuuming may be very effective. (Appropriate equipment must be used.)

To decontaminate the face, close eyes and plug ears. Carefully swab the face with non-abrasive, soft soap of slightly acid pH (5). Irrigate eyes with copious amounts of clean water followed by isotonic solution. The nose should be blown. If monitoring is available take a swab to ascertain the presence of material. If necessary, decontamine the surrounding area and instill saline. Collect the washing on tissue paper for later monitoring of radio-activity. Clean teeth/dentures. Shampoo the hair (any proprietary full strength brand), taking care not to spread the contamination to the eyes, nose, mouth, or ears, (the hairdresser's position is best, if practical). Do not shower when hair of scalp is contaminated.

Apply paper drapes to demarcate other anatomical areas/wounds. Wipe these areas clean using swabs lightly moistened with saline. Check the level of contamination in each area after cleansing. Irrigate open wounds with saline. Encourage bleeding. Debridement when appropriate, will reduce the contamination.

The irradiated patient

Irradiated patients present no risk to staff. These patients however, may develop nausea and vomiting. The early development of nausea and vomiting may indicate a high penetrating radiation dose that may progress to full radiation sickness syndrome. Patients who have been irradiated and who have received ordinary or radiation burns must undergo surgical or other conventional treatment for their injuries as early as possible. In cases of trauma associated with radiation, delaying treatment increases the risks. (In these patients it is vital that blood samples are taken early for lymphocyte count, HLA typing, chromosome and viral studies – which are essential to decisions on further treatment.)

At-risk patients should be referred to the nearest burns, oncology or specialist unit after discussion with the appropriate specialist(s).

All personnel involved should be decontaminated and be checked by NAIR staff before leaving any contaminated area.

Reference Document: Radiation Protection Dosimetry Vol. 41 No. 1 1992, ISBN 1870965 221.

BRITISH ASSOCIATION FOR ACCIDENT AND EMERGENCY MEDICINE GUIDELINES FOR THE MANAGEMENT OF CHEMICAL INCIDENTS

Reproduced with the permission of BAEM

Overview

Although most chemical incident plans are based on known risks such as large COMAH ('Control of Major Accident Hazards') sites such as oil refineries, accidents involving chemicals may occur off site during transportation, or involve low risk chemical sites with single or multiple chemicals. Incidents may also occur with rogue operators. On occasions an unrelated primary event may be lead to secondary events when chemicals are accidentally (or deliberately) released. These latter events may be triggered by construction/transport/fire/weather/terrorist incidents. Patients exposed to chemicals may present to the emergency services or hospital with a known exposure but may also seek medical treatment for vague conditions which subsequently turn out to involve chemicals. Exposure to chemicals may occur via oral ingestion, direct skin contact or via aerosol/gaseous inhalation. It is essential that all patients are assumed to have been exposed at the scene of an incident until proven otherwise. Emergency service staff and hospital staff must be aware of this issue. Hospital plans need to cater for large number of patients taking into account local risks. Incidents may be prolonged and may require activation of a 'medical' major incident plan (as opposed to a surgical/trauma incident plan). **Be prepared to be flexible and innovative.**

The European Council Directive (COMAH: Control of Major Accident Hazards regulations) covering premises which stock potentially hazardous substances will place a responsibility on both site operators and local authorities to prepare plans in respect of chemical hazards with effect from 2-2-1999. The quantity of chemical which will trigger a COMAH plan will vary depending on risk. Accident Departments will need to liaise with appropriate authorities when drawing up local plans as chemical incident casualty numbers may be few or very large.

On scene care

When an incident occurs involving known chemicals the emergency services will respond according to standard plans. The police have overall control of incidents. The Fire Service has a responsibility for making the area safe and rescuing the ill and injured. **Decontamination of the injured is an NHS role either on or off site.** Ambulance staff and medical teams must don protective clothing before undertaking emergency treatment. **It is essential that secondary casualties do not occur.**

1. Management aims:

- Ensure rescuer safety using safety clothing (i.e. TST suits).
- Remove the casualties to a safe well ventilated area.

- Decontamination will be carried out to **a limited extent on scene dependant on resources.**
- Remove all clothing. Use double blanketing to remove as much contamination as possible.
- Warm water may be used in copious quantities except with sodium and phosphorus.
- Injuries must be treated according to HAZCHEM ALS principles.
- Use 100% O_2 (except where contraindicated as in paraquat contamination). Do not use mouth to mouth technique for respiratory arrest.
- Any available information such as HAZCHEM/KEMMLAR data must be documented.

Accident and emergency department

1. Initial response of accident and emergency senior nurse/doctor:

Known incident	*Unknown incident*
Ensure: That the incident is adequately managed. Activate chemical incident plan. Involve all agencies. **Triage/decontaminate outside A/E if possible. Use separate areas and decontamination rooms.**	Patients may present before an incident is declared. Beware of odd symptoms or signs. The history of the incident or its site may be useful e.g. sewers. Assume the incident is chemical until proven otherwise. Establish control of the event in the department and activate the chemical incident plan.

2. Definitive accident and emergency care:

Facilities/procedures	*Clinical activities*
1. Departments should have a specific decontamination area with a separate ambulance door entrance and isolated ventilation equipment. The area being use for decontamination should be cordoned off from the rest of the department. Control points must be staffed to ensure orderly movements from dirty to clean areas. Impervious chemically resistant materials should cover the floor at these points to avoid transfer of contamination. Specific managers should be in place both within the decontamination and the clean areas of the department. 2. A shower system and/or decontamination bath should be in situ. 3. Appropriate equipment should be stocked and be easily available.	1. Assume the patient is still contaminated. Take precautions. Use clothing, boots, gloves and face mask/goggles to UK/EU standards (EN369/EN374/BS2092) or a TST suit. 2. Assess A/B/C. Clear the airway. Use 100% O_2 with non re-breathing mask. Ventilate if apnoeic. Monitor oxygen saturation. Beware of misleading oximeter results. 3. Decontaminate using a shower or bath. If patient is physiologically unstable removal of clothing and double blanketing will remove substantial amounts of chemicals. Soap and water are quite adequate. In the case of eye injuries substantial quantities of water may be required. Often it is easier to use local anaesthetic drops to allow this to go ahead.

4. Special blood and urine sampling equipment should be available
5. Links with public health departments should be in place.
6. Ensure that the rest of the department functions effectively.
7. Special ward areas including HDU should be used.

4. Establish IV access. Take blood samples for FBC, complete biochemistry screen including renal, liver and muscle enzymes levels, carbon monoxide levels, and ABGs, may also be needed. Urine and blood samples must be collected for long term storage.
5. Other investigation should include ECG, CXR, peak flow rate, and urinalysis.
6. **Patients who are symptomatic or who have abnormal results need admission.**
7. Patients should be observed for a few hours before discharge.
8. Most patients will need some follow up and monitoring by A/E, GP or medical OPD.

Reappraisal

Some patients may develop multi-system disease patterns following chemical exposure. Careful OPD monitoring including epidemiological input is essential. Some of the monitoring can be done in general practice, but must be collated centrally. Long term follow up is advisable. Some samples and all records will need to be kept. Some clinical syndromes are listed below but are not meant to be the only features that may develop. Children need paediatric follow up.

System	*Features*	*Investigations of value*
Neurological	Weakness, tingling, fits blackouts.	EEG, EMG, CT.
Neuromuscular	Weakness, myalgia, tiredness, dyspnoea.	EMG, CPK.
Respiratory	Dyspnoea, cough, haemoptysis.	Peak flow, Lung function tests, ABG.
Cardiac	Atypical chest pain, hypertension.	ECG, CKMB, Echo, Exercise testing.
Gastrointestinal	Nausea, vomiting, diarrhoea.	Cultures to exclude infection
Renal	Vague symptoms, hypertension.	Urinalysis, creatinine clearances. Renal opinion.
Haematological	Aplastic anaemia, bleeding, infection.	Haematological opinion.
Neuropsychiatric	Depression, anxiety, unemployment.	Psychological support.

Pitfalls

- Assume chemicals are involved
- Protect all staff
- Hospitals must have proper facilities and plans
- Incidents may be prolonged
- Whole populations may be affected
- This may be a medical major incident
- Long term monitoring is needed

BURNS

Mark Poulden

Each year in the UK burns account for around 600 deaths, 6000 admissions to burns units, 30 000 A&E attendances and unknown quantities of injuries treated in general practice and at home.

Burn wounds can be thermal, electrical or chemical, however early management of the patient follows the same principles of ABCs and:

1. Accurate history of time and nature of injury;
2. Identify the extent and depth of the burn;
3. Attention to airway wth O_2 and fluid resuscitation;
4. Baseline blood, ECG and X-ray investigations;
5. Analgesia;
6. Basic wound care including tetanus prophylaxis;
7. Consider catheter and NG tube;
8. Performing emergency escharotomy if required for deep circumferential burns;
9. Identifying and arranging transfer to a burns unit if required.

Stop the burning process

1. Remove from source of burn.
2. Remove all clothing if able.
3. Apply liberal amounts of cold water to initially cool the burnt area, as early cooling can reduce burn depth and reduce pain. Irrigation also helps removal of any chemicals.
4. However, once this is done remove wet soaks and keep the patient warm to prevent hypothermia.
5. Cover the burn with sterile towels or cling film.

Airway and breathing

Problems arise from airway compromise due to oedema, thermal lung injury or smoke inhalation with concomitant carboxyhaemoglobin or cyanide poisoning. Signs of these may not be initially apparent, so a high index of suspicion is required as complications develop rapidly. Indicators of potential problems include:

1. Facial burns;
2. Singeing of eyebrows and nasal vibrissae;
3. Carbon deposits or signs of inflammation in the oropharynx;
4. A hoarse voice;
5. Carbonaceous sputum;
6. History of impaired mental state or confinement in a burning environment;
7. History of explosion (beware other injuries);
8. Deep neck or thoracic wound causing obstruction or restriction to ventilation (consider escharotomy);
9. Carboxyhaemoglobin level >10% if patient involved in fire.

All patients should have high flow O_2 and be assessed by an experienced anaesthetist.

Circulation

Burnt patients lose plasma, fluid and electrolytes. Adults with greater than 15% burns and children with greater than 10% burns require intravenous fluids.

1. Site two wide bore, reliable lines peripherally. Alternative sites, cutdowns or intraosseous infusion may be required. If necessary venous access may be gained through burnt skin. The upper extremities are preferable.
2. Fluid resuscitation is guided by use of a burns formula. These assess fluid requirements from the time of injury. These are a guide only and frequent reassessment is necessary. Children require maintainence fluids in addition. Commonly used formulae include:

   - **Parkland/ATLS guidelines**
     2–4 ml/kg/%BSA in first 24 hours.
     Half in first 8 hours.
     Half over next 16 hours.
   - **Muir and Barclay formula**
     0.5 ml/kg/%BSA per period.
     Infused over 4, 4, 4, 6, 6, then 12 hours.

3. Insert urinary catheter to measure hourly urine output and monitor for myoglobinuria. Urine output should be 1 ml/kg/h.
4. Deep burns greater than 10% often require blood later (approx. 1 unit for each 10%).

Assessment of the burn

1. Calculate body surface area as follows:

- Lund and Browder Chart (adult or child);
- The 'rule of nines';
- Patients palm area approximates to 1% body surface area;
- Ignore simple erythema;
- With large burns subtract unburnt area from 100%.

2. Assess the depth as follows:

- Erythema – erythema only, blanches, no blisters;
- Superficial Partial Thickness – blisters, painful, underlying skin blanches;
- Deep Partial Thickness – painful, +/– blisters and decreased sensation, fixed patchy red staining;
- Full Thickness – pale and leathery or charred (may resemble normal skin initially), painless, insensate.

Investigations

1. ***Blood***

- Full bood count.
- Group and cross match.
- Urea and electrolytes.
- Glucose.
- Coagulation screen.
- Arterial gases including carboxyhaemoglobin.

2. ***Radiography***. Chest plus others as indicated.
3. ***ECG.***
4. ***Core temperature.***

Analgesia

The severely burnt patient will be restless and anxious from hypoxia and hypovolaemia, once these have been corrected analgesia should be titrated to the patients needs. Covering the burn can help reduce pain.

- Entonox is useful in the conscious patient, especially pre-hospital.
- Morphine intravenously (0.1–0.2 mg/kg), in small aliquots titrated to patients need.

Criteria for transfer

The following patients should be discussed with the regional burns centre for consideration of transfer:

- 10% BSA partial thickness burns in children or the elderly;
- 15% BSA partial thickness burns in adults;
- 5% BSA full thickness burns;
- Burns that involve face, hands, feet, genitalia, perineum or major joints;
- Circumferential burns of limbs or chest;
- Electrical burns, including lightening;
- Significant chemical burns;
- Inhalational injury;
- Burn injury with pre-existing medical condition which could complicate management;
- Burn injury with concomitant trauma;
- History or examination suggestive of NAI.

Complications

These can be summarized as immediate, early and late.

- Airway compromise.
- Inhalational injury.
- Hypovolaemia.
- Adult respiratory distress syndrome.
- Rhabdomyolysis, myoglobinuria and renal failure.

- Haemolysis, DIC and anaemia.
- Gastric stasis, gastric and duodenal ulceration (Cushings ulcer).
- Sickle cell syndrome.
- Wound infection and septicaemia.
- Glycosuria and hyperglycaemia.
- Tetanus.
- Multi organ failure.
- Scarring and contractures.
- Psychological problems and post-traumatic stress disorder.

Further reading

Advanced Trauma Life Support – Course and Manual.
Emergency Management of Severe Burns – Course and Manual.
Robertson C, Fenton O. ABC of Major Trauma. *British Medical Journal*, 1990; **301:** 282–286.
Settle JAD, *Burns Management.* London; Churchill Livingstone, 1996.

CALF PAIN – MUSCULOSKELETAL CAUSES

Musculoskeletal calf pain is common. The causes are usually benign. History and clinical examination will usually exclude a deep vein thrombosis (DVT). If the diagnosis of DVT cannot be excluded clinically then the patient should be assumed to have one until proven otherwise and investigated and treated as appropriate.

Rupture of the Achilles tendon

This is a significant injury both because of the functional deficit it may cause and because it is often missed on initial presentation. The history is of sudden onset of pain over the back of the lower calf which occurs during vigorous exercise or when running. The patient, most likely a middle-aged male, may complain of a sensation of being kicked in the back of the calf. The pain may cause the patient to fall over. The rupture is usually secondary to degeneration of the Achilles tendon. The patient will be unable to walk normally when weight-bearing. They will be unable to lift the heel fully from the ground and will complain of pain. Local injection of steroids (for Achilles tendinitis) or systemic steroids predispose to the condition.

Clinical examination will reveal a gap in the tendon 4–6 cm above the ankle, best appreciated when compared to the unaffected side. The absence of a gap does not exclude a rupture as blood rapidly fills the gap giving rise to a boggy swelling. There will be weakness, but not absence, of plantarflexion of the ankle (the long flexors of the foot are also weak plantarflexors of the foot). The only reliable and medicolegally defensible sign of continuity of the Achilles tendon is Simmonds test. The patient is asked to kneel on a chair with the ankle protruding over the edge. The belly of the gastrocnemius is squeezed. Plantar flexion of the foot confirms that the tendon is intact. Note: a positive Simmonds test indicates that plantarflexion has occurred when the calf muscles have been squeezed. In practice to avoid confusion it should be recorded in the notes that the Achilles tendon is intact and indicate that Simmonds test was performed.

If there is doubt about the integrity of the tendon (e.g. in partial rupture) an ultrasound examination may settle the debate.

Treatment is controversial. The tendon may be immobilized in a below knee plaster in full equinus to allow healing to occur. The plaster is changed on a regular basis gradually bringing the foot into the neutral position. Primary repair of the tendon may also be undertaken, particularly in the young athletic patient.

Achilles peritendinitis

This is common in athletes, particularly runners. The patient presents with pain in the back of the ankle exacerbated by activity and relieved by rest. The condition is caused by inflammation of the sheath of the tendon leading to fibrosis and thickening as healing occurs. Repeated episodes of inflammation cause progressive fibrosis and thickening thus leading to a chronic cycle.

Clinical examination reveals tenderness over the Achilles tendon and pain on dorsiflexion. Care should be taken to exclude a rupture of the tendon (see Simmonds test above).

Treatment in the early stages involves rest and analgesia. In the more chronic condition steroid injections into the sheath may help, but these may predispose to tendon rupture. In more intractable cases surgery may be undertaken to divide the adhesions and decompress the tendon.

Achilles tendinitis

This presents clinically in a similar fashion to Achilles peritendinitis but without the associated swelling. It may predispose to Achilles tendon rupture.

Treatment is as for peritendinitis. Severe cases may respond to immobilization in a plaster cast.

Gastrocnemius tear

Partial tear of the gastrocnemius, usually the medial head, is common in athletes, particularly the older, active sportsperson. The history is of sudden onset of severe localized pain in the back of the calf during exercise or other strenuous activity. The pain is exacerbated by walking.

Clinical examination reveals localized tenderness over the site of the tear. Walking is extremely painful. Swelling and bruising develop rapidly and the muscle belly may feel tense. Differentiation from DVT in severe cases may be difficult.

Rest and analgesia followed by gentle mobilization is the mainstay of treatment. Full recovery may take weeks or even months. Some patients develop an encapsulated haematoma at the site. This is best treated conservatively. Aspiration should be avoided as the haematoma may become infected. The haematoma usually resolves slowly. The rate of resolution may be increased by local ultrasound therapy.

Posterior tibial compartment syndrome

Pain in the calf following exercise is common. This pain usually settles spontaneously within a short time of cessation of exercise. It is recognized that some individuals, particularly athletes or walkers can develop a compartment syndrome in the posterior tibial compartment which mimics, but is more severe than, the normal pain. Measurement of compartment pressures when symptoms are present will confirm the diagnosis.

Osteochondritis of the Achilles tendon (Severs disease)

This, like all osteochondritides, affects older children and teenagers. It is due to traction on the insertion of the Achilles tendon into the calcaneum. Treatment is conservative, rest, analgesia followed by gentle mobilization. Resistant cases will respond to below knee plaster immobilization.

Further reading

Banerjee A. The assessment of acute calf pain. *Postgraduate Medical Journal*, 1997; **73** (856): 86–8.

Related topic of interest

Compartment syndrome (p. 100)

CARBON MONOXIDE POISONING

Carbon monoxide is an odourless, colourless, tasteless, non-irritant gas. It has been described as a 'silent killer' that each year causes the accidental death of around 50 people and results in the serious injury of another 200 in the United Kingdom. In 1996 there were 877 deaths from carbon monoxide poisoning in England and Wales; the majority were suicides due to car exhaust fumes. Poisoning by carbon monoxide is still an under-recognized problem.

Death may be secondary to cardiac toxicity, neurotoxicity, systemic acidosis or respiratory arrest.

The normal endogenous production of carbon monoxide is produced as a byproduct of haem breakdown. This leads to a normal baseline carboxyhaemoglobin (COHb) concentration of about 0.5%. In pregnancy and in haemolytic anaemias this can rise to 5%. Heavy smokers may have concentrations up to 13% and levels up to 20% have been recorded in urban joggers.

Children, pregnant women and their babies, and those with cardiovascular diseaes, are at an increased risk. Poisoning may result in chronic neuropsychiatric sequelae.

Sources

Carbon monoxide is produced by the incomplete combustion of carbon-containing fuel.

Causes of carbon monoxide poisoning include:

- Deliberate car exhaust fumes as a method of suicide (45%).
- Incomplete combustion of organic fuels – defective gas, oil, or solid fuel heating appliances (33%).
- Victims of house fires (20%).
- The hepatic metabolism of methylene chloride from paint stripper fumes – which is metabolized by the liver to form carbon monoxide.

Pathophysiology

- Carbon monoxide combines reversibly with the oxygen carrying sites of haemoglobin and has an affinity about 240 times greater than oxygen. Carboxyhaemoglobin is unavailable for oxygen transportation. This results in a hypoxic insult.
- Shift of the *oxygen dissociation curve to the left.* This effect reduced oxygen delivery to the tissues.
- Carbon monoxide is transported dissolved in plasma and binds to intracellular myoglobin and binds to mitochondrial cytochrome enzymes. Binding to cytochrome A3 is thought to play an important role in the toxicity.

Carbon monoxide may function as a local transmitter substance altering the permeability of the microvascular and may increase the adhesion of inflammatory cells and platelets to the capillary endothelium.

Carbon monoxide poisoning results in leakage of fluid across cerebral capillaries and thus to cerebral oedema.

Delayed neurological damage tends to focus on those parts of the brain lying at the boundaries of the field supplied by the arterial system, e.g. the basal ganglia. Neurological damage seems to be the result of free radical generation and lipid peroxidation.

Features

The diagnosis of carbon monoxide poisoning is not easy as it may simulate other illnesses. The onset is often insidious and may not be recognized by either the patient or the doctor.

1. ***Acute carbon monoxide poisoning.*** Usually recognized by the circumstance of the incident. Clinical features include:

- Headache (90%).
- Nausea and vomiting (50%).
- Dizziness/vertigo (50%).
- Weakness (20%).
- Altered level of consciousness (30%).
- Myocardial ischaemia, tachycardia, postural hypotension and hypotension.
- Increased muscle tone and hyper-reflexia.
- Skin blistering.
- Rhabdomyolysis.
- Retinal haemorrhages and papilloedema.
- *Neuropsychiatric deficits* – It is not necessary for the patient to have suffered severe or life-threatening poisoning for these effects to occur. The effects may be delayed occurring days or even weeks after exposure. The following have been described; lethargy, irritability, inability to concentrate, personality deficits, memory impairment, Wernickes aphasia, parkinsonian syndromes, cortical blindness, dementia, manic-depressive affect and hemiparesis.

The severity of poisoning depends on:

- The concentration of carbon monoxide breathed.
- The duration of exposure.
- The level of activity of the victim.
- The general health of the victim.

2. ***Chronic poisoning.*** May present with vague symptoms such as:

- Headache.
- Dizziness.
- Fatigue.
- Malaise.
- Abdominal pain.
- Flu-like symptoms.
- Symptoms suggestive of food poisoning or gastroenteritis.

History

Have a *high index of suspicion.* Obtain the following historical features:
Cause, duration of exposure, loss of consciousness (even if transient), other poisons (including alcohol), chest pain. Consider the possibility of chronic exposure which may have preceded the acute presentation.

1. Clinical assessment is more important than carboxyhaemoglobin levels.

2. 'Cherry red' discolouration of skin and mucous membranes is rarely seen in life.

3. Neurological signs. A neurological examination, including test of fine movement and balance (finger–nose movement, Rhomberg's test, normal gait and heel–toe walking), a mini mental state and testing of serial 7's and short-term memory are vital.

4. Myocardial effects. Tachycardia, hypertension arrhythmias, cardiac failure, myocardial ischaemia or myocardial infarction.

5. Associated injuries. Burns and smoke inhalation.

Investigations

1. ECG. Perform in all cases because ischaemic changes, ST depression or even ST elevation (due to myocardial toxicity and not secondary to thrombosis) can occur despite normal coronary arteries. ECG monitoring is also important looking for arrhythmias.

2. CXR. If smoke inhalation or inhalation of vomit is suspected.

3. Carboxyhaemoglobin. It is important to remember that blood carboxyhaemoglobin levels are poor guides to prognosis and the need for hyperbaric treatment. An increased level only indicates exposure. However, a normal carboxyhaemoglobin level does not rule out the presence of CO poisoning. Interpret with regard to timing of exposure and to oxygen therapy given.

The carboxyhaemoglobin concentration can be measured in venous or arterial blood (no significant difference in value obtained). Carbon monoxide can be measured in expired air. If such a device is used, it must be used quickly: there is little point taking a measurement if the patient has spent hours away from the source of carbon monoxide.

Carboxyhaemoglobin can be measured in venous blood. This equates to that measured in arterial sample and is less distressing for a patient. If however, a patient has signs of respiratory compromise arterial gases are necessary.

4. U & E. Look for hypokalaemia and anion gap.

5. Cardiac enzymes. Skeletal damage may cause rhabdomyolysis.

6. Arterial blood gases. These should be measured using a co-oximeter to assess oxyhaemoglobin and carboxyhaemoglobin and to measure pH.

A metabolic acidosis is a better guide than carbon monoxide levels to assess the severity and treatment requirements of carbon monoxide poisoning.

7. ***Measure for other toxins*** especially Paracetamol and alcohol.

8. ***Consider measurement of lactate.***

Treatment

1. ***Remove patients and relatives from the source of carbon monoxide.***

2. ***Oxygen therapy.*** Treat with the highest possible concentration of oxygen. Normobaric oxygen therapy should be administered. Ideally a tight-fitting face mask with a non-rebreathing reservoir bag aiming to achieve as high concentration as possible. To achieve 100% concentration an air-filled cushion-rimmed face mask, or an endotracheal tube with the cuff inflated is necessary. Consider treatment for 6 hours with 100% oxygen at ambient pressure. If any symptoms persist the oxygen should be continued and hyperbaric oxygen therapy considered.

3. ***Secure the airway*** and if necessary paralyse and ventilate.

4. ***Patients with reduced levels of consciousness*** perform blood glucose analysis to exclude hypoglycaemia.

5. ***Treat convulsions*** with a benzodiazepam or phenytoin.

6. ***Cerebral oedema.*** initial therapy is hyperventilation, mannitol (0.25–1 g/kg over 15 mins) or dexamethasone (6 mg/kg) dependent on the advice of the local hyperbaric chamber.

7. There is considerable debate about the added value provided by hyperbaric oxygen. To date randomized trials have disagreed on whether treatment with hyperbaric oxygen works in clinical practice. The latest study published by Scheinkestel and colleagues in the Medical Journal of Australia 1999 even suggested that hyperbaric oxygen might be harmful. Nonetheless, methodological questions arise in a number of the studies and there are still too many unresolved issues to discard hyperbaric oxygen as a treatment for acute carbon monoxide poisoning. Discuss the following for consideration of referral for hyperbaric therapy:

(a) Loss of consciousness at any stage since exposure.
(b) Carboxyhaemoglobin concentrations exceeding 20% at any time, regardless of CNS features.
(c) Neurological or psychiatric features, signs other than headache.
(d) *CO poisoning in pregnancy* – the fetal circulation is 10% higher than in the maternal and may result in a miscarriage or premature labour. A lower threshold for HBO therapy and consider if:

- The patient has neurological manifestations.
- The maternal COHb is >20%.
- There is evidence of fetal distress.

(e) *CO poisoning and ischaemic heart disease* – patients with IHD are at particular risk. May present with angina, MI, arrhythmias and cardiac failure. These patients should be referred for HBO therapy.

7. Always seek the advice of the local hyperbaric chamber team.

8. Arrange checking of applicances and flues and measurement of carbon monoxide concentration in the home before allowing anyone back.

Further reading

Cross M, Rogers M. *Carbon Monoxide: A Reference Document.* The Hyperbaric Medical Centre, DDRC – Plymouth. Freestyle Publications, 1997.

Henry JA. Carbon monoxide: not gone, not to be forgotten. *Journal of Accident and Emergency Medicine,* 1999; **16:** 91–103.

Scheinkestel CD, Bailey M, Myles PS, Jones K, Cooper DJ, Millar IL, Tuxen DV. Hyperbaric or normobaric oxygen for acute carbon monoxide poisoning: a randomised controlled clinical trial. *Medical Journal of Australia,* 1999; **170:** 203–10.

Turner M, Hamilton-Farrell MR, Clar RJ. Carbon monoxide poisoning: an update. *Journal of Accident and Emergency Medicine,* 1999; **16:** 92–6.

Related topics of interest

Burns (p. 74); Inhalation injuries (p. 192)

CEREBROVASCULAR SYNDROME – ACUTE

Acute stroke is a condition with 'rapidly developing clinical signs of focal (or global) disturbance of cerebral function, with symptoms lasting 24 hours or longer or leading to death, with no apparent cause other than of vascular origin'.

Ischaemic stroke is defined as stroke due to vascular insufficiency (such as cerebrovascular thromboembolism) rather than haemorrhage.

Stroke is the third commonest cause of death in the UK, accounting for 12% of all deaths, with over 100 000 first strokes occurring every year. The incidence of first ever stroke is 2 per 1000 population per year with over half the patients aged over 70 years.

1. Risk factors for stroke include:

- Hypertension.
- Hyperchlosterolaemia.
- Smoking.
- Increasing age.
- Male sex.
- Overweight.
- Diabetes.
- Oral contraception.

2. The main types of stroke are:

- Cerebral infarction (85%).
- Primary cerebral haemorrhage (10%).
- Subarachnoid haemorrhage (5%).

Prognosis depends on the underlying cause. In cerebral infarction the mortality is 10%. Of those who survive about 50% will experience some level of disability after 6 months. With intracranial haemorrhage 50% of patients die within 30 days.

The aim of treatment is to achieve rapid restoration and maintenance of blood supply to the ischaemic area in the brain and to minimize brain damage to reduce impairment disability and secondary complications.

Aetiology

There are numerous causes of stroke:

- Cerebral embolism e.g. carotid, vertebral and basilar arterosclerosis.
- Cardiac embolism e.g. post myocardial infarction, mitral valve and atrial fibrillation.
- Artherosclerosis.
- Hypercoagulable states, e.g. polycythaemia.
- Small vessel disease e.g. diabetes mellitus.

- Haemodynamic stroke, e.g. hypotension.
- Vasculitis.
- Subarachnoid haemorrhage.
- Primary intracerebral haemorrhage.

History

A history should establish the sudden onset of a focal neurological deficit and the associated risk factors such as heart disease and smoking.

Examination

The neurological examination may allow identification of the territory of the lesion whilst the general examination should concentrate on the aetiology of the stroke, such as heart murmurs, carotid bruits and atrial fibrillation. The blood pressure, both lying and standing and in both arms as a significant difference suggest aortic dissection or subclavian steal.

Differential diagnosis includes:

- Space-occupying lesions.
  (a) subdural haematoma;
  (b) cerebral tumour;
  (c) cerebral abscess.
- Multiple sclerosis.
- Focal epilepsy.
- Intracranial vascular lesion such as an arteriovenous malformation.
- Migraine.
- Hypoglycaemia.
- Hysteria.

Investigations

The following investigations should be considered:

- Blood glucose – to exclude hypoglycaemia or diabetes.
- Full blood count and ESR.
- Urea and electrolytes.
- Blood lipids – except the very elderly.
- Blood clotting tests – in all patients with cerebral haemorrhage. In young patients test for prothrombotic disorders including anti-cardiolipin antibodies, protein S and antithrombin III deficiency.
- Syphilis serology.
- Blood cultures – if suspicious of bacterial endocarditis.
- Autoantibody screening.
- Sickling tests – in appropriate ethnic groups.
- Cardiac investigations:

  (a) ECG;
  (b) Chest X-ray;
  (c) Echocardiography – indicated in patients with:

(i) abnormal cardiac findings on clinical examination, chest X-ray or ECG;
(ii) raised ESR or positive blood cultures, suggesting endocarditis;
(iii) stroke in a young patient (aged < 40 years) with no obvious cause.

(d) Carotid duplex scanning – indicated in those with:
   (i) Transient ischaemic attack or CT-confirmed ischaemic stroke with good recovery;
   (ii) Hemiparesis or monocular visual loss or aphasia (event in the carotid artery distribution);
   (iii) Patients fit for carotid surgery.

(e) Cerebral arterial angiography – in those with greater than 70% stenosis.

- CT scanning – this enables differentiation between ischaemic or haemorrhagic stroke and indications include:

   (a) doubt regarding the diagnosis;
   (b) need to exclude haemorrhage;
   (c) suspected cerebellar stroke with obstructive hydrocephalus – most commonly presents with acute onset of unsteadiness with rapid deterioration, but with no focal neurology. Neurosurgical intervention can be lifesaving.

Management

Admission to hospital in the acute phase of stroke allows appropriate investigation and treatment, however transient ischaemic attacks and mild strokes with rapid recovery can be investigated as outpatients.

There is no treatment that should routinely be given to most patients with acute stroke.

1. Aspirin. A systematic review of RCTs found that when aspirin is started within 48 hours of acute ischaemic stroke it reduces the risk of death and dependence as does the continued long-term use of aspirin. Patients who benefit are those in whom a CT has excluded intracranial haemorrhage.

Aspirin caused an excess of about two intracranial and four extracranial haemorrhages per 1000 people treated. The number needed to treat one extra patient to make a complete recovery from stroke was 91 (50–500). Common adverse effects such as dyspepsia are dose related. People unable to swallow safely after a stroke can be given aspirin as a suppository.

2. Thrombolytics. A systematic review of RCTs found that thrombolysis given soon after acute ischaemic stroke reduced overall risk of death and dependency, but this benefit was at the cost of an increased short-term risk of fatal intracranial haemorrhage. It remains unclear which people are most likely to benefit or be harmed.

3. Immediate systemic anticoagulation. One systematic review of RCTs has found that immediate treatment with systemic anticoagulants offers no short-term or long-term improvement in acute ischaemic stroke. The risk of deep venous thrombosis and pulmonary embolus is reduced, but this benefit is offset by a dose-dependent risk of intracranial and extracranial haemorrhage.

4. Blood pressure reduction. One systematic review of RCTs provides no evidence that blood pressure reduction has benefits after acute ischaemic stroke and suggests treatment is harmful in that acute blood pressure reduction may lead to increased cerebral ischaemia.

5. Surgical treatment for intracerebral haematomas. The balance between benefits and harm is not clearly established for the evacuation of supratentorial haematomas. There is no evidence from RCTs on the role of evacuation of infratentorial (cerebellar haematomas) whose conscious level is declining. However, current practice is based on the consensus opinion that they probably benefit from evacuation.

6. Neuroprotective agents. Calcium antagonists (nimodopine 60 mg 4 hourly) improve outcome after subarachnoid haemorrhage. A systematic review of nimodipine in patients with acute stroke showed no net benefit.

7. Others. Including glycerol, high-dose steroids and mannitol have shown no clear benefit.

Complications

1. Cerebral

- Oedema – if symptomatic use mannitol and hyperventilate.
- Haemorrhagic transformation – if symptomatic treat raised ICP and consider neurosurgical evacuation of haematoma.
- Seizures – anticonvulsants if repetitive or status.
- Depression – consider antidepressants.

2. Systemic

- Hyperglycaemia–maintain normoglycaemia as hyperglycaemia is harmful.
- Inappropriate ADH secretion – if symptomatic restrict fluid.
- Hypertension – if associated with hypertensive encephalopathy or the systolic is persistently >200 mmHg or diastolic >120 mmHg, consider cautiously lowering with oral agents such as labetolol and nifedipine.
- Pyrexia – exclude infection and reduce core temperature.
- Dysphagia – swallowing difficulties are best recognized to prevent aspiration.
- Deep vein thrombosis – consider prophylaxis in those patients who are high risk with subcutaneous low-dose heparin and antithromboembolism stockings.

3. Cardiac

- ECG repolarization changes – monitor for arrhythmias.
- Sudden cardiac death (6%).

Further reading

Brown M. Cerebrovascular disease. *Medicine International*, 1992; 4158–67.
Gubitz G, Sandercock P. Acute ischaemic stroke. *British Medical Journal*, 2000; **320:** 692–6.
Oppenheimer S, Hachinski V. Complications of acute stroke. *The Lancet*, 1992; **339:** 721–7.
Sandercock PA, Lindley RI. Management of acute stroke. *Prescribers' Journal*, 1993; **33:** 196–205.

Related topics of interest

Coma (p. 97); Diabetic emergencies (p. 117)

CERVICAL SPINE – ACUTE NECK SPRAIN

The term whiplash has been used to describe the injury resulting from a hyperextension injury to the neck, the symptoms that may be associated with such an injury and the mechanism of injury. Harold Crowe first used the term in 1928 to describe the mechanism of injury, namely hyperextension (not hyperflexion). The commonest cause of this injury is a rear shunt (20% of occupants affected), but the injury also occurs in front and side impacts. Of those who experience symptoms from such accidents, almost 50% will experience delay in onset of symptoms for 24 hours or more. The incidence of the injury has increased since the introduction of compulsory seat belt legislation in January 1983. This increase has been mirrored by a fall in the incidence of more serious injuries in car occupants over the same period. Front seat passengers are most likely to be affected (19%), followed by drivers (15%) and rear seat passengers (10%).

Presenting symptoms

- Neck pain (98%).
- Occipital headache (72%).
- Shoulder pain (36%).
- Low back pain (35%).
- Interscapular pain (20%).
- Arm and hand pain (12%).
- Arm and hand numbness (12%).
- Vertigo (8%).

Investigations

Standard cervical spine views are usually normal or may show loss of the normal lordosis on the lateral view due to muscle spasm. Flexion and extension views may show instability but these are rarely indicated in the acute situation. Patients with persistent symptoms may proceed to MRI scan which may reveal a range of soft tissue injuries from ligamentous tears to disc herniation.

Management

There is considerable debate as to how this injury should be managed. Most mild to moderate cases resolve with time irrespective of the treatment. The generally recommended regimen is rest and analgesia during the acute phase when pain is at its most severe, followed by gentle mobilization to maximize range of movement. The role of soft collars is controversial. Although they provide symptomatic relief in the early phase, continued use is likely to lead to restricted movement (a stiff painless neck as opposed to a mobile painful neck). Those with more severe or persistent symptoms may benefit from physiotherapy.

Prognosis

Prognosis is variable and depends on the population studied and the end point used. The majority of patients seen in A&E have mild to moderate symptoms where the prognosis for recovery is good. Those seen in physiotherapy or orthopaedic clinics tend to have symptoms at the more severe end of the scale where the prognosis for recovery is worse. That said the reported incidence of long-term symptoms varies from 26% at one year and 4% having continuous pain, to 44% with long-term symptoms and 10% being unable to work.

In general it is reasonable to give patients assurance that most symptoms improve considerably within a few weeks with the majority resolving within months.

It is commonly believed that litigation is associated with persistent symptoms. There is evidence to show that the end of litigation is not associated with a resolution of symptoms, suggesting that the symptoms are real and lead to litigation rather than the anticipated gain from litigation leading to persistence of symptoms.

There is a belief that those who have had whiplash are more likely to develop cervical spondylosis or have onset at an earlier age. There is no evidence to support this view.

Factors influencing prognosis

Various factors have been identified which are associated with poorer prognosis. These include:

- Reversal of the normal lordosis of the cervical spine on lateral cervical spine X-ray.
- Presence of objective (as opposed to subjective) neurological signs.
- Pre-existing cervical spondylosis.
- Thoracolumbar pain.

Further reading

Foy MA, Fagg PS. *Medico-Legal Reporting in Orthopaedic Trauma.* Churchill Livingstone, Edinburgh, 1996.

Hammercher ER, Van Werken C. Acute neck sprain. "Whiplash" reappraised. *Injury*, 1996; **27**(7): 463–6.

Johnson G. Hyperextension soft tissue injuries of the cervical spine – a Review. *Journal of Accident and Emergency Medicine*, 1996; **13:** 3–8.

Related topics of interest

Analgesia (p. 32); Spine and spinal cord trauma (p. 307)

CHRONIC OBSTRUCTIVE PULMONARY DISEASE

Chronic obstructive pulmonary disease (COPD) is a chronic, slowly progressive disorder characterized by airflow obstruction (reduced FEV_1 and FEV_1/VC ratio) that does not change markedly over several months. Most of the lung function impairment is fixed, although some reversibility can be produced by bronchodilator (or other) therapy.

Thus, a diagnosis of COPD in clinical practice requires:

- A history of chronic progressive symptoms (cough and/or wheeze and/or breathlessness).
- Objective evidence of airways obstruction, ideally by spirometric testing, that does not return to normal with treatment.

Usually a cigarette-smoking history of more than 20 years is obtained, although COPD does occur rarely in non-smokers.

In 1992 there were 26 033 deaths in England and Wales attributed to COPD, chronic bronchitis or emphysema which accounts for 6.4% of all male and 3.9% of all female deaths. In comparison, 1791 died of asthma.

COPD is a major cause of morbidity with frequent use of both GP and hospital services. The estimated annual health service workload due to chronic respiratory disease in an average UK health district of 250 000 people greatly exceeds that for asthma.

In a survey of all medical admissions to a UK health region 25% of admissions were due to respiratory diseases and over half of these were COPD.

Goals of the COPD guidelines

- Early and accurate diagnosis.
- Best control of symptoms.
- Prevention of deterioration.
- Prevention of complications.
- Improved quality of life.

Management of an acute exacerbation of COPD

1. Deciding whether to treat an acute exacerbation at home or in hospital. The more of the following referral indicators that are present suggest the need for admission to hospital:

- Inability to cope at home.
- Severe breathlessness.
- Poor, deteriorating general condition.
- Poor level of activity or confined to bed.
- Cyanosis.
- Worsening peripheral oedema.
- Impaired level of consciousness.
- Already receiving long-term oxygen therapy.
- Living alone, not coping.

- Acute confusion.
- Rapid onset of symptoms.
- Arterial pH less than 7.35.
- Arterial PaO_2 less than 7 kPa.

2. If a patient is to be discharged from the A&E Department the following safeguards should be considered:

- The patient should have adequate support to be able to cope at home.
- The patient (or carer) should understand the treatment prescribed and the use of any delivery devices.
- Sufficient medication should be supplied to last until the next opportunity for consultation with the GP (or specialist).

History

1. Record the following:

- The patient's exercise tolerance (including the patient's level of independence).
- Current therapy including the use of nebulizers and long-term oxygen therapy.
- Time course of the current exacerbation.
- Patient's social circumstance and quality of life, especially whether living alone/alone with support/with family. Also suitability of their accommodation.
- Previous admissions including ITU.
- Smoking history.

Signs

1. Signs suggesting a significant deterioration include:

- Infection (pyrexia, purulent sputum).
- Severe airways obstruction (audible wheeze, tachypnoea, use of accessory muscles).
- Peripheral oedema.
- Cyanosis.
- Confusion.

Investigations

Urgent investigations should always include measurement of arterial blood gas (noting the inspired oxygen concentration and a chest radiograph). Other investigations should include:

- Full blood count.
- Urea, electrolytes.
- ECG.
- FEV_1 and/or peak flow.
- Blood cultures.
- Sputum.

Treatment

1. *Oxygen.* The aim of treatment with oxygen is to achieve a PaO_2 of greater than 6.6 kPa without a fall in pH less than 7.26 (secondary to a rise in $PaCO_2$).

- In patients with a history of COPD aged 50 years or more, do not give an FiO_2 of more than 28% via a Venturi mask or use nasal cannulas (2 litres per minute) until the arterial gas tensions are known.
- Check blood gases within 60 minutes of initiating oxygen or changing the inspired oxygen concentration.
- If the pO_2 is responding and the effect on pH is modest, increase the inspired concentration of oxygen until the PaO_2 is greater than 7.5 kPa.
- Monitoring by pulse oximetry may be acceptable if the arterial blood gas measurements have shown the $PaCO_2$ and pH are both normal and the patient remains stable with no fall in SaO_2.

2. *Bronchodilators.* Nebulized bronchodilators should be given on arrival and at 4–6 hourly intervals. They may be used more frequently if required. The nebulizer should be driven by compressed air if the $PaCO_2$ is raised and there is respiratory acidosis. Oxygen can continue to be given by nasal prongs.

For moderate exacerbations a beta agonist (Salbutamol 2.5–5 mg or Terbutaline 5–10 mg) or an anticholinergic drug (Ipratropium bromide 0.25–0.5 mg) should be given.

For severe exacerbations or if the response is poor they both can be administered.

If the patient is not responding intravenous methylxanthines by continuous fusion (aminophylline 0.5 mg/kg/hour) should be considered. If given, blood levels of theophylline should be measured on a daily basis.

3. *Antibiotics*

- Antibiotics have been shown to be effective if two or more of the following are present:

  (i) Increased breathlessness.
  (ii) Increased sputum volume.
  (iii) Development of purulent sputum.

In addition, all patients with acute or chronic respiratory failure (pH less than 7.35) should receive antibiotics.

The four most likely pathogens in order of importance are:

(i) *Haemophilus influenzae*;
(ii) *Streptococcus pneumoniae*;
(iii) *Moraxella catarrhalis*;
(iv) *Chlamydia pneumoniae*.

- Common antibiotics will usually be adequate; the newest brands are rarely appropriate. Thus, amoxycillin or tetracycline are first choice unless used with poor response prior to admission.
- For more severe exacerbations, or if there is lack of response to the above agents, several second-line alternatives can be considered including a broad-spectrum cephalosporin or one of the newer macrolides.

- Oral antibiotics rather than intravenous should be used unless there is a contraindication to oral therapy.
- If the chest radiograph shows evidence of pneumonia the patient should be treated according to the British Thoracic Guidelines on pneumonia.

4. ***Corticosteroids.*** Whether corticosteroids alter the course of an acute exacerbation remains unclear. It is common practice to use a 7–14-day course of systemic corticosteroids (Prednisolone 30 mg per day, or Hydrocortisone 100 mg if the oral route is not possible). This approach is justified if:

- The patient is already on oral corticosteroids.
- Previously documented response to oral corticosteroids.
- The air-flow obstruction fails to respond to bronchodilators.
- The first presentation of airway obstruction.

5. ***Diuretics.*** Diuretics are indicated if there is peripheral oedema and/or a raised jugular venous pressure.

6. ***Anticoagulants.*** It is probable that pulmonary emboli are more common than is usually recognized in severe COPD but the benefit of prophylactic anticoagulation has not been evaluated.

The Thromboembolic Risk Factors Consensus Group recommend prophylactic subcutaneous heparin for patients with acute on chronic respiratory failure.

Intermittent positive pressure ventilation

Ventilatory support either as non-invasive intermittent positive pressure ventilation (NIPPV) or invasive intermittent positive pressure ventilation (IPPV) should be considered in a patient with a pH of less than 7.26 and a rise in $PaCO_2$ failing to respond to supportive treatment. NIPPV has been shown in randomized controlled trials to reduce the number of patients required IPPV and the length of stay in hospital and to be of most value if used earlier than recommended. Confused patients and those with a large volume of secretions are less likely to respond well to NIPPV.

The decision to institute or withhold ventilatory support must be made by a senior clinician.

1. ***Factors to encourage use of IPPV***

- A demonstrable remedial reason for current decline – for example, radiographic evidence of pneumonia or drug overdosage.
- The first episode of respiratory failure.
- An acceptable quality of life or habitual level of activity.

2. ***Factors likely to discourage use of IPPV***

- Previously documented severe COPD that has been fully assessed and found to be unresponsive to relevant therapy.
- A poor quality of life – for example, being housebound, in spite of maximal appropriate therapy.
- Severe co-morbidities – for example, pulmonary oedema or neoplasia.

Misconceptions about the difficulty of weaning patients from a ventilator should not preclude intubation and IPPV. The mean survival of patients who are hypercapnic on admission but who later became normocapnic was 2.9 years.

3. Doxapram therapy. This supportive therapy acts as a respiratory stimulant and may be considered in patients with an acidosis (pH less than 7.26) and/or hypercapnia and hypoventilation. It may tide a patient over for 24–36 hours until an underlying cause such as infection is controlled.

Further reading

BTS Guidelines for the Management of Chronic Obstructive Pulmonary Disease. *Thorax*, 1997; **52**(5): S1–S28.

COMA

Coma (Greek for a deep sleep) is defined as a prolonged state of unconsciousness. Consciousness is maintained by activity of the reticular formation in the brain stem and thus coma is due to global suppression of nerve function or a lesion in the brainstem.

Coma is best assessed using the *Glasgow Coma Scale* and a total score 8 or less indicates coma. Since all patients in coma have their eyes closed and do not speak, the nature of the motor response is the best guide to the depth of coma.

Common causes of coma

1. ***Structural brain damage***
   - Tumour.
   - Haematoma (traumatic, spontaneous).
   - Trauma.
   - Infarction.
   - Infection (abscess, encephalitis, meningitis, cerebral malaria).

2. ***Metabolic disorders***
   - Hypoxia.
   - Hypoglycaemia and hyperglycaemia.
   - Renal and hepatic failure.
   - Hypothermia and hyperthermia.

3. ***Drugs***
   - Alcohol.
   - Sedatives, narcotics and hypnotics.
   - Carbon monoxide.

4. ***Endocrine***
   - Diabetic coma.
   - Hypopituitarism.
   - Hypothyroid.
   - Adrenal cortical failure.

5. ***Miscellaneous***
   - Epilepsy.
   - Hysteria.
   - Hypertension.

History

As full a history as available is taken but the unconscious patient requires treatment prior to attempting diagnosis. Whatever the aetiology, the patient may suffer further deterioration due to airway obstruction, respiratory depression or circulatory failure.

Examination

1. ***Respiratory pattern***
   - *Cheyne–Stokes* suggests bilateral hemisphere lesions, high brain stem lesion.
   - *Sustained deep breathing* suggests mid-brain lesion.
   - *Irregular breathing* with deep sighing breaths suggests pontine or medullary lesions.

2. ***Head*** – examine for evidence of head injury.

3. ***Neck*** – look for signs of meningism, except in cases of suspected cervical injury.

4. ***ENT*** – examined for signs of a basal skull fracture or infection.

5. ***Tongue*** – which may have been bitten during an epileptic fit.

6. ***Breath*** – may reveal alcohol, acetone, uraemia, or hepatic foetor.

7. ***Skin*** – examine for:
   - Injection sites of addict or diabetic.
   - Pupura of meningococcal septicaemia.
   - Spider naevi, palmar erythema, jaundice of liver failure.
   - Pigmentation of Addisons.
   - Cherry-red colour of carbon monoxide poisoning.
   - Coarse, dry skin of myxoedema.
   - Fine, supple skin in hypopituitarism.

8. ***Neurological:***
   - Focal neurology is examined for:
     (i) Facial asymmetry.
     (ii) Limb weakness.
     (iii) Plantar response.
     (iv) Corneal reflexes.
     (v) Deep tendon reflexes.

   - *Pupils* – examine pupil size and reaction to light.
     (i) *Fixed dilated pupils* – irreversible brain damage e.g. drugs, hypothermia, epileptic seizures.
     (ii) *Unilateral dilatation with fixed pupil*, e.g. tentorial herniation, III nerve palsy, rapidly expanding ipsilateral lesion, e.g. subdural.
     (iii) *Pinpoint fixed pupils* – opiate poisoning, barbiturates, organophosphates, metabolic disorders.
     (iv) *Small reactive pupils* – metabolic disorders, pontine lesion.
     (v) *Fixed mid-size pupils* – high mid-brain lesion.

   - *Fundi:*
     (i) Papilloedema.
     (ii) Hypertensive retinopathy.
     (iii) Sub-hyaloid haemorrhage.

- *Eye deviation* – in cerebral lesions the eyes deviate towards a destructive lesion and away from an irritative lesion. In brain-stem lesions, the eyes deviate away from a destructive lesion.

Investigations

1. Hypoglycaemia. The blood glucose must be checked immediately using a BM stix test in every unconscious patient. Hypoglycaemia is reversed with intravenous glucose or glucagon. A plasma glucose is taken prior to treatment to confirm the diagnosis.

2. Arterial blood gases.

3. Drug screen. A rapid drug screen is appropriate for alcohol, aspirin and paracetamol. Sedative drugs and hypnotics are probably best taken for estimation, and kept for analysis later if required. Specifically consider *opiate toxicity. Naloxone* should be given as a trial to those patients with suspected opiate toxicity and those with meiosis and respiratory depression make one suspect opiate poisoning.

4. Others. U/E, plasma osmolality, FBC, LFTs, blood smears for parasites, blood ammonia, urinary metabolic screen and other drug analysis may be required according to patients' circumstances. *Chest X-ray* and/or *CT* may be required.

Outcome

Recovery is often complete from life-threatening coma secondary to metabolic disorders or drugs. Structural lesions have a poorer prognosis. Prevention of secondary brain damage from hypoxia, hypotension, hypoglycaemia is important so as not to worsen prognosis.

Further reading

Jennett B. Coma. Medicine International 1992: 4120–3.

Related topics of interest

Diabetic emergencies (p. 117); Trauma scoring and injury scaling (p. 329)

COMPARTMENT SYNDROME

Compartment syndrome is defined as a condition in which high pressure within a closed fascial space (muscle compartment) reduces capillary blood perfusion below the level necessary for tissue viability, may be acute or chronic (exertion) and be secondary to a variety of causes.

The leg and forearm muscles are most frequently involved, with 45% due to fractures.

The lower extremity consists of four compartments:

- Anterior (most commonly affected).
- Lateral.
- Deep posterior.
- Superficial posterior.

The forearm consists of two compartments:

- Volar (most commonly affected).
- Dorsal.

However any limited osseofascial space may be affected including the hand, foot, thigh, shoulder and buttocks.

Causes

1. ***Decreased compartment size***
   - Tight fitting dressing and/or POP.
   - Thermal injury and frostbite.
   - MAST suit application.

2. ***Increased compartment size***
   - *Primarily oedema accumulation*
     - (i) Post-ischaemic swelling.
     - (ii) Drug overdose or other unconscious limb compression.
     - (iii) Thermal injury and frostbite.
     - (iv) Intensive muscle use (exercise, seizures).
     - (v) Venous disease.
     - (vi) Venomous snakebite.
   - *Primarily haemorrhage accumulation*
     - (i) Coagulation disorders, e.g. DIC haemophilia.
     - (ii) Anticoagulation.
     - (iii) Arterial injury.
   - *Combination of oedema and haemorrhage*
     - (i) Fracture.
     - (ii) Soft tissue injury or muscle tear including crush injuries.

Pathophysiology

The compartments are confined by osseofascial boundaries. Within this compartment, tissue perfusion is dependent upon the balance of hydrostatic and oncotic pressures across the capillary membranes. Significant pathophysiologic changes occur when intracompartmental pressures are greater than 30–40 mmHg. This compromises the circulation which leads to ischaemic changes in the muscles and nerve. Anoxic capillary damage with resultant leakage is the major cause of post-ischaemic swelling. When the damaged area is reperfused, large quantities of fluids can leak into the compartment. Myoglobin and potassium released from dying muscle cells will be absorbed and may lead to renal failure and/or cardiac dysfunction. Eventually various amounts of muscle regenerate and fibrous tissue replacement occurs leading to a contracture deformity.

The precise pressure and time thresholds for irreversible nerve or muscle injury are not defined and thus criteria for surgical decompression are controversial.

Diagnosis

Diagnosis on clinical grounds is difficult, therefore, a high index of clinical suspicion required. Early findings of acute compartment syndrome can be summarized by the '*six Ps*'.

Additionally swelling, tenseness and tenderness on palpation of the involved compartment may be present.

1. ***Pain.*** Is the most important and is a deep, aching and unrelenting feeling of pressure. The pain is frequently out of proportion to the primary injury, and is often exacerbated by passive stretch of the affected muscle group.
2. ***Pressure.***
3. ***Paresis.***
4. ***Paraesthesia.*** A common early finding whilst anaesthesia is a later finding.
5. ***Pink colour.***
6. ***Pulse.*** Pulses are generally present because central arterial flow is rarely occluded.

Differential diagnosis includes:

1. ***Vascular occlusion.***
2. ***Neuropraxia or other nerve injury.***

Investigation

Objective measurement of the intracompartment pressure is essential for accurate diagnosis. The normal resting compartment pressure is 4 ± 4 mmHg.

Most methods involve the transmission of intramuscular hydrostatic pressure in a fluid medium to a pressure transducer.

There are four types of device:

- The needle manometer technique.
- The slit catheter technique.
- The wick catheter technique.
- An electronic digitalizer fluid pressure monitor.

Indications for fasciotomy are debatable:

- Greater than 30 mmHg represents a relative indication for immediate fasciotomy in normotensive patients.
- The other view is based on a critical differential between blood pressure and compartment pressure, which is necessary for a compartment to be adequately perfused (delta P). delta P = Mean arterial blood pressure (MABP) – Compartment pressure. A safe delta P is 40–50 mmHg.

Treatment

Aims to reduce the intracompartment pressure and improve tissue perfusion.

1. Remove any compressive element which may itself be adequate to decompress the limb.

2. Measure compartment pressure if suspicion exists. Repeated or continuous measurement may be necessary. Extreme elevation of the limb should be avoided as this may result in decreased distal arterial pressure and diminished tissue perfusion.

3. Check:
- serum potassium;
- U+E;
- Urine for myoglobin.

4. Keep the patient well hydrated monitor for systemic effects such as renal impairment or cardiac dysfunction.

5. Surgery must be definitive and adequate to decompress the entire compartment and intra-operative compartment pressure measurement may be useful to assess adequacy.

Further reading

Murbarak SJ *et al.* Compartment syndrome. *Current Orthopaedics*, 1989; **3:** 36–40.
Ward KR. Compartment syndrome. *Critical Decisions in Emergency Medicine*, **16**: 125–33.

Related topics of interest

Electrical injury (p. 143); Fractures – principles of treatment (p. 155)

CORE CURRICULUM

This curriculum has been developed jointly by the Specialist Advisory Committee (SAC) for Accident & Emergency Medicine and the Faculty of Accident & Emergency Medicine.

The content is not meant to be exhaustive but to highlight areas of clinical knowledge, skills and attitudes relevant to higher specialist training in Accident and Emergency Medicine. Training should emphasize proficiency in resuscitation, assessment, initial management and appropriate referral of patients as well as responsibilities for organizational and administrative aspects of an A&E service.

Overview of accident and emergency medicine

1. Principles of emergency care.

- Organizational issues and quality standards.
- Manpower and skill mix.
- Resuscitation, recognition of threats to life and limb.
- Triage of the emergency department patient.
- Understanding of 'timeliness' and documentation.
- Interface with primary/community care.
- Therapeutics and pain control.
- Patient dignity and privacy.
- Ethical issues and confidentiality.

2. Emergency medical services.

- Pre-hospital care and the ambulance service.
- Paramedic training and function.
- Major Incident planning/procedures/practice.

3. Epidemiology of accidents and emergencies.

4. Accident prevention and health promotion.

Training is based on the acquisition of *knowledge*, *skills* and *attitudes* and can be broadly outlined as follows.

Knowledge base

1. Cardiovascular diseases.

- Cardiopulmonary resuscitation.
  - (a) One and two-rescuer CPR.
  - (b) Choking victim.
  - (b) Infant CPR.

- Advanced cardiac life support (certification is expected).
  - (a) Treatment of ventricular fibrillation/ventricular tachycardia/asystole/electromechanical dissociation/bradyarrhythmias.
  - (b) Protocols, drugs and pacing.
  - (c) Resuscitation team leadership.

- Chest pain
  (a) Ischaemic heart disease.
  (b) Myocardial infarction and thrombolysis.
  (c) Angina pectoris.
  (d) Pulmonary embolism.
  (e) Aortic dissection.

- Heart failure and pulmonary oedema.
- Supraventricular and ventricular tachycardias.
- Hypertensive emergencies.
- Cardiac pacemaker function/failure.
- Peripheral vascular disease.

2. Trauma – recognition and resuscitation room management.

- Advanced trauma life support (certification is expected).
  (a) Primary survey/resuscitation.
  (b) Secondary survey.
  (c) Definitive care.
  (d) Transfer arrangements.

- Head and facial trauma.
- Chest and cardiac trauma.
  (a) Blunt/penetrating.
  (b) Tension pneumothorax.
  (c) Cardiac tamponade.
  (d) Massive haemothorax.
  (e) Open chest wound.
  (f) Ruptured aorta.
  (g) Blast injury.
  (h) Flail chest/lung contusion.

- Abdominal trauma.
  (a) Blunt/penetrating.
  (b) Special investigations.

- Genito-urinary trauma.
- Extremity trauma.
  (a) Hand injuries – accurate diagnosis of bony, tendon and nerve injuries.
  (b) Skeletal trauma.
  (c) Vascular trauma.
  (d) Soft tissue injury.

- Spinal trauma. Immobilization/log-rolling techniques.
- Paediatric trauma.
- Trauma in pregnancy.

3. Anaesthesia.

- Principles of airway management.
- Rapid sequence induction.
- Pain relief.

- General, regional, local anaesthesia.
- Interface with intensive care.

4. ***Shock.***

- Clinical findings and differential diagnosis.
- Fluid resuscitation.
- Blood/blood products.

5. ***Pulmonary emergencies.***

- Acute respiratory failure.
- Asthma.
- Chronic obstructive airways disease.
- Foreign body.
- Pneumothorax.
- Chest infection.
- Thermal/chemical injury.
- Evaluation of dyspnoea.
- Poisoning.

6. ***Gastrointestinal conditions.***

- Acute GI bleed.
- Vomiting, diarrhoea and dehydration.
- Abdominal pain evaluation.
- Foreign body ingestion.

7. ***Ophthalmology.***

- The red eye.
  (a) Foreign body/corneal abrasion.
  (b) Conjunctivitis.
  (c) Acute glaucoma.
- Trauma.
  (a) Chemical burns.
  (b) Hyphaema and blow-out fracture.
- Causes of visual impairment.
- Orbital cellulitis.

8. ***Metabolic emergencies.***

- Hypoglycaemia.
- Ketoacidosis/hyperosmolar coma.
- Electrolyte abnormalities.
- Acid–base abnormalities.

9. ***Gynaecology and obstetrics.***

- Urinary tract infections.
- Pelvic inflammatory disease/lower abdominal pain.

- Ectopic pregnancy.
- Antenatal bleeding.
- Emergency delivery.

10. Genito-urinary medicine.
- Sexually transmitted diseases.
- Epididymitis.
- Testicular torsion.
- Sexual assault.
- Nephrolithiasis.

11. Infectious diseases.
- Hepatitis.
- HIV/AIDS.
- Tuberculosis.
- Malaria.
- Childhood illnesses.
- Pyrexia of undetermined origin.

12. Toxicology emergencies.
- Recognition of clinical syndromes.
- Initial treatment of poisoning.
- Agent-specific therapy.
- Role of poison centres.
- Decontamination facilities/procedures (including radio-activity).

13. Childhood emergencies.
- Advanced paediatric life support (certification is expected).
- Developmental paediatrics.
- Croup/epiglottitis.
- Asthma.
- Fever.
- Dehydration/gastrointestinal disorders.
- Meningitis/septicaemia.
- Seizures.
- Congenital/inherited illness.
- Pain relief.
- Parasuicide in adolescents.
- Child abuse.

14. Environmental emergencies.
- Burns.
  (a) Grading/resuscitation.
  (b) Smoke inhalation.
  (c) Outpatient treatment.
- Heat illness.
- Hypothermia.
- Near drowning.

- Electrical injury (including lightning).
- Bites.
  - (a) Snake/dog/cat/human/arthropod.
  - (b) Rabies/tetanus prophylaxis.
- Anaphylaxis.

15. ENT conditions.

- Epistaxis/septal haematoma.
- Foreign bodies.
- Infections.
- Upper airway obstruction.
- Dental emergencies.

16. Neurological emergencies.

- Coma.
- Headache/subarachnoid haemorrhage.
- Meningitis.
- Seizures.
- Stroke.

17. Musculo-skeletal conditions.

- Orthopaedic and neurovascular extremity examination.
- Strains/sprains/fractures.
- Dislocations.
- Septic joint.
- Soft tissue injury/infection.
- Nerve entrapment syndromes.
- Back pain.
- Locked joint.
- Rheumatological disorders.

18. Behavioural emergencies.

- Mental state examination.
- Organic illness manifest as behavioural disorders.
- Acute psychosis.
- Deliberate self-harm.
- Suicidal and homicidal evaluation.
- Alcohol misuse.

19. Geriatric emergencies.

- Psycho-social assessment.
- Mental state examination.
- Mobility assessment.
- Multi-system pathology.

20. Social emergencies.

- Overall care of the patient.
- Frequent attenders.

- Homelessness.
- Alcohol-related problems.
- Hospital hopper.
- Drug misuse.

21. ***Haematological emergencies.***
- Haemoglobinopathies.
- Haemophilia.

22. ***Legislation/statutory circulars.***
- Common law and confidentiality.
- Children's Act.
- Mental health Act.
- Health and Safety at Work Act.
- Road Traffic Act.
- Data Protection Act.
- Access to Health Records Act.
- Patients' Charter.
- NHS and Community Care Act.
- Role of the coroner.
- Organ/tissue donation.
- Hospital Complaints Procedure.
- Equal opportunities.

Clinical skills

1. ***Wound management.***
- Types of wounds/extremity examination.
- Wound preparation.
- Wound closure techniques.
- Foreign bodies.
- Extensor tendon repair.
- Incision of abscesses and pulp space infections.
- Flexor tendon sheath infections (including palmar spaces).
- Finger tip injuries.
- Dressing techniques.
- Plaster techniques.
- Joint aspiration, soft tissue injection.
- Anaesthetic techniques.

2. ***Cardiopulmonary resuscitation and megacode training (i.e. ALS).***
- Cardioversion/carotid sinus massage.
- Emergency thoracotomy.
- Breaking bad news.

3. ***Major trauma management (i.e. ATLS) and team leader function.***

4. ***Airway (C-spine control).***
- Basic airway management.

- Advanced airway management (tracheal intubation/alternatives).
- Surgical airway.

5. ***Breathing.***
- Needle/tube thoracotomy.
- Ventilation techniques.

6. ***Circulation.***
- Central venous access.
- Arterial access.
- Cut-down techniques.
- Femoral vessel cannulation.
- Pericardiocentesis.
- Intraosseous access.
- CVP monitoring.

7. ***Diagnostic peritoneal lavage.***
8. ***Splinting/immobilization.***
- Spinal immobilization.
- Limb splinting/traction splints.
- Logrolling.

9. ***ENT.***
- Indirect laryngoscopy.
- Nasal packing.

10. ***Maxillo-facial.***
- Dental anaesthesia.
- Dental socket suture.
- Plastic surgery techniques.

11. ***Reduction of fractures/dislocations (local and regional anaesthetic techniques/pain relief).***
12. ***Gastric lavage.***
13. ***Slit lamp.***
14. ***Emergency delivery.***
15. ***Interpretation of radiographs (CT/MRI included).***
16. ***Transportation of patients.***

Communication skills

1. ***Professional relationships.***
- Patients and relatives.
- Colleagues.
- Other staff.

2. ***Bereavement care.***

Managerial skills

1. ***Department policies/procedures.***
2. ***Staff management (manpower/personnel procedures).***

3. *Equipment (choosing to ordering).*
4. *Resource management/clinical budgeting.*
5. *Contracting/standards setting.*
6. *Information technology.*
7. *Clinical audit/quality monitoring.*
8. *Compliments/complaints.*
9. *Medico-legal statements.*
10. *Committee working.*
11. *Liaising with other agencies.*
12. *Public relations/media.*
13. *Major incident planning/exercises.*

Teaching skills

1. *Lecture preparation.*
2. *Small group techniques.*
3. *Presentation techniques.*
4. *Teaching critique.*
5. *Departmental teaching programme.*
6. *Professional development (self-directed learning).*

Research skills

1. *Literature survey.*
2. *Scientific study design.*
3. *Data evaluation/statistics.*
4. *Preparing publications.*

Attitudes

1. *Leadership.*
2. *Reliability.*
3. *Teamwork.*
4. *Self-motivation.*

CPR – NEWBORN

The 1998 European Resuscitation Council Guidelines for resuscitation of babies at birth have been based on the International Liaison Committee on Resuscitation (ILCOR). They estimate that worldwide there is the potential to save 800 000 babies per year from morbidity or mortality from newborn asphyxia by using simple airway interventions. A relatively small number of newborn babies need resuscitation beyond gentle stimulation to breathe. Of the few that do need supplemental help the majority only require assisted ventilation for a short period of time, the remaining minority will need advanced interventions including circulatory support and drug administration.

The British Paediatric Association (1993) recommends that every delivery, wherever it takes place, there should be at least one person who is responsible for giving basic care to the baby, initiating resuscitation if necessary and summoning more help if needed.

Conditions in which neonatal resuscitation may be needed

- Fetal distress.
- Thick meconium staining of amniotic fluid.
- Vaginal breech deliveries.
- Gestation of <32 completed weeks.
- Serious congenital abnormality.
- Concern of attending staff.

Preparation

Before delivery check that the correct equipment is present and functioning. The room should be warm (25°C) and the radiant heat source switched on and pre-warmed towels available. Surgical gloves should be worn over clean hands to protect the baby and healthcare worker. The baby should be assessed after birth.

The Apgar scoring system has been widely used as an indicator for the need for resuscitation at birth. The need for resuscitation can however be more accurately assessed by evaluating the heart rate, respiratory activity and colour than by the total Apgar score. Since even a short delay in initiating resuscitation may result in a long delay in establishing spontaneous and regular respiration, resuscitation should be started immediately when indicated and not delayed for the assessment of the one minute score.

Apgar scores for different signs in newborns

Sign	*Score*		
	0	*1*	*2*
Heart rate	Nil	< 100	> 100
Respiratory effort	Absent	Gasping or irregular	Regular or crying
Muscle tone	Flaccid	Some tone	Active
Response to stimulation	None	Grimace	Cry or cough
Colour	White	Blue	Pink centrally

Cover the baby with a warm, dry towel at all times. Most babies will breathe or cry within 90 seconds of birth; suction of the pharynx is not usually necessary, nor is supplemental oxygen. These babies should be handed direct to the mother. If the baby is not breathing adequately the ABC of resuscitation should be followed.

Classification according to initial assessment

On the basis of the initial assessment babies can be divided into four groups:

- Fit and healthy, vigorous, effective respiratory efforts, centrally pink and heart rate greater than 100 beats per minute. This baby requires no intervention other than drying, wrapping in a warm towel and handing to the mother.
- Breathing inadequately or apnoeic. Central cyanosis. Heart rate greater than 100 beats per minute. This group of babies may respond to tactile stimulation and/or facial oxygen, but often needs basic life support.
- Breathing inadequately or apnoeic. Pale or white due to poor cardiac output and peripheral vasoconstriction. Heart rate less than 100 beats per minute. These babies sometimes improve with initial basic life support, but normally require immediate intubation and positive pressure ventilation.
- Breathing inadequately or apnoeic. Pale or white due to poor cardiac output and peripheral vasoconstriction. No detectable heart rate. These babies require immediate ventilation, chest compressions and full advanced life support, including resuscitation drugs.

Basic life support

1. Airway. Position baby face upwards with the head supported in a neutral position. Look, listen and feel for respiratory efforts. Clear the airway by gentle suction of the mouth and nares if obstructed.

2. Breathing. If respiratory efforts are shallow, or slow and no meconium is present, stimulate gently and offer supplementary oxygen if the baby is cyanosed. If the heart rate is less than 100 beats per minute, or decreasing, start lung inflation via a mask. If there is no response prepare to perform tracheal intubation and call for help if necessary.

3. Circulation. Evaluate the heart rate and colour of the baby. Monitor the heart rate by auscultation or palpation of the base of the cord. If it is greater than 100 beats per minute continue monitoring, but if it is less than 100 beats per minute and decreasing, start or continue positive pressure ventilation.

If the heart rate is less than 60 beats per minute, start external chest compression and consider drugs and volume expansion.

External chest compression

Place the thumbs over the lower third of the sternum with the hands around the chest, or apply pressure with two fingers. The sternum should be compressed about 2–3 cm in a term baby at a rate of about two compressions per second and the lungs should be re-inflated with oxygen after every three compressions.

Drugs and fluids

Epinephrine (Adrenaline) should be given initially, followed by sodium bicarbonate if necessary.

Hypovolaemia should be considered when there is evidence of acute bleeding or a poor response to resuscitation.

Naloxone should be reserved for the apnoeic baby whose mother has received opiate analgesia up to 4 hours before delivery. Do not give Naloxone to the baby of an opiate-dependent mother as this will precipitate a severe withdrawal crisis.

1. (Adrenaline)

- *Preparation:* 1 in 10000 dilution (100 µg/ml).
- *Dose:* 1st and 2nd dose 10 µg/kg (0.1 ml/kg); 3rd dose 100 µg/kg (1 ml/kg).
- *Route:* 1st dose, tracheal tube (provided that lungs are inflated); 2nd and 3rd doses, umbilical venous catheter.

2. Sodium bicarbonate

- *Preparation:* 4.2% (0.5 mmol/ml) or 8.4% (1 mmol/ml) solution with equal volume of dextrose.
- *Dose:* 1–2 mmol/kg (2–4 ml/kg of 4.2% solution) via umbilical venous catheter; 2 doses may be given.

3. Volume expanders

- *Preparations:* Plasma, or group O Rh negative blood that is not crossmatched; 4–5% human albumin.
- *Dose:* 10–20 ml/kg via umbilical venous catheter over 5–10 minutes (may be repeated).

4. Naloxone hydrochloride

- *Dose:* 100 µg/kg (0.25 ml/kg) intramuscularly.

Meconium

If the amniotic fluid is lightly stained and the baby is well it is not necessary to intubate.

If there is particulate meconium aspirate the mouth and nostrils gently as soon as the head is delivered. If the baby is vigorous and pink intubation is of no benefit and may cause later complications. If the baby is not vigorous intubate and aspirate meconium from the trachea by applying suction directly to the tracheal tube while withdrawing and removing the tube, or through a wide-bore suction catheter passed down a large tracheal tube. Ventilate the baby when as much meconium as possible has been removed.

Indications for discontinuing resuscitation

The decision to abandon resuscitation efforts should be taken by an experienced member of staff.

Resuscitation efforts should usually be abandoned if there is no spontaneous cardiac output after 15 minutes, or if the baby is failing to make any respiratory efforts despite Naloxone therapy by 30 minutes. Those who make independent respiratory efforts but are unable to maintain adequate tidal exchange should be transferred to a Neonatal Unit for further respiratory support and reassess after 24–48 hours.

Further reading

European Resuscitation Council Guidelines for Resuscitation. The 1998 European Resuscitation Council Guidelines for Resuscitation of Babies at Birth. 101–116.

Hamilton P. Care of the newborn in the delivery room. *British Medical Journal*, 199; **318:** 1403–6.

CS GAS INJURY

CS gas is a white crystalline solid whose chemical name is 2-chlorobenzylidene malononitrile but commonly called CS from the initials of Carson and Stoughton who were the first to synthesize the substance in 1928.

The CS spray unit is a registered firearm and in Britain the spray used by police contains a 5% concentration of CS in a solvent, methyl isobutyl ketone (MIBK). CS is now being used by various police forces in the UK as an incapacitant and also used as a weapon, although its sale is illegal in Britain.

In a statement on CS spray a report published by the Department of Health in 1999 by the Committees on Toxicity, Mutagenicity and Carcinogenicity of Chemicals in Food, Consumer Products and the Environment concluded that it did not in general raise major health concerns. They did however caution that follow-up studies in humans needed to be performed.

The particles are highly soluble in water and produce a pronounced local reaction within seconds of contact on mucous membranes. CS gas is rapidly broken down in the body (1.5–5 seconds) to a non-irritant compound. Thus symptoms are self-limiting and short-lived and generally cease in 10–30 minutes. However, occasionally ocular and mucous membrane effects can last for up to 24 hours. Systemic symptoms would be only expected after exposure to a high concentration. Remember that panic and hysteria can supervene but be vigilant when dealing with patients with eye and respiratory complications.

Side effects

1. ***General.*** CS gas has a peculiar odour and a disgusting burning taste. If saliva containing CS gas is swallowed nausea and vomiting may result. Hypersensitivity reactions have been reported.

2. ***Eyes.*** Pain, blepharospasm and lacrimation. Conjunctival inflammation and oedema and peri-orbital oedema. There may also be physical injury to the eye by the pressure jet from the cannister. Photophobia and reduced visual acuity may also result.

3. ***Nose.*** Discomfort, pain and rhinorrhoea.

4. ***Skin.*** Burning and erythema which usually settles within 24 hours. Erythema or blistering may develop later. Prolonged exposure, particularly when clothing is wet, may result in chemical burns. Allergic contact dermatitis with vesicles, blisters and crusting may occur.

5. ***Respiratory tract.*** Sore throat, tight chest, coughing, sneezing and increased secretions. Bronchospasm and laryngospasm may occur. Pulmonary oedema has been described following excessive exposure in a CS gas factory worker. Patients with pre-existing respiratory disease may be more at risk of severe effects. Rarely, secondary pneumonia may develop 24–36 hours after exposure. Apnoea has also been reported.

Management

Hospital treatment is rarely needed. In most cases effects resolve spontaneously within 15–30 minutes after exposure and treatment in hospital is often not required. Staff should wear impermeable gloves, masks, close fitting goggles and gown. The patient should be placed in a well-ventilated area, preferably where there is a free flow of air to ensure rapid evaporation and dispersal of gas. Remove contaminated clothing (dry if possible) and place in plastic bags and seal. Do not allow water to come into contact with clothing as it may cause the gas to evaporate.

Eye contamination

Remove contact lenses. Hard lenses may be washed and returned. Soft lenses should be discarded.

Usually tear secretions are sufficient to remove chemical from the eye. The current recommendation in Britain for treating ocular exposure is to 'blow-dry air directly onto the eye'. The recommendation of the manufacturers of CS in the US is to perform copious ocular irrigation to dislodge, dilute and wash away the irritant. Where ocular effects persist irrigate with normal saline or water.

Afterwards test pH and stain with fluorescein and examine with a slit lamp. Normally the epithelium is intact asides mild punctate staining with associated conjunctival irritation. Patients should be prescribed a short course of topical broadspectrum antibiotic. If any concerns or symptoms persist refer to an ophthalmologist.

Problems are particularly pronounced when the CS gas is fired at close range; powder infiltration of the conjunctiva, cornea and sclera may occur. Forces can be so great that conjunctival tearing may result. Corneal stromal oedema and later deep vascularization may ensue and a multitude of complications have been reported, including, pseudoterygium, infective keratitis, trophic keratopathy, posterior synechia, secondary glaucoma, cataracts, hypaema, vitreous haemorrhage and traumatic optic neuropathy.

Skin contamination

Wash skin with soap and water. Further treatment is usually unnecessary. Treat as chemical burn. Clothing may be decontaminated by washing several times in a washing machine with normal powder or liquid.

The solvent may cause erythema and blistering of the skin. The onset may be delayed for up to 8 hours and can persist for up to one week. This is thought to be related to the solvent in which the CS is held in the particular formulation.

Treatment is symptomatic with the use of an emollient cream if the skin is dry. Topical steroids may be used for contact dermatitis.

Inhalation

Remove from exposure. Give oxygen if necessary. Look for signs of respiratory distress. If symptoms persist observe for bronchospasm, especially in patients with underlying respiratory disease. Symptomatic and supportive treatment only .

Further reading

Breakell A, Bodiwala GG. CS gas exposure in a crowded night club: the consequences for an accident and emergency department. *Journal of Accident and Emergency Medicine*, 1998; **15:** 56–64.

Committees on Toxicity, Mutagenicity and Carcinogenicity of Chemicals in Food, Consumer Products, and the Environment. *Statement on 2-chlorobenzylidene malononitrile (CS) and CS spray.* London: Department of Health, 1999. www.doh.gov.uk/pub/docs/doh/csgas.pdf

Yih JP. CS gas injury to the eye. *BMJ*, 1995; **311:** 276.

DIABETIC EMERGENCIES

Diabetes mellitus is present in 3–7% of the population. The diagnosis is usually made on clinical grounds with biochemical confirmation.

In *symptomatic patients* (symptoms include polyuria, polydipsia and weight loss) a single fasting (overnight and for more than 10 hours) or random venous plasma glucose level is often diagnostic.

1. ***The patient is diabetic if:***
   - Fasting plasma glucose ≥ 7.8 mmol/l or
   - Random plasma glucose ≥ 11.1 mmol/l.
2. ***In asymptomatic patient's diabetes is unlikely if:***
   - Fasting glucose < 5.5 mmol/litre or
   - Random glucose ≤ 7.8 mmol/litre.
3. ***The classification is:***
   - *Insulin-dependent diabetes mellitus.*
   - *Non-insulin-dependent diabetes mellitus.*
     (a) Non-obese.
     (b) Obese.
   - *Malnutrition-related diabetes mellitus.*
   - *Secondary.*
     (a) Pancreatic disease.
     (b) Hormonal aetiology.
     (c) Drug induced.
     (d) Abnormalities of insulin or its receptors.
     (e) Genetic.
     (f) Other.
   - *Gestational diabetes mellitus.*

Hypoglycaemia

A 1 year survey of admission to an Accident & Emergency department resulted in 200 admissions resulting from hypoglycaemia: 96 had one admission, 34 were admitted on 104 occasions.

Hypoglycaemia risk is related to the level of diabetic control. In the UK Prospective Diabetes Survey, mild hypoglycaemia was reported in 37% of patients on insulin after 3 years and 2.3% had experienced a severe attack.

Symptoms and signs

Symptoms and signs are secondary to the neuroglycopenia neurohumoral (autonomic) responses.

1. ***Symptoms include:***
   - *Autonomic*
     (a) Tremor.
     (b) Sweating.
     (c) Anxiety.
     (d) Nausea.
     (e) Palpitations.
     (f) Hunger.
   - *Neuroglycopenia*
     (a) Confusion/odd behaviour.
     (b) Tiredness.
     (c) Speech difficulties.
     (d) Impaired concentration.
     (e) Drowsiness.
     (f) Visual disturbance.
   - *Non-specific*
     (a) Weakness.
     (b) Dizziness.
     (c) Headache.
     (d) Paraesthesia.

2. ***Signs include:***
   - Sweating.
   - Pallor.
   - Tachycardia.
   - Tremor.
   - Aggressive/irrational behaviour.
   - Decreased conscious level.

3. ***Neurological sequelae include*** seizures and focal defects. Permanent neurological sequelae may occur after prolonged hypoglycaemia. Recurrent severe hypoglycaemic episodes may impair intellectual function.

4. ***Precipitants of hypoglycaemia include:***
   - Missed, delayed or inadequate meal.
   - Excess exercise.
   - Timing error or excess dose of insulin.
   - Alcohol intake.

Hypoglycaemic unawareness occurs in 25% of longstanding diabetics and is due to impaired adrenergic responses. There is no current evidence to suggest that human insulin increases this phenomenon.

Sulphonylureas (stimulate insulin secretion), those drugs with a long half-life (e.g. chlorpropamide), a prolonged action on the beta-cells (e.g. glibenclamide) or drugs excreted via the kidneys (if there is renal impairment) are prone to cause hypoglycaemia.

The UK Prospective Diabetes Survey reported that 17% of patients experienced mild clinical hypoglycaemia per year whilst on sulphonylureas.

Treatment

If hypoglycaemia is clinically suspected, rapidly check the blood sugar with a BM stix and treat if hypoglycaemia, having first taken a blood specimen for formal estimation. Hypoglycaemia is unusual unless the plasma glucose is less than 2.5 mmol/l, however the threshold varies from patient to patient, e.g a diabetic who has prolonged hyperglycaemia may get symptoms if the plasma glucose is rapidly lowered towards the normal level. Rapidly reverse the hypoglycaemia. After reversal the aetiology of the episode is sought and appropriate advice given.

1. Mild episodes are treated by the patient taking a sugared drink (e.g. 3 or 4 lumps of sugar with a little water), which may be repeated in 10–15 minutes. This will raise blood glucose rapidly and should be followed by some biscuits to maintain the blood sugar.

With increasing severe hypoglycaemia eventually coma will develop which can lead to irreversible brain injury.

2. Severe episodes may be treated using:

- *Glucose gel* applied to the buccal lining.
- *Glucagon* – mobilizes hepatic glycogen stores and thus is not effective in the starved patient. Useful in the combative patient or other patients with poor venous access.
  (a) *Dose:* 1 mg either i.v., i.m. or s.c.
  (b) *Contraindications:* insulinoma, phaeochromocytoma and glucagonoma.
  (c) *Side effects:* nausea, vomiting, rarely hypersensitivity reactions.
- *Glucose*
  (a) *Dose:* Glucose 50% i.v., up to 50 ml, into a large vein which may need to be repeated. An infusion of 5% or 10% glucose needed to maintain normoglycaemia.
  (b) *Side effects:* hypertonic and may cause venous irritation and thrombophlebitis.

3. Hypoglycaemia. secondary to sulphonylurea ingestion should be admitted to hospital as prolonged hypoglycaemia is likely.

4. Children are treated with 10% glucose 5 ml/kg, so as to avoid hyperglycaemia with higher concentrations of glucose.

Complications of diabetes

1. Ocular. Retinopathy, cataracts, vitreous haemorrhage.

2. Neurological. Peripheral neuropathy, mononeuritis multiplex, autonomic neuropathy and cerebrovascular accident.

3. Renal. Hypertension, nephropathy, pyelonephritis and renal failure.

4. Vascular. Small and large vessel disease may cause ischaemia of the myocardium, brain, kidneys and feet.

5. Dermatological. Fat atrophy, fat hypertrophy, ulcers, infections, xanthomata and necrobiosis lipoidica diabeticorum.

6. Infections. Urinary tract infections, candida, pneumonia, TB, and cutaneous infection.

DIABETIC KETOACIDOSIS

This is a complication of diabetes mellitus that may result from failure to take adequate doses of insulin or as the first manifestation of diabetes. The patients are typically hyperglycaemic but not always. The mortality in specialist units is <5% and causes of death include hypokalaemia, cerebral oedema and the precipitating illness (such as an infection, aspiration or myocardial infarct).

The differential diagnoses includes alcoholic ketoacidosis, hyperglycaemic hyperosmolar coma and hypoglycaemic coma.

Signs and symptoms

Polydipsia, polyuria and unexplained weight loss are the cardinal symptoms. The patient is dehydrated, due to the osmotic diuresis, with Kussmaul's breathing and acetone on the breath. The patient may have a depressed level of consciousness or be in coma (10%).

Nausea, vomiting and abdominal pain may result.

Hypothermia may be an associated finding. Signs of infection or other precipitant should be sought.

Complications include:

- Cerebral oedema.
- Venous thrombosis.
- Rhabdomyolysis.
- Aspiration.

Investigations

1. ***Plasma glucose***. This is typically elevated about 25 mmol/l but may be normal.

2. ***Urinalysis.*** Marked glycosuria and ketonuria.

3. ***Acid–base balance.*** Arterial blood gases should be measured. Acidosis with an elevated plasma anion gap is expected. To confirm the identity of the anion, serum ketones should be measured. The nitroprusside test (Acetest or Ketostix on plasma or urine) measures aceto-acetate and acetone, but not hydroxybutyrate. If ketones are not present, then diagnoses such as renal failure, poisoning with methanol or ethylene glycol need to be considered.

4. ***Electrolytes.***
   - *Sodium* concentration is expected to be low, due to the shift of water out of the ICF due to the osmotic effects of glucose. The Na^+ concentration is expected to fall by 2.4 mmol/l for every 10 mmol/l rise in the plasma glucose. If, after this correction, the Na^+ concentration is below 140 mmol/l, free water should be restricted. If it is higher, care must be taken to avoid hypernatraemia.
   - *Potassium* concentration is usually around 5 mmol/l. There is however, an overall total body deficit of K^+ due to the osmotic diuresis.

- *Urea and creatinine* may be altered due to pre-renal effects, or pre-existing diabetic nephropathy. Creatinine may be falsely elevated in some assays.

5. ***Blood, urine and sputum cultures.***
6. ***Chest X-ray.***
7. ***ECG.***

Treatment

Attention to the ABCs and monitor in a high-dependency area.

1. ***ECF volume replacement.*** Initially rapidly infuse 1–2 litres of normal saline over the first hour, and then according to clinical assessment. A CVP may be required. Large volume deficit may be present but once the tissues are adequately perfused, half strength normal saline is required.

2. ***Hyperglycaemia.*** In the absence of hypokalaemia, soluble insulin should be added to the intravenous fluids as an initial bolus of 0.1 units/kg, followed by an infusion of 0.1 units/kg/hour. Once the glucose is <14 mmol/l, glucose (5–10%) with insulin infused to maintain plasma glucose 10–14 mmol/l.

3. ***Potassium.*** Supplements are required once the K^+ falls below 4.5 mmol/l or 5 mmol/l if the patient is excreting urine rapidly. It is given as 10–40 mmol/l initially. Once insulin is started and the patient is passing urine, potassium can be given at the following hourly rate:

   - 20 mmol/l if K^+ 4–5 mmol/l.
   - 40 mmol/l if K^+ 3–4 mmol/l.
   - 40–60 mmol/l if K^+ 3 mmol/l.

4. ***Acidosis.*** The use of bicarbonate is controversial and should be decided by the specialist team. The dangers include hypokalaemia, Na^+ load, increased CO_2 production, late metabolic acidosis and cerebral oedema.

5. ***A nasogastric tube*** in the nauseated, vomiting or unconscious patient. Gastric atony and retention are common.

6. ***A urinary catheter*** is required in the comatose, incontinent or patient who has not passed urine.

7. ***Treat any underlying cause*** such as sepsis, myocardial infarction, trauma etc.

Hyperosmolar non-ketotic coma

- Typically occurs in non-insulin-dependent diabetics. Often associated with a precipitant such as sepsis, and drugs such as diuretics.
- Dehydration is very severe, and profound hyperglycaemia with an associated hyperosmolar state but without ketosis and acidosis distinguish the condition from ketoacidosis.

- Treatment is initially the same as ketoacidosis but:
  (a) Dehydration is more profound but careful fluid balance is essential.
  (b) Hypotonic saline is preferred.
  (c) Less insulin is required.
- Thrombotic events are common and prophylactic anticoagulation is necessary.

Further reading

Amiel SA. Hypoglycaemia in diabetes mellitus. *Medicine International*, 1993: 279–81.
Goguen JM, Josse RG. Management of diabetic ketoacidosis. *Medicine International*, 1993: 275–78.

Related topics of interest

Coma (p. 97); Endocrine emergencies (p. 147)

DROWNING AND NEAR-DROWNING

Drowning is suffocation due to submersion in liquid. The term near-drowning implies survival for at least a short period after the event. It is the third most common cause of accidental death in childhood. Children under the age of four account for half of all deaths with boys predominating. Drowning also occurs in adults when the predisposing factors include, alcohol, drugs, suicide, trauma, epilepsy or acute illness causing loss of consciousness or incapacitation (myocardial infarction or stroke).

Two distinct types of drowning are recognized, dry drowning and wet drowning. Two other conditions also associated with drowning are immersion syndrome and secondary drowning.

Dry drowning (15%)

The entry of a small quantity of water into the larynx causes intense laryngospasm. The laryngospasm persists after the onset of involuntary apnoea. Death is due to cardiac arrest secondary to hypoxia.

Wet drowning (85%)

There may or may not be initial laryngospasm, if there is it resolves prior to the onset of involuntary apnoea. Reflex gasping leads to aspiration of water which results in hypoxia by three main mechanisms: decreased pulmonary compliance due to dilution of surfactant; intrapulmonary shunting and alveolar obstruction by fluid and debris. As with dry drowning death is due to cardiac arrest secondary to hypoxia.

Although in the past great emphasis was placed on the difference between fresh and salt water drowning, in practice, with the relatively small volumes of water aspirated, this makes little difference to the initial management.

Immersion syndrome

Cardiac arrest may result from submersion in intensely cold water due to increased sympathetic flow to the heart and increased vasomotor tone leading to myocardial ischaemia and ventricular fibrillation or vagally mediated bradycardia and peripheral vasoconstriction (the diving reflex).

Secondary drowning

Occurring from a few minutes up to 72 hours after a near-drowning event, secondary drowning is due to the adult respiratory distress syndrome (ARDS). Up to 15% of those reaching the A&E department alive after a near-drowning episode will succumb to ARDS.

Management

1. At the scene. The first priority is to ensure ones own safety. Help should be sought and the victim removed from the water if it is safe to do so. The possibility of cervical spine injury should be kept in mind and adequate cervical immobilization maintained.

The patient should be assessed and basic life support initiated if appropriate. There is no need to attempt to remove water from the lungs. Most of the water in the lungs would have been absorbed. Attempts to remove water from the lungs can lead to regurgitation and aspiration of water from the stomach thereby exacerbating the effects of previously inhaled water.

As water has approximately 100 times the conductive power as air the body temperature will fall rapidly. The patient should be kept as warm and as dry as possible en route to hospital.

If spontaneous breathing returns the patient should be managed in the recovery position to reduce the risk of further aspiration (taking care to protect the cervical spine).

2. *In hospital.* The patient is re-assessed. Basic life support is carried out as required. Administer 100% oxygen, via endotracheal tube if the patient is not breathing spontaneously. A nasogastric tube is inserted to empty the stomach after the airway is protected.

If hypoxia persists, in the spontaneously breathing patient apply CPAP (continuous positive airways pressure) via face mask. In the intubated patient apply PEEP (positive end-expiratory pressure).

Active steps should be taken to prevent hypothermia or reverse existing hypothermia. This may include peritoneal or pleural lavage with warm saline. Although cardiopulmonary bypass is advocated, in practice this can rarely be arranged outside of a cardiothoracic centre.

3. *Investigations*

- Core temperature (usually by low reading rectal thermometer or oesophageal probe).
- Arterial blood gases.
- Baseline laboratory investigations: FBC, U&E, blood glucose, LFTs, cardiac enzymes, clotting studies.
- ECG.
- Chest X-ray.
- Monitor urine output.

4. *When to stop resuscitation.* As a general rule resuscitation should be carried out until the temperature is over 32°C. This may require several hours of resuscitation even with active rewarming. There are several reports of good survival after prolonged resuscitation in such circumstances. The difficulty is knowing when to stop resuscitation. If the body temperature does not rise after several hours with active rewarming and resuscitation then the outlook is poor, although the decision as to when to stop resuscitation should be made on a case by case basis.

5. *Post-resuscitation care.* All but the most mild cases of near-drowning require hospital admission for a minimum of 24 hours to exclude late onset ARDS. In the mildest of cases it is recommended that the patient is observed for 6 hours and discharged only if they have a normal respiratory system examination, a normal chest X-ray and normal blood gases. The majority of patients will require a period of monitoring on the intensive care unit and/or high dependency unit.

Although often administered, there is no evidence that prophylactic antibiotics, steroids or barbiturates improve outcome.

Outcome

In those surviving to hospital admission, particularly if there is evidence of spontaneous respiratory effort the outcome is generally good. Factors that predict better outcome are:

- Age (children generally do better than adults).
- Duration of immersion (shorter immersion times have a better outcome than longer immersion times).
- Water temperature (cold immersion has a better outcome that warm immersion).
- Time to initiation of basic life support (shorter time to BLS improves outcome).
- The absence of associated medical conditions.

It should be remembered that these prognosticating factors are inter-related. So for instance a victim with a short period of immersion in warm water may have a poorer prognosis than a similar victim having a longer period of immersion in cold water.

Further reading

Sachdeva RC. Near Drowning. *Critical Care Clinics*, 1999; **15:** 281–96.

Simcock T. Immediate care of drowning victims. *Resuscitation*, 1999; **41:** 101–4.

Thanel F. Near drowning. Rescuing patients through education as well as treatment. *Postgraduate Medicine*, 1998; **103:** 141–4, 149–53.

EAR, NOSE AND THROAT

Non-traumatic ear conditions

Otitis externa

This is an inflammation of the skin of the external ear. It presents as localized pain and swelling of the external auditory meatus, with discharge and erythema. The patient may complain of deafness on the affected side which will be conductive in nature. The following predispose to this condition:

- Heat.
- Humidity.
- Swimming.
- Trauma.

1. ***Causes include.***

- Bacterial infection (*Pseudomonas*, *Staphylococcus aureus*, *Proteus* or *Streptococcus pyogenes*).
- Fungal infection.
- Viral infection.
- Secondary to other skin conditions such as eczema or psoriasis.
- Presence of a foreign body.

2. ***Treatment.*** Simple cases involve local aural toilet, analgesia and topical antibiotics (often combined with a topical steroid). Topical Neomycin is contraindicated in cases where the tympanic membrane is ruptured (or rupture cannot be confidently confirmed by direct examination) as its use is associated with sensorineural deafness. The ears should be kept dry during treatment. Severe cases may require oral antibiotics (e.g. flucloxacillin) and referral for an ENT opinion.

The differential diagnosis includes:

- Furuncle (usually a staphylococcal infection).
- Impetigo.
- Herpes simplex.
- Herpes zoster (Ramsey Hunt syndrome).

A rare complication of otitis externa is *malignant otitis externa*. This is a condition in which osteomyelitis supervenes and may spread to involve the skull base and temporal bone. Cranial nerve involvement may be the first indication of this complication. Meningitis, brain abscess and death may result. Urgent referral for an ENT opinion is required.

Otitis media

This is caused by blockage of the Eustachian tube often secondary to a viral upper respiratory tract infection. The majority of cases occur in children under the age of five. The clinical features are of:

- Earache.
- Pyrexia.
- Conductive deafness.

In younger children the pain may not be localized to the ear, hence the importance of examining the ears of any pyrexial child.

In simple viral cases the tympanic membrane will appear red with dilated vessels. However, the eardrums are red or infected with fever, crying and viral upper respiratory tract infections. It is usually bilateral.

In bacterial cases (usually *Streptococcus pneumonia* or *Haemophilus influenzae*) the tympanic membrane will appear dull with loss of the normal light reflex. This progresses to bulging and in some cases a perforation of the drum with discharge of pus. In mycoplasma the ear drum may have haemorrhagic blisters (myringitis bullosa haemorrhagica).

In mild cases with the appearance of a red drum, simple analgesia is all that is required, over 50% settling within 24 hours. In more severe cases or in cases that do not settle oral (not topical) antibiotics are required. The antibiotic of choice is amoxycillin or erythromycin.

The most common complication of otitis media in children is glue ear when there is a persistent middle ear effusion. Many cases resolve spontaneously. For those cases that do not resolve *grommets* may be inserted to promote drainage.

Mastoiditis

An uncommon complication of otitis media caused by extension of the infection into the mastoid air sinus. This presents as swelling behind the ear with erythema and localized tenderness. The pinna may be displaced downwards and forwards. Patients should be referred for admission and intravenous antibiotics.

Earache

Earache may be the main presenting complaint of pathology from structures other than the ear including the teeth (abscess or caries), temperomandibular joint, cervical nodes, throat (tonsillitis or quinsy), tongue (carcinoma of the posterior third), pharynx or larynx.

Traumatic conditions affecting the ear

Subperichondrial haematoma

This results from local trauma to the pinna (commonly in boxers and rugby players). The haematoma which is located between the pericondrium and pina cartilage requires drainage either by aspiration under local anaesthesia or under general anaesthesia. Following drainage a pressure bandage is applied to prevent recurrence. Failure to drain the haematoma may result in necrosis of the cartilage and the associated cosmetic deformity known as 'cauliflower ear'.

Foreign body

Usually occurs in children but may present in adults (often the end of a cotton bud). The foreign body may be difficult to remove in children without endangering the ear drum. Without the appropriate equipment and a good light source, or without relevant experience it is often better to refer to the ENT team for removal. This is especially true in a child who may be frightened and unco-operative. The ENT team will often perform procedures in children under general anaesthetic.

Barotrauma

Barotrauma usually results from scuba diving or air travel.

- *External ear barotrauma* results if the external auditory canal is occluded (e.g. cerum plug).
- *Middle ear barotrauma* is characterized by localized pain and occasionally bleeding from the affected ear. If the drum is ruptured there will be a conductive hearing deficit. Inspection of the drum will reveal either reddening or frank rupture.
- *Inner ear barotrauma* is rupture of the round or oval window. A perilymphatic fistula results. Referal to ENT is advised. Features are characterized by:
  (a) Tinnitus.
  (b) Vertigo.
  (c) Sensorineural hearing deficit.

For middle ear barotrauma the treatment is simple analgesia and decongestants. Antibiotics should be prescribed when there is tympanic membrane rupture, previous infection or after diving in polluted water. ENT follow up should be arranged. If caused by scuba diving the patient should be advised not to dive until complete healing has occurred.

Patients with signs suggestive of inner ear barotrauma should be discussed immediately with the ENT department as the symptoms resemble those of the more serious labyrinthine decompression sickness ('the staggers'), and decompression treatment may be required.

Non-traumatic nose conditions

Epistaxis

Epistaxis in children is often the result of minor trauma (e.g. nose picking) or spontaneous. In adults trauma is a common cause. Other causes include:

1. *Local*
   - Idiopathic.
   - Trauma – including post-surgical and foreign body.
   - Inflammatory.
   - Infective.
   - Tumours.

2. *General*
   - Atherosclerosis.
   - Bleeding disorders – congenital, acquired, renal/liver disorders, anticoagulants, haematopoietic disorders.
   - Hereditary e.g. haemorrhagic telangiectasia.
   - Pregnancy.

The condition can conveniently be subdivided into anterior and posterior according to the location of the site of bleeding.

Anterior epistaxis

This is usually due to bleeding from *Little's area* on the anterior portion of the nasal septum. The bleeding area can be inspected by slightly elevating the tip of the nose. A small clot often reveals the location of the bleeding point. In the spontaneous cases the area looks hyperaemic. The bleeding is usually easy to control and stopped by applying direct pressure to the side over the nose overlying the bleeding point (not as is commonly taught by applying pressure over the bridge of the nose). During this manoeuvre the patient is sat forward to prevent swallowing of the blood. When the bleeding has stopped the patient is advised not to pick the nose or to blow the nose forcibly. Additionally advise the application of vaseline to the anterior septum twice a day for a few weeks. In a few cases local cautery may be required to control the bleeding. In the few cases where local pressure or cautery fail to control the bleeding, anterior nasal packing or balloon tamponade may be required. If the nose requires packing or balloon tamponade the patient should be admitted for observation under ENT.

Posterior epistaxis

This usually occurs in the elderly. The patient may become profoundly shocked. An i.v. line should be set up and blood sent for FBC (including platelet count), group and save and clotting studies.

The bleeding can usually be controlled by posterior nasal packing or balloon tamponade. The patient should be admitted and observed for signs of shock. Rarely these simple measures fail to control the bleeding and surgical control may be required by clipping the maxillary or ethmoid artery or ligating the external carotid artery.

Traumatic conditions affecting the nose

Nasal fracture

Nasal fracture is generally a relatively minor injury resulting from local trauma to the nose. It may however be associated with more extensive facial fracture or intracranial injury. The mechanism of injury and clinical examination should suggest the presence of associated injuries. The injury is usually closed, although open fractures may occur.

On history enquire regarding previous nasal deformity and the patient may complain of:

- Pain.
- Nasal deformity.
- Epistaxis.
- Nasal obstruction.

In simple nasal fracture the nose is examined for evidence of swelling, deformity (either lateral deformity or depression), crepitus or abnormal mobility of the nasal septum and septal deviation and septal haematoma. Treat associated epistaxis. In minor injuries with minimal swelling, no deformity, septal deviation or septal haematoma, the patient can be reassured and treated with simple analgesia. They should be advised to return in 5–7 days when the swelling has settled if they have trouble breathing or notice any deformity (minor degrees of deformity can be difficult to assess in the presence of swelling). Patients with definite deformity or septal deviation should be referred to the ENT clinic within 5–7 days. Correction of any deformity or septal deviation should be carried out within 10 days. Septal haematoma should be referred immediately for drainage as necrosis of the septal cartilage following by collapse of the nasal bridge may occur. Treatment of the wound or associated abrasions require cleaning and antibiotic cover in open fractures.

In younger patients in whom a fracture may prove difficult to detect and can have serious long-term effects on mid-face development, specialist referral is recommended.

X-ray examination of the nose is not required in the A&E department.

Complications include:

- Cosmetic deformity.
- Epistaxis.
- Septal haematoma.
- Septal deviation.
- Secondary wound infection.
- Anosmia.
- CSF leak.

Foreign body

As with foreign body of the ear children are most commonly affected. The foreign body is often visible within the nose. As with the ear an attempt should only be made to remove the foreign body in the A&E department if the operator is experienced and is confident that they can remove it. Often only one attempt will be possible, if there is any doubt the patient is best referred to ENT. If the foreign body is successfully removed a careful examination for a second foreign body should be made.

Throat

Tonsillitis

Commonly viral in origin the majority settle with simple analgesia. There are no clinical features which reliably differentiate between bacterial and viral tonsillitis.

The commonest bacterial pathogen implicated in tonsillitis is the beta haemolytic *Streptococcus*. The treatment consists of simple analgesia. A throat swab may be taken. If the symptoms fail to settle after 48 hours (or at this stage if the throat swab returns as positive) a presumptive diagnosis of bacterial tonsillitis may be made and Penicillin V prescribed. If the organism is a beta haemolytic *Streptococcus* a 10-day course is recommended to eradicate the organism. Amoxycillin should be prescribed with caution as they will cause a maculopapular rash if the underlying cause is glandular fever. If glandular fever is suspected a monospot test will confirm the diagnosis.

Always consider adult epiglottitis as this is a serious pathology and may compromise the airway.

Quinsy (peri-tonsillar abscess)

An uncommon complication of tonsillitis. The patient is systematically unwell. The characteristic appearance allows the diagnosis to be made. In tonsillitis the lateral margin of the tonsil can be clearly demarcated from the soft palate. In quinsy the whole of the tonsillar bed and soft palate of the affected side is enlarged. Treatment is referral to ENT for drainage.

Foreign body

In adults, bones (usually fish or chicken) are probably the commonest foreign body seen, in children, coins. The commonest sites for oesophageal foreign bodies to impact are at the level of:

- The cricopharyngeus muscle.
- Left main bronchus.
- The cardia.

Foreign bodies that fail to progress down the oesophagus will require removal. Generally foreign bodies that have entered the stomach will transit the gut freely.

1. Bone. The patient will complain of discomfort, pain on swallowing or the inability to swallow at all. They are usually able to accurately indicate the level at which the foreign body has lodged. A fish bone will often be seen to be lodged in the tonsil or posterior part of the tongue. This can easily be removed with forceps. If the foreign body cannot be seen on direct inspection, a lateral soft tissue X-ray of the neck will often reveal it or may show retropharyngeal swelling or air. If the foreign body cannot be seen on direct inspection or on X-ray the patient should be referred for indirect laryngoscopy.

2. Coin. Again discomfort, pain on swallowing or inability to swallow is often the presenting complaint. A child is less likely to be able to identify the level at which the foreign body has lodged. If a metal detector is available and the operator has experience in its use then failure to detect the coin above the umbilicus can be taken as good evidence the coin has passed into the stomach. If the metal detector indicates the coin is above the umbilicus then lateral soft tissue X-ray of the neck and/or chest should be performed to determine the level of the coin.

Further reading

Suoza De. Textbook of the Ear, Nose and Throat. 1995, Sangam Books Ltd.

Related topic of interest

Maxillofacial injury (p. 226)

ECLAMPSIA

The incidence of eclampsia is approximately 1 in 2000 maternities. Sixty-eight per cent of seizures occur in hospital. The UK Eclampsia Trial definition consisted of: Seizures occurring in pregnancy or within 10 days of delivery and with at least two of the following features documented within 24 hours of the seizure:

1. ***Hypertension*** diastolic blood pressure (DBP) of at least 90 mmHg (if DBP less than 90 mmHg on booking visit) or DBP increment of 25 mmHg above booking level.
2. ***Proteinuria*** one 'plus' or at least 0.3 g/24 hours.
3. ***Thrombocytopenia*** less than 100 000/μl.
4. ***Raised aspartate amino transferase*** (AST) greater than 42 IU/l.

Pre-eclampsia

Pre-eclampsia is a multisystem disorder that is usually associated with raised blood pressure and proteinuria but, when severe, can involve the woman's liver, kidneys, clotting system, or brain. The placenta is also involved with increased risk of poor growth and early delivery for the baby. It is a relatively common complication of pregnancy, and can occur at any time during the second half of pregnancy or the first few weeks after delivery.

For many women who have mild pre-eclampsia the outcome is good, but severe disease can lead to death or serious problems for the woman and/or her baby.

Predicting who is at risk of an eclamptic fit is difficult, as only around 1–2% of those with even very severe pre-eclampsia will fit.

Features

- Hypertension.
- Proteinuria.
- Generalized oedema occurring after 20 weeks gestation.
- Haemoconcentration.
- Hypoalbuminaemia.
- Hepatic dysfunction.
- Coagulation problems.
- Hyperuricaemia.

Indicators of severe pre-eclampsia

- Systolic blood pressure >160 mmHg.
- DBP >110 mmHg.
- Proteinuria ++ or +++.
- Serum creatinine >1.2 mg/dl.
- Platelets <100 000/μl.
- Increased AST or ALT.

- Epigastric pain.
- Headache, other cerebral or visual symptoms.
- Retinal exudates, haemorrhages, or papilloedema.
- Pulmonary oedema.

Pathophysiology

- Eclampsia is thought to result from abnormal placental development.
- Placental ischaemia and alterations in the ratio of prostacyclin and thromboxane occur with platelet aggregation, thrombin activation and fibrin deposition.
- Seizures are thought to be as a result of cerebral vasospasm and endothelial damage leading to ischaemia, microinfarcts and oedema.

Pre-disposing factors

- Nulliparity.
- Multiple gestations.
- Extremes of age.
- Diabetes mellitus.
- Hydatidiform mole.
- Fetal hydrops.
- Family history of eclampsia.

Presentation of eclampsia (UK Eclampsia Trial)

1. ***Features documented at most recent antenatal visit:***

- Proteinuria alone (10%).
- Hypertension alone (22%).
- Proteinuria and hypertension (57%).
- Neither proteinuria or hypertension (11%).

2. ***Symptoms preceding seizure (occurred in 59% of cases):***

- Headache (50%).
- Visual disturbances (19%).
- Epigastric pain (19%).
- All of the above (4%).

Complications

In the UK cerebral haemorrhage is the most common cause of death in eclampsia. Overall one in 14 offspring of women with eclampsia die.

1. ***Major complications.*** A total of 35% had at least one major complication.

- Required ventilation (23%).
- Disseminated intravascular coagulation (9%).
- HELLP (7%).
- Renal failure (6%).
- Pulmonary oedema (5%).
- Acute respiratory distress syndrome (1.8%).
- Cerebrovascular accident (1.8%).
- Cardiac arrest (1.6%).
- Death (1.8%).

Management

- Summon senior A&E and obstetric staff.
- Secure airway and administer high-flow oxygen.
- Place wedge under right hip or nurse in left lateral position.
- Secure intravenous access and draw blood for FBC, U&Es, LFTs, clotting screen, cross match, and Kleihauer test if abruption suspected.
- Control seizures.
- Control hypertension.
- Monitor vital signs including BP, ECG, RR, SaO_2 and fetal heart rate.
- Catheterize bladder, monitor urine output, and test urine for protein.
- Arrange urgent transfer to Obstetric Unit for delivery.

Drug treatment

Drug	*Dose*	*Onset*	*Side effects*
Seizure control			
Diazepam or Lorazepam	5–10 mg slow i.v. bolus 2–4 mg slow i.v. bolus		
Magnesium sulphate	4–6 g slow i.v. bolus over 5 minutes then 1–2 g/h i.v. infusion		Loss of patellar reflexes Drowsiness Slurring of speech Flushing Muscle weakness Respiratory depression Rarely respiratory or cardiac arrest
Blood pressure control			
Hydralazine	5 mg slow i.v. bolus every 20–30 min	10 min	Headache, tremor, nausea, vomiting, tachycardia
or			
Labetolol	10 mg slow i.v. bolus doubling every 10–20 min to max 300 mg total or 1–2 mg/min i.v. infusion	5–10 min	Bradycardia (fetal), maternal flushing, nausea
Fluids			
Crystalloid	1–2 ml/kg/h with monitoring of urine output		

Further reading

Duley L, Gulmezoglu AM, Henderson-Smart DJ. *Anticonvulsants for women with pre-eclampsia.* The Cochrane Library.

The Eclampsia Trial Collaborative Group. Which anticonvulsant for women with eclampsia? Evidence from the Collaborative Eclampsia Trial. *Lancet*, 1995; **345:** 1455–63.

ECSTASY

Ecstasy, or MDMA (3-4 Methylenedioxymethamphetamine) is an amphetamine derivative. In general, most cases of MDMA toxicity result only in mild symptoms. However, severe toxicity may develop after typical recreational doses. Death from MDMA was first reported in 1987 in the USA and in 1991 in Britain. It was first synthesized in 1914 for use as an appetite suppressant and in the 1950s as a psychotherapeutic drug because of its mood-modifying ability. Its clinical use was banned in the USA in 1985 because of its neurotoxicity and its potential for misuse. In the UK, MDMA has been listed since 1977 as a Class A drug under the Misuse of Drugs Act, 1971.

It is a 'designer' drug and is popular with the 'rave' scene. It is estimated that about half a million people have experimented with MDMA in Britain. Street MDMA range from 50–100% purity, with variable contaminants and cost between £10–15 per tablet (MDMA dose of 30–150 mg).

Synonyms of ecstasy include XTC, E, Adam, Denis the Menace, White Dove, MDMA and White Burger.

Mild toxicity

Most cases of MDMA toxicity result in mild symptoms:

- Mild increase in body temperature.
- Trismus (jaw-clenching).
- Bruxism (grinding of teeth).
- Sweating.
- Dilated pupils/blurred vision.
- Tachycardia/hypertension.
- Agitation/anxiety.
- Anorexia.
- Nausea, vomiting/abdominal pain and diarrhoea.
- Increased respiratory rate.
- Muscle aches/stiffness/spasms.

Severe toxicity

Toxicity may produce varied effects which can be broadly classified as follows:

1. Hyperthermia. Severe and sometimes fatal reactions may occur following ingestion of recreational doses previously tolerated without any problems. This is usually due to excessive exertion without adequate fluid replacement, leading to a syndrome resembling heat-stroke with the cardinal symptoms being:

- Fulminant hyperthermia (over 39°C).
- Convulsions.
- Disseminated intravascular coagulopathy.
- Rhabdomyolysis with myoglobinaemia and acute renal failure.
- Cardiovascular collapse.

- Hepatocellular necrosis.
- Adult respiratory distress syndrome (ARDS).

2. Cardiovascular effects
- Sudden death.
- Hypertension.
- Tachycardias.
- Arrhythmias – ventricular tachycardia/ventricular fibrillation.
- Peripheral ischaemia.
- Cardiac failure.
- Chest pain.

3. Renal effects
- Rhabdomyolysis results in myoglobinuria and creatine phosphokinase (CPK) release – may result in acute tubular necrosis and renal failure. This is exacerbated by hypovolaemia.
- Bladder neck constriction can lead to urinary retention.

4. Hyponatraemia. A proportion of patients develop hyponatraemia which is usually after drinking excessive amounts of water in the absence of sufficient exertion to sweat off the fluid. The syndrome of inappropriate antidiuretic hormone secretion may be present with excess vasopressin secretion. Deaths have been reported from this syndrome.

5. Respiratory effects
- Increased respiratory rate.
- Pneumomediastinum.
- Retropharyngeal emphysema.
- Pulmonary oedema and ARDS may occur.
- Aspiration pneumonia.

6. Hepatotoxicity. Acute fulminant liver failure has been reported. Consider ecstasy as a cause of unexplained jaundice or hepatomegaly in young people.

7. Neurotoxicity. The following have been described:
- Agitation/delirium.
- Confusion.
- Dystonia.
- Hypertonia/hyper-reflexia.
- Seizures.
- Cerebral infarction.
- Cerebral haemorrhage.
- Cerebral venous sinus thrombosis.
- Subarachnoid haemorrhage.
- Cerebral oedema.
- Nystagmus.
- Coma.
- Myoclonus/clonus.

8. ***Psychiatric disorders***

- Anxiety.
- Antisocial behaviour.
- Emotional instability.
- Hallucinations.
- Compulsive behaviour.
- Acute confusional state.
- Depression.
- Panic attacks.
- Flashbacks.
- Acute paranoid psychoses.

Little is known regarding the long-term effects of ecstasy abuse. Long-term psychiatric problems including depression have been reported due to serotoninergic neurotoxicity.

Laboratory abnormalities

- Hyponatraemia.
- Elevated creatine phosphokinase (CPK).
- Hyperglycaemia or hypoglycaemia.
- Syndrome of inappropriate ADH – low serum osmolality and high urine osmolality.
- Neutrophil leucocytosis.
- Thrombocytopaenia.
- Coagulopathy.
- Hyperkalaemia.
- Metabolic acidosis.
- Renal abnormalities.
- Liver abnormalities.

Treatment

Initial treatment is supportive. Patients with severe toxicity will require intervention such as intubation and ventilation and intensive care management.

1. Airway and breathing. The patient's airway would be cleared and ventilation assessed. High-flow oxygen would be given via an oxygen mask. Depending on the patient's clinical state and result of arterial blood gases he may require to be ventilated.

2. Circulation. The patient's circulatory status would be assessed and if there were signs of circulatory failure he would require administration of intravenous fluids in the first instance.

If after appropriate fluid boluses the blood pressure was still low then consideration would be given to invasive monitoring, e.g. central venous pressure and administering pressor agents. This would normally be carried out on an Intensive Care or High Dependency Unit.

3. Disability. The patient's conscious level would be assessed. If unconscious his blood sugar would be checked and if found to be hypoglycaemic intravenous glucose would be administered. Epileptic fits and agitation can be controlled with bolus doses of diazepam.

4. Exposure. The patient would be exposed and examined and his temperature taken.

5. Hyperthermia. In severe cases management should be aggressive. Minimize physical activity, sponge the patient with tepid to cool water, use fans to maximize evaporative heat loss. Place the patient in a hypothermic blanket. If the temperature exceeds 40°C other methods include an infusion of cooled intravenous fluids, ice packs, ice water baths, gastric lavage, bladder or rectal lavage, or peritoneal dialysis with cold dialysate.

If this was ineffective the patient would be paralysed and ventilated and transferred to an Intensive Care Unit.

Dantrolene is controversial but can be considered. This inhibits the calcium ion release from the sarcoplasmic reticulum thus uncoupling the excitation–contraction process. If given the dosage is 1 mg/kg intravenously over 10–15 minutes. If no response was imminent repeat doses would be given every 15 minutes to a maximum of 10 mg/kg.

6. Rhabdomyolysis. Elevated CPK and myoglobinuria. If present the patient would require aggressive fluid management to encourage fluid diuresis to prevent damage to the kidneys. Consider bicarbonate and mannitol (alkaline diuresis) to prevent acute renal failure.

7. Blood clotting. Measurements would be taken to check the clotting of the blood as in some cases this can be prolonged and associated with disseminated intravascular coagulopathy. If this is present the patient may require clotting factors and other blood products to treat bleeding complications.

8. Hyponatraemia. A measurement of the patient's plasma sodium will confirm the diagnosis.

Treatment for hyponatraemia developed after ecstasy is that initially fluids should not be given. The syndrome of inappropriate anti-diuretic secretion may be present and this will need confirming by measuring serum and urine osmolality and urinary sodium. In severe cases of hyponatraemia consider infusion of isotonic (0.9%) saline or hypertonic saline.

9. Hypertension. If the patient was hypertensive then this may have required treatment with an anti-hypertensive drug (e.g. nifedipine). Consider the use of an α-blocker (e.g. phentolamine or labetalol).

10. Metabolic acidosis. If there is an associated metabolic acidosis and this was not able to be corrected by correction of hypoxia and fluid balance then sodium bicarbonate administration would be considered.

11. Renal and liver failure. Measurements would be taken to monitor the renal and liver function of the patient and appropriate action taken.

12. Prevention of drug absorption. Consideration would also be given to preventing absorption of the drug and the drug known as activated charcoal may be given by nasogastric tube if the drug had been taken within one hour post-ingestion. An adult dose would be 50 g of activated charcoal.

Further reading

Henry JA, Jeffreys KJ, Dowling S. Toxicity and deaths from 3,4-methylenedioxymethamphetamine ("ecstasy"). *Lancet*, 1992; **340:** 384–7.

O'Connor B. Hazards associated with the recreational drug "ecstasy". *British Journal of Hospital Medicine*, 1994; **52:** 507–14.

ECTOPIC PREGNANCY

An ectopic pregnancy is a gestation in which the fertilized ovum implants outside the uterine cavity. Each year approximately 11 000 women in the UK suffer from an ectopic pregnancy. The incidence has been increasing and now occurs in one in every hundred pregnancies in the UK. Most women have an ectopic pregnancy presenting around the sixth week. Left untreated a tubal ectopic pregnancy can lead to rupture of the fallopian tube and life-threatening haemorrhage. Ectopic pregnancy is the commonest cause of maternal deaths in the UK (8%).

The confidential enquiry into maternal deaths in England and Wales stated that, 'Any woman presenting with unexplained abdominal pain with or without vaginal bleeding should not be allowed home until every means available had been used to exclude an ectopic pregnancy'.

Improvements in management have led to a fall in the mortality rate which is now approximately 0.4 per 1000.

Site

The majority (96%) implant in the fallopian tube. Other sites include the ovary (1%), cervix (1%) and the abdominal cavity (1%). Rarely an intrauterine pregnancy will co-exist with an ectopic pregnancy (heterotopic gestation).

Risk factors

The following factors predispose to ectopic pregnancy:

- Previous ectopic pregnancy (10%).
- Tubal surgery, including sterilization.
- Pelvic inflammatory disease.
- Contraception; intra-uterine contraceptive device or progestogen only pill.
- Infertility treatment.
- Endometriosis.
- Congenital anatomical uterine variants.
- Ovarian and uterine cyst/tumours.
- Increasing maternal age.

Symptoms

The classic presentation of sudden onset of unilateral severe abdominal pain accompanied by collapse and fresh vaginal bleeding may occur. However, this condition not uncommonly becomes a medicolegal complaint as it is easy to miss in its more subtle presentations.

The cardinal symptoms are:

- Amenorrhoea.
- Lower abdominal pain, usually unilateral.
- Abnormal vaginal bleeding (85%).
- Collapse/syncope.
- Shoulder-tip pain (due to sub-diaphragmatic irritation).
- Cullen's sign (rarely seen).

Examination

- Look for signs of hypovolaemic shock.
- Abdominal tenderness ranging to acute peritonism may be present.
- Bimanual vaginal examination may reveal tender adnexa and sometimes a mass, but should only be performed by a specialist.
- Speculum inspection usually reveals vaginal blood.

Diagnosis

The aim is to diagnose the condition before tubal rupture occurs.

- Pregnancy test – Almost always positive. Serum beta-HCG levels are lower than expected for a normal pregnancy.
- Transabdominal ultrasound may be useful in demonstrating an intra-uterine pregnancy or adnexal mass. In cases of ectopic rupture free fluid may be seen.
- Transvaginal ultrasound scan can detect a uterine pregnancy within five days of a missed period in experienced hands. This is the preferred method of scanning when ectopic pregnancy is suspected.

Treatment

- Give oxygen.
- Insert two large cannulae.
- Cross match 6 units blood.
- Request rhesus and antibody status; anti-D Ig may be required.
- Fluid resuscitate as appropriate.
- Referral to gynaecological team.
- Non-responders require urgent surgery.
- The traditional treatment for tubal ectopic pregnancy is laparotomy with salpingectomy (removal of the conceptus with the fallopian tube in which it has implanted).
- Newer approaches include the use of laparoscopy and techniques that allow the fallopian tube to be preserved.
- Salpingotomy (in which an incision is made into the tube) allowing the conceptus alone to be removed.
- Medical treatment aiming to terminate the pregnancy.
- Expectant management in which there is no active intervention until the end of pregnancy.

ELECTRICAL INJURY

Electrical injuries are arbitrarily divided into *high voltage* (>1000 volt) and *low voltage.* More than 90% of cases occurring in young males. Electric burns account for less than 5% of admissions to major burn units. The mortality (3–15%) and morbidity (20%) is high.

The spectrum of injury ranges from a transient unpleasant sensation to instant cardiac arrest. The mechanism of tissue damage is complex, and not completely defined but includes the *direct effects* of current on cell membranes of nerves, blood vessels and muscles, and the conversion of electric energy into *heat energy* as current passes through the body.

High-voltage injuries are generally more serious although fatal electrocution may occur with low-voltage household current (110 V). Most household and commercial electrical sources are alternating current at 60 cycles/second and may cause tetanic contractions and prevent the victim from releasing themselves.

Factors that determine the nature and severity of electric trauma include:

- amperage;
- voltage;
- resistance to current e.g. reduced by water;
- type of current;
- duration of contact;
- current pathway.

Basic life support

- Rescuer safety is paramount and only after the power is switched off by an authorised person or the source is safely cleared may the victims cardiopulmonary status be determined. Additionally consider the possibility that high-voltage electricity can arc or pass through the ground.
- If the victim is located above ground, rescue breathing should be started at once and the victim lowered to the ground as soon as possible.
- Associated trauma may be a feature so spinal protection is required.

Arrhythmias are treated as per European Advanced Life Support Resuscitation Council guidelines. Patients with electrical burns of the face, mouth and neck may require special airway techniques, as extensive soft tissue swelling may develop and compromise the airway.

Cardiac effects

- VF, asystole or VT progressing to VF are the arrhythmias most likely to occur.
- Alternating current increases the likelihood of precipitating VF. Direct current is more likely to induce asystole. Transthoracic current flow (hand-to-hand) is more likely to be fatal than a vertical (hand-to-foot) or straddle (foot-to-foot) current path.
- ECG changes include ST and non-specific ST-T wave changes.

- Systemic hypertension is common with high voltage injuries and possibly due to catecholamine release.
- Dysrythmias and conduction defects may occur.
- Myocardial damage occurs rarely.
- Hypovolaemia secondary to fluid and blood loss into the tissues.
- Major vessel thrombosis, delayed rupture of large vessels and aneurysms have been reported.

Respiratory effects

Respiratory arrest – may occur due to:

- inhibition of medullary centre by direct effect;
- tetanic contraction of diaphragm and chest wall muscles;
- prolonged paralysis of respiratory muscles.

Trauma related

1. Skeletal muscle. This tends to dominate the clinical picture of electrical injury and is often the 'hidden' tissue damage that accounts for the greatest morbidity, functional impairment and cosmetic disfigurement. Skeletal muscle cells are particularly vulnerable to injury. A massive release of intracellular contents, with cell lysis occurs.

- Fluid requirements are often massive.
- Devascularization over the next 3–4 days is caused by injured blood vessels which thrombose.
- Compartment syndrome and compressive neuropathies – may require escharotomy and fasciotomy.
- Infection may occur.
- Amputation may be required.
- Chronic effects include muscle atrophy and fibrosis.
- Release of K+.
- Release of muscle enzymes resulting in myoglobinuria and renal failure.
- At initial operation necrotic muscle is difficult to distinguish and it is often necessary to re-inspect and debride necrotic tissue every 48 hours.

2. Fractures.

3. Dislocations.

4. Haemorrhage. Spleen, liver, bladder.

5. Head injury.

Cutaneous effects

1. Entry and exit wounds – usually the current path in electric shocks is predictable however:

- a skin contact may serve as both an entry and exit point;
- it is possible in very high voltage shocks to have several entry and exit points.

2. Burns. Gross inspection of the cutaneous injury does not give any indication of the extent of involved underlying tissue damage.

- Electrothermal burns – low voltage, limited, rarely more than 10%.
- Arc burns – treat as thermal burns (temperature 2000–4000°C), mostly involve a very small area (<1%) and are caused by low-voltage shock.
- Mixed burns – high voltage, often extensive and cause major sequalae.

Neurological effects

1. ***Acute***
   - Coma.
   - Epilepsy.
   - Motor and sensory deficits.
   - Headache.
   - Dizziness, lassitude, mood and personality disturbances.

2. ***Delayed***
   - Peripheral nerve injury.
   - Sensory, motor, and vasomotor nerve injury.
   - Spinal cord injury rarely.

Occular effects

- Conjunctivitis.
- Corneal burns.
- Retinal burns (may cause decreased vision).
- Cataract (rare) – delayed onset weeks to years and associated with electrical contact with head.

Auditory effects

- Ruptured eardrums.
- Delayed tinnitus.
- Reduced hearing.

Lightning

A high voltage direct current shock. Around five people are killed in England and Wales annually from lightening. For every fatality, four or more are injured.

1. ***Hills*** open country and open stretches of water are dangerous places in thunderstorms – and included in this category are golf courses. The advice to take is to get indoors or inside a car. If caught outdoors, throw away any metal or conductive object – a golf club, a carbon fibre fishing rod, a gun or umbrella. Do not shelter under a tree, especially an isolated tree.

2. ***A warning sign*** of impending strike is hair standing on end. If this occurs crouch into a ball with your legs together. Indoors, unplug your TV aerial and do not use the telephone.

3. ***Complications*** – patients who do not suffer cardiorespiratory arrest have an excellent chance of recovery.

- Primary cause of death is cardiac arrest due to asystole or ventricular fibrillation.

- Respiratory arrest may occur due to respiratory muscle spasm or suppression of the respiratory centre.
- Transient loss of consciousness, and temporary blindness or deafness may occur.

Further reading

Lee RC *et al. Electrical Trauma. The Pathophysiology, Manifestations and Clinical Management.* Cambridge University Press, 1992.

Smith T. On Lightning. *British Medical Journal*, 1991; **303:** 1563.

Related topics of interest

Burns (p. 74); Compartment Syndrome (p. 100)

ENDOCRINE EMERGENCIES

Acute adrenal crisis

Acute adrenal crisis may occur in either *primary or secondary adrenal insufficiency*. The acute event is often precipitated by acute stress, e.g. infection, trauma in a patient with pre-existing chronic adrenal insufficiency or abrupt cessation of glucocorticoid therapy in patients with adrenal atrophy, secondary to chronic steroid administration.

Acute destruction of the adrenal cortex due to haemorrhage is most commonly caused by septicaemia in children (Waterhouse–Friderichsen syndrome) and anticoagulant therapy in adults. The diagnosis should be considered in cases of hypotension, collapses, non-specific abdominal pain, confusion and cases of spontaneous hypoglycaemia.

Signs and symptoms

1. ***Primary adrenal insufficiency (Addison's disease)***:

- Hyper-pigmentation of skin creases, buccal mucosa and scars.
- Weakness and fatigue.
- Nausea, vomiting and diarrhoea.
- Anorexia and weight loss.
- Postural hypotension or hypotension.
- Decreased level of consciousness.

2. ***Secondary adrenal insufficiency*** may be preceded by symptoms of hypopituitarism, hypogonadism, hypothroidism and symptoms of hypothalmic or pituitary tumour (headaches, visual defects).

3. ***Biochemical features***

- Hyponatraemia.
- Hyperkalaemia.
- Raised blood urea.
- Hypoglycaemia.
- Plasma cortisol of <600 nmol/l in the acutely ill patient.

4. ***Treatment***

- Correct hypoglycaemia.
- Replace fluid volume with normal saline (1 litre over the first hour) and thereafter according to clinical state. Correct electrolyte deficits e.g. serum potassium – initial serum K^+ is increased, however there is a deficit of total body K^+ and replacement should be started when serum K falls after hydration and cortisol administration.
- Give Hydrocortisone – 100 mg i.v. then 100 mg 6 hourly.
- Mineralocorticoid replacement with fludrocortisone will be required for those with primary adrenal insufficiency.
- Treatment of underlying cause, e.g. infection.
- Look for associated conditions such as hypothyroidism and panhypopituitarism.

Thyroid crisis

This is a life-threatening emergency usually precipitated by stress, e.g. infection or trauma in a poorly treated or untreated thyrotoxic patient. Death occurs from hypovolaemic shock, coma, congestive cardiac failure and tachyarrythmias.

Signs and symptoms

1. ***General.*** Fever, sweating, warm skin and dehydration.

2. ***Cardiovascular.*** Hyperdynamic circulation, wide pulse pressure, sinus tachcardia, atrial arrhythmias, congestive cardiac failure, myocardial ischaemia and infarction.

3. ***Central nervous.*** Agitation, tremor, weakness, proximal myopathy, confusion, psychosis and coma.

4. ***Abdominal.*** Nausea, vomiting, diarrhoea, abdominal pain and jaundice.

Investigations

- Take blood for T3 + T4, plasma glucose, electrolytes and FBC.
- ECG monitoring and 12 lead ECG.

Treatment

1. ***General.*** Parenteral fluids, treatment of arrhythmias or cardiac failure, antipyretics and identify precipitant such as underlying infection.

2. ***Specific***

- *Block hormone action – Beta blockers* block the peripheral effects of the thyroid hormone e.g. propranolol (1–5 mg i.v.) or 20–80 mg orally, to control tachycardia, fever, tremor and restlessness.
- *Block hormone synthesis – Propylthiouracil* (600–1200 mg loading dose) blocks thyroid hormone synthesis and peripheral conversion of T4 to T3.
- *Block hormone release – Iodine compounds* in high dose decrease thyroid hormone release. T3 to be given 2–4 hours after propylthiouracil.

3. ***Plasmapheresis*** can be considered.

4. ***Give hydrocortisone*** (100 mg i.v.) to treat relative adrenal insufficiency, which may be present.

Myxoedema coma

Due to thyroid hormone deficiency that results in encephalopathy. Can develop insidiously or precipitated by exposure to cold, infection, drugs (phenothiazines) or other stress. Mortality high (50%) especially in the elderly.

Signs and symptoms

1. ***General.*** Cold intolerance, dry skin, constipation, weakness, lethargy, slow speech, weight gain. Facial puffiness, coarse dry skin, yellow pigmentation (carotenaemia), hair loss, thinning of eyebrows, enlarged tongue.

2. *Central nervous.* Disorientation, progress to coma, grand-mal epilepsy, ataxia, myxoedema madness (psychosis).

3. *Cardiovascular.* Bradycardia, cardiomegaly, distant heart sounds.

4. *Biochemical features*
- Core temperature – hypothermia.
- Arterial blood gases – hypoxaemia, hypercapnia and respiratory or mixed acidosis.
- Hyponatraemia.
- Hypoglycaemia.
- Low thyroid hormones and elevated TSH.
- Hypercholesterolaemia.
- Elevated CPK.

5. *CXR.* May reveal cardiomegaly and a pericardial effusion.

6. *ECG.* Bradycardia, low voltage changes, flat or inverted T waves and J waves.

7. *Treatment*
- Treat respiratory failure as necessary.
- Correct hypoglycaemia.
- Treat hypotension with crystalloid.
- Treat hypothermia with passive rewarming.
- Insert a nasogastric tube and urinary catheter.
- Administer cortisol.
- Correct hyponatraemia.
- Identify and treat precipitant.

8. *Specific.* Initial replacement of thyroid hormone is given as liothyroxine sodium, by slow intravenous injection of 5–20 micrograms. Care with patients when known IHD as may precipitate arrhythmias, angina or MI.

Hyponatraemia

Asymptomatic hyponatraemia is often benign. Symptomatic hyponatraemia with CNS manifestations (hyponatraemic encephalopathy) require treatment to prevent brain damage that is due to brain oedema, respiratory insufficiency and hypoxaemia. The morbidity is most closely related to the age and sex of the patient (highest in children and menstruant women) rather than the magnitude or duration of the hyponatraemia.

Causes of hyponatraemia

- Postoperative.
- Intravenous hypotonic fluid administration.
- Inappropriate ADH secretion.
  - (a) Lung and cerebral tumours.
  - (b) Adrenal insufficiency.
  - (c) Hypothyroidism.

- Drugs including diuretics, sedatives, oral hypoglycaemic, etc.
- AIDS.
- Psychogenic polydipsia.

Signs and symptoms

1. ***Early hyponatraemic encephalopathy***

- Headache.
- Nausea/vomiting.
- Weakness.

2. ***Advanced hyponatraemic encephalopathy***

- Reduced level of consciousness.
- Bizarre behaviour.
- Visual/auditory hallucinations.
- Incontinence.
- Hypoventilation.

Very advanced hyponatraemic encephalopathy results in manifestations secondary to increased intracranial pressure and include focal or grand mal epilepsy, coma and respiratory arrest.

3. ***Treatment*** – ideally treat the underlying cause and:

- *Asymptomatic hyponatraemia* generally does not require aggressive treatment with hypertonic saline, as symptomatic measures combined with fluid restriction are usually sufficient. In volume-depleted patients isotonic (154 mM) sodium chloride is usually the fluid of choice.
- *Symptomatic hyponatraemia* is best treated with hypertonic (usually 514 mM) sodium chloride, often in conjunction with a loop diuretic. Aim to raise the sodium to around 130 mmol/l, but by about 1 mmol/l/h. This is best performed in the ITU, where neurological, respiratory, and haemodynamic monitoring can be made.

Further reading

Anonymous. *Endocrine Emergencies.* Bailliere's Clinical Endocrinology and Metabolism. 1992; **6:** 1–228.

Arieff AI. Management of hyponatraemia. *British Medical Journal*, 1993; **307:** 305–8.

Related topic of interest

Diabetic emergencies (p. 117)

FACTITIOUS DISORDERS

Factitious disorders are characterized by physical or psychological symptoms produced by an individual under voluntary control. An essential characteristic is that there is no apparent goal other than to assume the patient role, the most florid example being *Munchausen's syndrome.*

Factitious disorders should be distinguished from malingering, in which symptoms are also under voluntary control but the goal is personal gain (e.g. narcotics, compensation).

The diagnosis can be confirmed only by the patient's confession, and careful history taking and gentle confrontation may be effective in securing this. Factitious illness is often misdiagnosed but should be considered in patients with perplexing clinical problems and in dramatic presentations with no obvious organic cause.

It can be difficult to diagnose in the setting of the A&E department; an incorrect diagnosis of factitious illness may prove costly to both patient and doctor. It must not be forgotten that the patient who suffers from factitious illness is still at risk from organic disease.

Munchausen syndrome

The Munchausen syndrome was coined by Asscher (1951) to describe patients who repeatedly presented to hospitals with dramatic symptoms suggesting serious physical illness. It is most frequently seen in men.

1. Common presentations include:

- Patients who feign surgical illness, hoping for a laparotomy (*laparotimorphilia migrans*).
- Patients with alarming symptoms of bleeding (*haemorrhagica histrionica*).
- Patients who present with curious fits (*neurologica diabolica*).
- Patients who present with false heart attacks (*cardiopathia fantastica*).

Other evidence of deception, (i.e. the use of many aliases and addresses) may be discovered. Occasionally extreme measures to deceive doctors are used.

Patients presenting with simulated illness should be confronted tactfully and offered referral to a psychiatrist. Unfortunately psychiatric treatment is seldom helpful and the patient will often self-discharge when confronted with the diagnosis.

2. Munchausen's syndrome by proxy is a form of child abuse in which a parent (usually the mother) fabricates symptoms and signs in the child.

Neurological

1. Pseudocoma. May result in patient intubation. Spontaneous flickering of the eyelids and resistance to passive attempts at opening them, and the upward eye sign (with upward rolling of the eye and gaze avoidance) are suggestive of pseudocoma.

2. Pseudoseizures. There is often bizarre motor activity, with unusual precipitants, but no loss of consciousness.

Metabolic

1. ***Hypoglycaemia.*** Often related to self-administration of insulin or oral hypoglycaemic drugs, especially in diabetics, health care professionals or relatives of diabetics.

2. ***Brittle diabetic.*** Some patients with brittle diabetes may be factitious.

3. ***Phaeochromocytoma.*** Can be simulated by administration of catecholamines and present with palpitations, sweating and hypertension.

4. ***Thyrotoxicosis.***

5. ***Diuretic abuse.***

6. ***Water intoxication.***

Cardiac

1. ***Chest pain.*** May present with myocardial type chest pain and demand analgesia. May have signs of previous investigations such as cardiac catheterization.

2. ***Arrhythmias.*** Both bradycardias and tachycardias which have resulted in cases requiring pacemakers or cardioversion.

Respiratory

- *Asthma.*
- *Upper airway obstruction with stridor.*
- *Haemoptysis.*

General

1. ***Dermatitis artefacta*** – skin lesions are produced deliberately.

2. ***Factitious PUO*** – the patient produces symptoms of a febrile illness and will even tamper with the recording of the temperature.

3. ***Factitious AIDS*** – a recently described condition in which patients feign AIDS.

Further reading

Asher R 1972 Talking sense. Pitman.

Sutherland AJ, Rodin GM. Factitious disorders in a general hospital setting: clinical features and a review of the literature. *Psychosomatics*, 1990; **31:** 392–9.

FEBRILE CONVULSION

A febrile convulsion is a seizure associated with a fever in the absence of evidence of intracranial infection and with no other obvious cause. They are common, affecting approximately 3–5% of all children. The majority occur between the ages of 3 months and 6 years, with a peak incidence at 18 months. The history is characteristically of a child with a febrile illness, usually a viral respiratory tract infection, who has a major seizure. The seizure is generally tonic/clonic, not focal in nature and short-lasting (less than 10 minutes) and recovery is rapid and complete.

Treatment

Attention as always is paid to the *A*irway, *B*reathing and *C*irculation.

Until recently the mainstay of treatment for convulsions was diazepam. Recently a consensus view has determined that lorazepam has advantages over diazepam. The guidelines below are based on those recommendations.

Status Epilepticus Protocol
APLS 3rd edition update

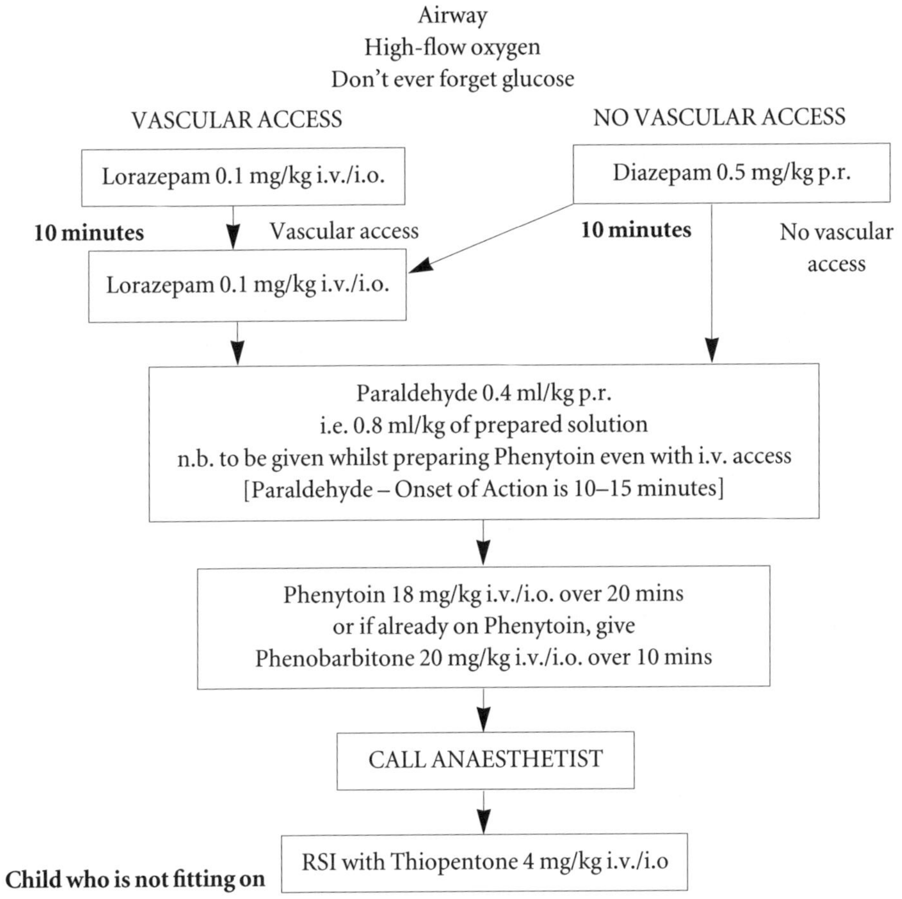

If the child has stopped fitting then attention should be paid to protecting the airway. In the majority of cases the child will recover rapidly once the convulsion has stopped and specific manoeuvres to protect the airway are not required. If the child remains unconscious they should be placed in the recovery position until they have woken up.

The parents should be reassured and allowed to stay with and hold the child if appropriate. The nature of the fit and prognosis should be explained (this explanation should be repeated and expanded on later).

If the child is conscious oral paracetamol should be given, if not the rectal route can be used. The child should be uncovered to allow cooling. Care should be taken not to allow the child to become hypothermic.

Investigations

The first and most important investigation is a blood glucose. A stick test should be used initially to exclude hypoglycaemia at the bedside. A laboratory result will confirm the reading. Hypoglycaemia should be treated with 10% glucose at a dose of 5 ml per kg. The blood sugar should be rechecked to gauge response.

Urine should be obtained to exclude a urinary tract infection.

In uncomplicated febrile convulsion in the absence of a definite indication neither a lumbar puncture nor a chest X-ray is routinely indicated (although local protocols vary).

FBC, blood cultures and clothing screen should be performed if indicated.

Neither CT scan nor EEG is routinely required in a simple febrile fit.

All children having their first febrile convulsion need admission to hospital for evaluation and appropriate investigation.

Prognosis

The majority (60–70%) of children have only a single fit. Approximately 3% of children will go on to have epilepsy. Parents should be warned that subsequent administration of the pertusiss vaccination should be accompanied by oral paracetamol for 72 hours.

Further reading

Behrman RE, Kliegman RM. *Nelsons Textbook of Paediatrics.* 1999, WB Saunders .

Related topic of interest

Meningitis (p. 231)

FRACTURES – PRINCIPLES OF TREATMENT

A fracture is a break in the continuity of a bone. A long bone consists of four regions: diaphysis, metaphysis, epiphyseal plate and epiphysis.

Diaphysis

The shaft of the bone.

Metaphysis

The often splayed end of the bone between the diaphysis and epiphyseal plate.

Epiphyseal plate

The growing cartilaginous part of the bone invisible on X-ray and seen as a black line in childrens X-rays but not seen in adults.

Epiphysis

The end of the bone distal to the epiphyseal plate.

Pathology

Fractures may be open or closed.

1. ***Closed (simple) fracture.*** A fracture with no communication with the exterior of the body. A fracture may be associated with a wound, but if the two do not communicate then the fracture is not compound. Infection in such an instance can only arise by haematogeneous spread. This is rare. The haematoma in a closed fracture is contained and blood loss is minimized.

2. ***Open (compound) fracture.*** A fracture which communicates with the exterior of the body via a wound. The communication may occur because the bone fragment has pierced the skin (within-out) or because an external object has opened the wound up down to the level of the fracture (without-in). Open fractures may become infected due to entry of organisms from the exterior. Because blood can exit via the wound, blood loss may be significant.

Aetiology

Fractures may occur in an otherwise normal bone as a result of:

1. ***Direct violence.*** Application of a force directly to the bone which exceeds the strength of the bone, e.g. crush injury to a terminal phalanx.

2. ***Indirect violence.*** Transmission of a force which exceeds the strength of a bone, e.g. a fall onto the outstretched hand resulting in a fracture of the surgical neck of humerus.

3. ***Fatigue (stress) fractures.*** Repeated application of forces to a bone beyond the limit of the bone may result in a fatigue or stress fracture, e.g. a march fracture of the second metatarsal.

4. Pathological fracture. A fracture through a diseased bone (e.g. bone cyst or secondary deposit) may occur after application of minimal force.

Patterns of fractures

Fractures are described as simple if only two fragments result from the injury and comminuted if more than two fragments result. Fractures are described as complex if they involve structures such as major nerves or blood vessels. The shape or pattern of a fracture may be used in its description.

1. Hairline. Fractures resulting from a force sufficiently large to fracture the bone but not to cause displacement of the fracture ends.

2. Greenstick. The resilience of children's bones can result in a partial fracture which buckles the bone. In such fractures the periosteum usually remains intact.

3. Intra-articular. Fractures may partially or completely involve the articular surface of a joint. Complete anatomical correction is required to prevent late osteoarthritis.

4. Others. Transverse, spiral, oblique compression, avulsion and depressed fractures are as their name suggests.

Deformity

The following terms describe the types of deformity seen in fractures.

1. Displacement (translation). Shift in position of the distal fragment of a fracture in relation to the proximal fragment (e.g. undisplaced, posteriorly displaced, anteriorly displaced, etc.).

2. Angulation. The degree of tilt of the distal fragment in relation to the long axis of the proximal fragment.

3. Axial rotation. The degree of rotation of the distal fragment around the long axis of the proximal fragment.

Fractures involving an epiphysis: the Salter–Harris classification

1. Type I. Fracture through the epiphyseal plate. This may result in obvious widening of the plate or may not be radiologically evident.

2. Type II. A fracture involving both the epiphyseal plate and a fragment of the metaphysis (75% of all epiphyseal plate fractures).

3. Type III. A fracture involving the epiphyseal plate and extending into the epiphysis.

4. Type IV. A fracture involving the epiphyseal plate, metaphysis and epiphysis.

5. Type V. A crush fracture of the epiphyseal plate. This may not be evident on X-ray and can present late as a disturbance or arrest of growth.

Management

1. ***History.*** The mechanism of injury should be elicited. This will indicate the force of injury, the likely type of fracture and the likelihood of associated injuries (e.g. multiple fractures, foreign bodies in wounds).

In children the possibility of non-accidental injury (NAI) should always be considered. The factors which suggest that NAI may be a possibility include delayed presentation, injury out of proportion to the force applied, multiple injuries and fracture type or pattern uncommon for that age group. It is the responsibility of the assessing doctor to raise the suspicion of NAI and then to refer to a physician experienced in managing such cases to determine whether NAI is likely to have occurred.

2. ***Examination.*** The clinical signs of fracture are pain, swelling, loss of function and deformity. The injured part should be examined to look for evidence of deformity, open fracture, nerve or major vessel involvement and other injuries (e.g. dislocated elbow in association with Colles fracture).

3. ***Treatment.*** The treatment for a particular fracture depends on the fracture type, degree of deformity, whether the fracture is open or closed and major nerve or vessel involvement. The general principles for management of any fracture are, initial resuscitation, reduction, immobilization (e.g. plaster, splintage, traction or internal fixation) and rehabilitation to achieve the optimum end point of return to normal function.

Attention should be paid to pain relief. This may be achieved with analgesia, reduction, immobilization and/or nerve block. In practice a combination of these techniques will be used.

Further reading

McRae R. Practical Fracture Treatment: 3rd edn. Edinburgh, Churchill Livingstone, 1994.

Related topics of interest

Compartment syndrome (p. 100); Scaphoid fracture (p. 183); Wrist injury (p. 337)

GAMMA-HYDROXYBUTYRATE (GHB)

GHB ($HOOC-CH_2-CH_2-CH_2OH$) is a naturally occurring metabolite of γ-aminobutyric acid (GABA). It is found in the central nervous system, kidney, heart, skeletal muscle and brown fat. It was synthesized in the 1960s and used as a sedative pre-medicant and an intravenous anaesthetic induction agent. Its side effects include vomiting and epileptic features precluded its use. It has also been used for the treatment of narcolepsy and experimentally for the treatment of alcohol dependance and opiate withdrawal. In the 1990s in the United States it was used illicitly and banned by the FDA. It became available in the UK in nightclubs since 1994. It is not controlled under the Misuse of Drugs Act and therefore it is not an offence to consume this drug. It is used in the rave scene for its euphoric effects and increased libido. It is a colourless, odourless, liquid with a mild, soapy, salt taste. It is usually taken orally but may also be injected.

It has been used illicitly by body builders and has been attributed to improve athletic performance and increase muscle mass whilst decreasing fat. It has also been quoted as being used as a 'date rape' drug as it is easily masked when put into party drugs. The recipe is available on the internet and it can be prepared at home by mixing sodium hydroxide and butyrol lactate at the correct pH and heating gently.

Synonyms include GHB, liquid X, liquid ecstasy, Georgia homeboy, easy lay, fantasy and soap.

Pharmacokinetics

GHB is rapidly absorbed from the gastrointestinal tract within 15 minutes of oral ingestion. There is therefore no role for gastric decontamination. It is metabolized to carbon dioxide and water. Peak plasma concentrations are reached in under 2 hours after ingestion. Effects usually resolve spontaneously within 96 hours.

The effects are potentiated by alcohol, benzodiazepines, opiate analgesics and other psychoactive drugs.

It is not detected by routine toxicological tests. It can be measured in urine and blood.

Side effects

1. ***Mild–moderate***

- Nausea, vomiting and diarrhoea.
- Headache, ataxia, dizziness, confusion, agitation, euphoria, hallucinations, tremor and myoclonus and amnesia.
- Urinary incontinence.
- Hypothermia.
- Increased libido.

2. ***Severe***

- Cheyne Stokes respiration and respiratory depression.
- Bradycardia and hypotension.
- Coma and seizures.

Laboratory abnormalities

- Metabolic respiratory acidosis.
- Hypernatraemia.
- Hypokalaemia.
- Hyperglycaemia.

Treatment

- Respiratory support.
- Atropine for persistent symptomatic bradycardia.
- Patients typically regain consciousness within 5 hours of the ingestion.
- Naloxone has been shown to reverse some of the effects in animals.
- Diazepam for convulsions.
- All patients should be observed for a minimum of 2 hours.
- Chronic use will probably be shown to be associated with withdrawal.

Further reading

Thomas G *et al.* Coma induced by abuse of γ-hydroxybutyrate (GBH or liquid ecstasy): a case report. *British Medical Journal*, 1997; **314:** 35–6.

Chin R *et al.* Clinical course of γ-hydroxybutyrate overdose. *Annals of Emergency Medicine*, 1999; **31:** 716–22.

Li J *et al.* A tale of novel intoxication: A review of the effects of γ-hydroxybutyric acid with recommendations for management. *Annals of Emergency Medicine*, 1999; **31:** 728–33.

Adverse events associated with ingestion of gamma-butyrolactone. *Morbidity and Mortality Weekly*, 1999; **48** (7).

GASTROINTESTINAL HAEMORRHAGE – UPPER

District hospitals admit each year 50–80 cases of upper gastrointestinal haemorrhage per 100 000 of the population, of whom more than two-thirds are aged over 60 years.

Peptic ulcers account for 50% of bleeds and about one-third of patients have recently taken NSAIDs. Eighty per cent of patients' bleeding stops spontaneously without therapeutic intervention. Mortality rises with age but the overall death rate has been reported at 4% in the UK national audit. Causes of death are most commonly related to coexisting disease, post-operative deaths, underlying disease or exsanguination.

Patients with massive lower GI bleeding should be considered as possibly having upper gastrointestinal bleeding and undergo endoscopy of the upper tract as up to 11% of patients are bleeding from the upper gastrointestinal tract.

Accurate diagnosis is essential and flexible endoscopy is the mainstay of diagnosis. Radionuclide scanning and arteriography have a place in diagnosis when endoscopy fails.

Aetiology

- Duodenal ulcer/duodenitis.
- Gastric ulcer/gastritis/gastric erosions.
- Oesophagitis/oesophageal ulcer.
- Mallory–Weiss tear.
- Varices.
- Upper gastrointestinal malignancy.
- Polyps.
- Angiodysplasia.

History and examination

Important *historical features* include:

- PMH of peptic ulcer.
- PMH of previous bleed.
- PMH of bleeding disorder.
- Liver disease.
- Alcohol intake.
- Aspirin or NSAIDs intake.
- History of vigorous retching or vomiting (Mallory–Weiss syndrome).

The patient's examination includes general condition regarding cardiorespiratory systems and assessment of blood loss. Examine for signs of hepatic disease and alcohol abuse.

Severity of GI haemorrhage

1. ***Mild to moderate haemorrhage defined as:***

- Patient is aged <60 years.
- No PMH.
- No hypovolaemia.
- Haemoglobin >10 g.

2. ***Life-threatening haemorrhage defined as:***

- Patient >60 years.
- Hypovolaemic (systolic blood pressure, 100 mmHg or diastolic blood pressure falls on sitting and standing).
- Haemoglobin <10 g.
- Severe disease e.g. liver, cardiovascular, respiratory.

Investigations

- Full blood count.
- Urea and electrolytes.
- LFTs.
- Coagulation screen.
- HbsAg in liver disease.
- Blood group and save serum if haemoglobin normal or if bleed is considered mild or moderate.
- Cross-match blood if haemoglobin <10 g, or with a life-threatening bleed.

Management

1. ***Mild to moderate haemorrhage***

- Admit to medical ward.
- Fluids only on day one, food thereafter. Nil by mouth 6 hours pre-endoscopy.
- Observe for continued haemorrhage or re-bleeding.
- Endoscopy on next routine list.

2. ***Severe haemorrhage***

- Restore blood volume; consider using CVP line.
- Admit to HDU.
- Inform consultant physician and consultant surgeon.
- Observe for continued bleeding or rebleeding.
- Sips of water only until endoscopy, preferably done within 12 hours of bleed.
- If liver disease present, avoid sedation; clear bowel with magnesium sulphate mixture 10 ml tds or lactulose 20 ml tds or an enema; 20 g protein diet per day.

3. ***Transfusion***

- Oxygenate with high flow oxygen.
- A large bore intravenous cannula is inserted.
- If there is supine or postural hypotension, tachycardia or reduced capillary refill, a plasma expander, followed by whole blood should be given as soon as possible.

- CVP measurement should guide replacement, especially those with cardio vascular disease.
- A urine catheter and measurement of hourly urine output are required in patients with shock.
- Packed cells may be required if there is anaemia but a normal or increased blood volume.
- Group O Rh– blood may be required in emergencies.

Investigations

1. Endoscopy. Flexible endoscopy should be the first diagnostic test in patients who present with upper GI bleeding. Endoscopy allows accurate diagnosis of the cause of bleeding in up to 90% of patients when undertaken within 48 hours of a bleeding episode, but only 33% accurate when performed more than 48 hours. The procedure should be performed in the stable patient within 48 hours, but if bleeding is severe, and continued, then early endoscopy is indicated.

If signs of recent bleeding from an ulcer are present at endoscopy, haemostasis may be achieved using laser therapy, thermal coagulation or direct injection of a vasoconstrictor and/or sclerosant. There is a reduction of about one-third in the death rate after such procedures.

Surgery

Operation is the mainstay for the treatment of patients with persistent bleeding from peptic ulcer disease. It may not always be possible to pinpoint the source of upper GI bleeding before operation but endoscopy should be attempted prior to surgery either in the endoscopy suite or in theatre, depending on the urgency of the case.

Delayed operation usually results in greater blood loss, higher morbidity and mortality rates in patients aged >60 years but early operation in the younger patients leads to unnecessary operations.

Consider emergency surgery for patients with a bleeding peptic ulcer if:

- A patient requires more than 4 units of whole blood to maintain blood volume over 24 hours.
- A patient continues to bleed or re-bleeds.

Acute variceal bleeding

Oesophageal varices account for 2–4% of bleeds but carry a 30% mortality. Upper GI bleeding associated with cirrhosis and accompanying liver compromise, carries a high mortality rate. There is a high recurrence rate, so long-term therapy such as repeated sclerotherapy, propranolol therapy, shunt surgery and liver transplantation are considered.

1. Management. Patients should be managed in a HDU-type setting.

- Resuscitate patient.
  (a) 2 large-bore venflons.
  (b) Transfuse blood and fresh frozen plasma if there are clotting abnormalities.
  (c) Colloid should be given whilst awaiting blood.

Crystalloids are best avoided. Do not over replace fluids.

- Checking clotting, FBC, urea and electrolytes and cross match 6 units of blood.
- Give metoclopramide 20 μg as an i.v. bolus followed by i.v. octreotide infusion.
- Arrange endoscopy with sclerotherapy once stable. If bleeding is very profuse then obtain the help of an anaesthetist to protect the airway.
- If bleeding continues despite sclerotherapy or profuse haemorrhage, pass a Sengstaken–Blakemore tube.
- Transfer to a HDU for intensive nursing care.
- Re-check clotting and correct any abnormalities with blood/FFP/platelets and 10 mg of i.v. vitamin K daily.
- Give omeprazole 10–20 mg bd to prevent bleeding from sclerotherapy ulcers.
- Monitor and treat liver and renal function.
- Arrange for further endoscopy and sclerotherapy.
- *Injection sclerotherapy* – this is the best method of arresting the acute bleed with a success rate of 80%. If bleeding is severe obtain assistance from an anaesthetist to protect the airway.
- *Sengstaken–Blakemore or Minnesota balloon tamponade* – in those of whom injection sclerotherapy is hampered by too massive haemorrhage, balloon tamponade is carried out immediately until the patient's condition is stabilized, followed by sclerotherapy (keep the tube refrigerated).

- *Medical control*
  (a) Nitroglycerin.
  (b) Vasopressin (pitressin).
  (c) Somatostatin and its analogues (e.g. i.v. octreotide 50 μg/h with an initial 50 μg bolus). Continue infusion for 24–48 hrs (500 μg in 250 mg normal saline at 25 ml/h).

- *Surgery* – operative intervention is reserved for those patients who are not controlled by sclerotherapy. Oesophageal stapling and portosystemic shunts should be reserved for the 5–10% of patients in whom sclerotherapy fails to control the bleeding, but carries a high mortality.

Further reading

Report of a Joint Working Group of the British Society of Gastroenterology, the Research Unit of the Royal College of Physicians of London and the Audit Unit of the Royal College of Surgeons of England. Guidelines for good practice in and audit of the management of upper gastrointestinal haemorrhage. *Journal of the Royal College of Physicians of London*, 1992; **26:** 281–9.

Related topics of interest

Intravenous fluids (p. 200); Shock (p. 291)

GENITOURINARY TRAUMA

Renal injuries

Ninety per cent of renal injuries are due to blunt abdominal trauma, with associated injuries occurring in 40% of cases. Children are more prone to renal injuries which may be due to the relative lack of perinephric fat.

Few renal injuries need immediate treatment and 95% can be treated non-operatively. The urinary tract is evaluated as part of the secondary survey.

1. *Classification*

- *Minor* (85%) – contusions/superficial lacerations with an intact capsular and pelvicaliceal system.
- *Major* (10%) – deep lacerations with associated capsular tear and/or pelvicaliceal system involvement.
- *Critical* (5%) – renal fragmentation or renal pedicle injury.

2. *Clinical signs.* Renal injury should be suspected if there is a history of injury to the flank and the patient complains of loin pain.

Clinical signs include:

- Soft tissue injury to flank or penetrating injury.
- Loin tenderness.
- Loss of loin contour.
- Loin mass.
- *Haematuria* – not an accurate sign as to the severity of renal injury i.e. a renal pedicle injury may present with only microscopic haematuria or macro scopic haematuria need not be due to severe damage.

3. *Investigations*

- A CT scan documents the presence and extent of a blunt renal injury and is becoming more common as part of an abdominal CT scan.
- The stable patient can be assessed first with a *KUB*.

The presence of the following suggests potential renal damage:

(a) Scoliosis (with concavity towards the side of the injury).
(b) Loss of psoas shadow.
(c) Enlarged renal outline.
(d) Displaced bowel.
(e) Elevation of the ipsilateral diaphragm.
(f) Fractured ribs or transverse processes.

Intravenous urography – indicated in patients with:

(a) Macroscopic haematuria.
(b) Microscopic haematuria and systolic BP < 90 mmHg (after completion of the primary survey).

(c) Patients with microscopic haematuria and haemodynamic stability probably have minor renal injuries. The decision to investigate will be based on clinical judgement and discussion with a urologist.

Abnormal IVU features include:

(a) Delayed excretion.
(b) Extravasation.
(c) Disruption of renal outline.
(d) Calyceal distortion.
(e) Filling defect in the collecting system.
(f) Non-visualization.
(g) Hydronephrosis.

- Non-visualization or extravasation of contrast necessitates further evaluation by *arteriography*, but only if the patient remains stable.

4. Management

- ABCs.
- Stage renal injury radiologically.
- Treat most patients with minor/major renal injuries expectantly.
- Operate on patients with cortical and unstable major injuries.

5. Complications of renal trauma include:

- Hypertension.
- AV fistula.
- Hydronephrosis.
- Pseudocyst and calculus formation.
- Chronic pyelonephritis.
- Loss of renal function.

Bladder injuries

Comprise approximately 22% urologic injuries due to blunt trauma in 86% of cases. There are often associated injuries in addition to the commonly found pelvic fracture.

1. Classification and clinical signs

- *Injuries:*
  (a) Contusion.
  (b) Extraperitoneal rupture.
  (c) Intraperitoneal rupture.
  (d) Both intra- and extraperitoneal rupture.

- *Rupture is caused by:*
  (a) Penetration of a bone spicule.
  (b) Compression of a distended bladder.

- *Suspicion of a bladder injury where there is a:*
  (a) Pelvic fracture.
  (b) Lower abdominal trauma (blunt or penetrating).
  (c) Gross haematuria.
  (d) Inability to void.

2. *Investigations*
(a) *KUB.*
(b) *Cystography* if no urethral injury suspected (to include post-micturition film).

3. *Treatment.* *Treatment* is by a urologist.

Urethral injury

1. *Classification and clinical signs*

- More common in males. Injuries are usually either:
  (a) *Bulbar* – usually caused by straddle injuries.
  (b) *Membranous* – caused by pelvic fracture or penetrating trauma.

- *The suspicion of urethral injury is raised if:*
  (a) Pelvic fracture or deep perineal laceration with gross haematuria.
  (b) Blood at the meatus.
  (c) Perineal bruising.
  (d) Abnormal voiding or inability to void.
  (e) High riding or boggy prostate.
  (f) Vaginal bleeding or laceration.

2. *Investigation.* An anterior retrograde urethrogram, followed by a cystogram.

3. *Treatment.* An option is to place a suprapubic catheter and withhold further investigation until a urologist is available. A urethral catheter must not be placed as it risks the creation of a false passage or completion of a partial tear.

If no sign of urethral injury exists, an attempt is made to pass a well-lubricated Foley catheter. If any difficulty is encountered, the procedure must stop and further investigation undertaken.

Further reading

Skinner D *et al.* ABC of major trauma. *British Medical Journal*, 1991.
Talbot-Stern JK. Urinary Tract Injuries. *Critical Decisions in Emergency Medicine*, Lesson 5. pp. 35–40.

Related topics of interest

Abdominal trauma (p. 4); Head injury (p. 173); Maxillofacial injury (p. 226); Spine and spinal cord trauma (p. 307); Thoracic trauma (p. 321)

GYNAECOLOGY

The common presenting symptoms of gynaecological problems to the A&E department are vaginal bleeding, pelvic pain and vaginal discharge. Bleeding and pelvic pain associated with pregnancy are covered in the section on obstetric emergencies. Patients will also present to the A&E department for emergency contraception (the morning after pill).

A negative ßHCG pregnancy test virtually excluded a viable pregnancy.

Vaginal bleeding

Vaginal bleeding can be sub-divided into bleeding related to the menstrual cycle and bleeding unrelated to the menstrual cycle.

1. ***Conditions causing bleeding related to the menstrual cycle:***

- Dysfunctional uterine bleeding.
- Endometriosis.
- Toxic shock syndrome (see below).
- Uterine fibroids.

2. ***Conditions causing bleeding unrelated to the menstrual cycle:***

- Cervical polyps.
- Malignancy.
- Urethral lesions (e.g. caruncle).
- Uterine polyps.

3. ***Management.*** A full history is taken specifically asking about contraception use and date of last menstrual period and normal menstrual pattern. If the patient is stable routine referral to the gynaecology clinic should be arranged for investigation and follow up.

Pelvic pain

In addition to surgical causes for pelvic pain (e.g. acute appendicitis) gynaecological causes for pelvic pain include:

- Pelvic inflammatory disease.
- Pelvic abscess.
- Rupture or haemorrhage into an ovarian cyst.
- Torsion of an ovarian cyst.
- Menstruation.
- Ovulation.
- Endometriosis.
- Malignancy.

1. ***Management.*** History and examination will usually suggest the possibility of a surgical cause of pelvic pain. If the cause is unclear then ultrasound examination will confirm the diagnosis in many cases of gynaecological origin. If pelvic inflammatory disease is suspected referral for definitive diagnosis and treatment should be

made. Antibiotics should not be prescribed upon a clinical diagnosis made in the A&E department.

Vaginal discharge

A vaginal discharge is normal. The colour and consistency varies with age and during pregnancy. The investigation and management of an abnormal discharge included speculum inspection and swabbing (including a wet slide preparation) for *Trichomonas vaginalis*, *Candida*, *Gonococcus* and *Chlamydia*. In addition a cervical smear is taken. The management of vaginal discharge is generally outside the scope of the A&E department. Patients presenting with a discharge should be referred for proper investigation and management. Antibiotics should not be prescribed until a firm diagnosis has been made.

Toxic shock syndrome

This is characterized by pyrexia associated with diarrhoea and erythematous rash in the presence of shock. It is due to an endotoxin produced by *Staphylococcus aureus* and is associated with the use of tampons. The initial management is removal of the tampon, fluid resuscitation and intravenous antibiotics (e.g. Flucloxacillin).

Emergency contraception

Local protocols on the prescribing of post-coital contraception vary. Because the treatment can be commenced within 72 hours of intercourse some departments feel that it is best prescribed by primary care where the relevant counselling and follow up can be arranged. The commonest regimen involves taking two doses of a combined oestrogen and progesterone pill separated by twelve hours. The treatment acts by preventing implantation. Follow up should be arranged at about three weeks post-treatment to ensure that normal menstruation has taken place. If menstruation has not occurred then a pregnancy test is performed. The failure rate of the technique is quoted at 2–5%. Contraindications to this regimen include pregnancy and a history of thrombo-embolic disease.

Insertion of an intra-uterine contraceptive device (IUCD) is an alternative method but is outside the scope of A&E departments.

Further reading

Stevens L, Kenney A. Emergencies in Obstetrics and Gynaecology. Oxford, Oxford University Press, 1994.

Related topics of interest

Abdominal pain (p. 1); Genitourinary trauma (p. 164); Obstetric emergencies (p. 250); Shock (p. 291); Urological conditions (p. 334)

HAEMATOLOGICAL CONDITIONS

D Burke

Haemoglobinopathies

These fall into two distinct groups. Those resulting from structural abnormalities in the globulin molecule of haemoglobin, e.g. sickle cell disease and those resulting from an imbalance in the production of globin molecules (which are usually otherwise normal) leading to the thalassaemias. The thalassaemias rarely present as acute emergencies to the A&E department.

Bleeding disorders

1. Inherited. There are three common inherited bleeding disorders, Haemophilia A (factor VIII deficiency), Haemophilia B (factor IX deficiency) and von Willebrands disease (von Willebrand factor deficiency, produced in endothelial cells and megakaryocytes). Most patients with inherited bleeding disorders are aware of their condition and tend to seek help at their local unit rather than presenting to the A&E department. It is essential when to seek expert help early when managing these patients.

2. Drug induced

- *Warfarin.* When managing a patient on warfarin presenting with an acute bleed, the beneficial effects of reversing the effects of warfarin on the acute bleed versus the potential complications due to the underlying condition for which anticoagulation has been prescribed should be borne in mind. Before a decision to reverse the effects of anticoagulation is made the matter should be discussed with the clinician responsible for managing the patients warfarin therapy (the patients anticoagulant card should have details of the condition for which the warfarin has been prescribed, a contact number and the most recent INR). If the responsible clinician is not available the matter should be discussed with a clinical haematologist.

  The anticoagulant effects of warfarin may be reversed by the administration of vitamin K or coagulation factors. The onset of action of vitamin K (oral or i.v.) is several hours but the effect may last for several weeks. FFP or factor IX concentrate have a more immediate but shorter-acting effect.

  Even with an INR in the therapeutic range, bleeding can occur if there are local predisposing factors (e.g. ulcer).
- *Thrombolytic therapy* (streptokinase, t-PA, urokinase). Thrombolytic agents cause destruction of fibrinogen and consumption of plasminogen and α_2-antiplasmin. As well as leading to clot lysis, this predisposed the recipient to the risk of severe bleeding.

  Localized bleeding (e.g. from cannula sites) can be controlled by local pressure. More severe or inaccessible bleeding should be treated initially by stopping the infusion. If this fails to control the bleeding an infusion of cryoprecipitate to reverse the effects of the thrombolytic therapy may be required. In more severe or intractable cases platelet infusions or tranexamic acid may be required. When treating bleeds associated with thrombolytic therapy, advice should be sought from a haematologist. Monitoring of treatment and response using fibrinogen levels and APTT will be required.

- *Disseminated intravascular coagulation* (DIC). This condition is characterized by consumption of platelets and clotting factors and widespread fibrin deposition leading to activation of fibrinolysis. The result is haemorrhage associated with small vessel occlusion leading to tissue ischaemia. The mortality is dependent on both the severity of DIC (in severe cases over 80%) and to the prognosis of the underlying condition. There are many precipitating factors including:

  (a) Tissue damage. Trauma, burns, shock, hypoxia.
  (b) Infection. Gram positive (e.g. pneumococcal) and gram negative (e.g. meningococcal) septicaemia.
  (c) Pregnancy. Amniotic fluid embolus, abruptio placentae, eclampsia, retained products.
  (d) Proteolytic activation of coagulation factors. Snake bites, pancreatitis.
  (e) Incompatible blood transfusion.

3. Management. The management of DIC is complex and controversial. Expert advice should always be sought. Basic principles of management are:

- Identify and if possible remove precipitating factors.
- Resuscitation (oxygen and fluid).
- Monitor and replace as necessary platelets and blood factors (cryoprecipitate, FFP).
- Heparin infusion.

Idiopathic thrombocytopaenia purpura. This occasionally presents to the A&E department as either a bleeding disorder (epistaxis, purpura or post dental extraction) or as an incidental find on an FBC. In children it is usually preceded by a viral illness and spontaneous resolution occurs in 90% of cases within 3 months. In adults spontaneous resolution occurs in only 5% of cases. Severe bleeding at presentation is uncommon. All cases should be referred on for investigation and follow up.

Haematological malignancy. This may present first to the A&E department. They may present as a manifestation of marrow failure (bleeding, infection), as lymphadenopathy or in the case of acute leukaemia as bone pain. An FBC will usually indicate the possibility of a malignancy except in the case of lymphadenopathy associated with lymphoma.

Further reading

Provan D, Chisholm M, Duncombe A, Singer C, Smith A. Oxford Handbook of Clinical Haematology. Oxford, Oxford University Press, 1998.

HEAD INJURY

There are approximately one million patients who present and 150 000 admitted to hospitals in the UK each year with head injuries. Almost half of them are aged under 16 years old. Fifty percent of all trauma deaths result from head injuries. Of deaths that occur in patients who reach hospital alive, two-thirds are due to head injury and these head-injured patients are the most common cause of life-long disability. Approximately 8 severe, 18 moderate and 280 minor head injuries occur per year per 100 000 population in England and Wales. The annual incidence of disability in adults with head injuries admitted to hospital is 100–150 per 100 000. The most common causes of injury are falls (41%), assaults (20%) and road traffic accidents (13%).

Damage to the brain can occur directly as a result of the original injury (*primary brain damage*) or indirectly due to other factors (*secondary brain damage*).

Primary brain damage is instantaneous, irreversible and results from shearing and pressure forces that cause diffuse axonal injury, microcirculatory disruption, tissue haemorrhage, lacerations and contusions.

Secondary brain damage is due to increased intracranial pressure (ICP), reduced cerebral blood flow (CBF) and hypoxic blood. Potentially avoidable deaths are often the result of delayed, inappropriate or inadequate treatment of secondary brain damage.
Causes include:

- Hypoxia.
- Hypercapnia.
- Hypotension.
- Cerebral oedema.
- Intracranial haemorrhage.
- Intracranial infection.
- Epilepsy.

Head injury severity

The Glasgow Coma Scale (GCS) can be used to categorize patients. Coma is defined as a GCS of 8 or less.

- *Severe* GCS less than 9.
- *Moderate* GCS 9 to 12.
- *Mild* GCS 13 to 15.

A deterioration in GCS is the most significant sign of the development of increased ICP and a hallmark of secondary brain damage, hence the importance of repeated neurological assessment. The Glasgow Coma Scale itself can be used to categorize patients.

Risk of an operable intracranial haematoma in head-injured patients

GCS	*Risk*	*Other features*	*Risk*
15	1 in 3615	None	1 in : 31 300
		PTA	: 6700
		Skull fracture	: 81
		Skull fracture & PTA	: 29
9–14	1 in 51	No fracture	1 in : 180
		Skull fracture	: 5
3–8	1 in 7	No fracture	1 in : 27
		Skull fracture	: 4

Focal signs or fits increase the likelihood of presence of intracranial haematoma.

History

- Accident mechanism and details (RTA, fall etc.).
- Clinical condition of the patient.
- Baseline GCS at accident scene and record of the same.
- ***A***llergies
  Medications
  Past medical history
  Last meal
  Events leading up to injury.
- Specifically alcohol history, anticoagulants, epileptic, diabetic history.
- Symptoms of nausea, vomiting, headache, fits, diplopia, amnesia.

Examination

- AVPU and Glasgow Coma Scale.
- Pupil size and response to light.
- Examination for basal skull fracture.
- Examine for a compound head injury or depressed skull fracture.
- Lateralized extremity weakness, sensation (include sacral region), deep tendon reflexes and plantar responses.

Basal skull fracture

These fractures are not apparent on skull X-rays but intracranial air or an opaque sphenoid sinus suggests their presence. More important are the following physical findings:

- Racoon eyes (bilateral periorbital haematoma) with cribriform plate fracture.
- Subhyaloid haemorrhage.
- Scleral haemorrhage without a posterior limit.
- Haemotympanum, rhinorrhoea and otorrhoea.
- Battles sign (bruising over the mastoid process).

Management

Guidelines for the initial triage of head injuries

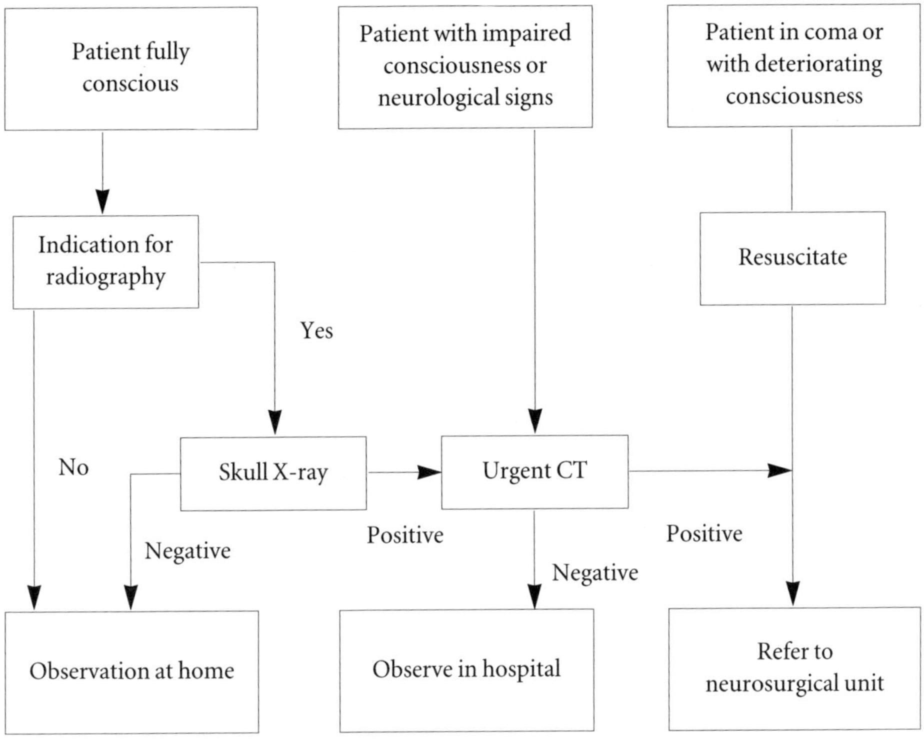

The ABCs are followed.

1. ***The indications for intubation and ventilation after head injury are:***
    - Coma.
    - Loss of protective laryngeal reflexes.
    - Inadequate ventilation.
      Hypoxaemia (PaO_2 < 9 kPa on air or < 13 kPa on oxygen) hypercarbia ($PaCO_2$ > 6 kPa).
    - Spontaneous hyperventilation causing $PaCO_2$ < 3.5 kPa.
    - Respiratory arrhythmia.
    - Reduction of ICP by inducing hypocarbia.
    - Failure to control seizures by conservative methods.

2. ***Indications for SXR after recent head injury include:***
    - *Orientated patient*
      (a) History of loss of consciousness or amnesia.
      (b) Suspected penetrating injury.
      (c) CSF or blood loss from nose or ear.
      (d) Scalp laceration (to bone or >5 cm long) bruise or swelling.

(e) Violent mechanism of injury.
(f) Persisting headache and/or vomiting.
(g) In a child, fall from a significant height (which depends in part on the age of the child).
(h) And/or onto a hard surface; tense fontanelle; suspected non-accidental injury.

- *Patient with impaired consciousness or neurological signs*
  (a) All patients unless urgent CT is performed or transfer to neurosurgery is arranged.

Note: Skull X-ray is not necessary if CT is to be performed.

3. ***Indications for admission to a general hospital:***
   - *Orientated patient*
     (a) Skull fracture or suture diastasis.
     (b) Persisting neurological symptoms or signs.
     (c) Difficulty in assessment (e.g. suspected drugs, alcohol, non-accidental injury, epilepsy, attempted suicide).
     (d) Lack of responsible adult to supervise patient.
     (e) Other medical condition (e.g. coagulation disorder).
   - *All patients with impaired consciousness*

   Note: Transient unconsciousness or amnesia with full recovery is not necessarily an indication to admit in an adult, but may be so in a child.

4. ***Additional indications for computed tomography in a general hospital:***
   - Skull fracture or after a fit.
   - Confusion or neurological signs persisting after initial assessment and resuscitation.
   - Unstable systemic state precluding transfer to neurosurgery.
   - Diagnosis uncertain; or
   - Tense fontanelle or suture diastasis in a child.

   Note: CT should be performed urgently, within 24 hours of admission.

5. ***Additional indications for referral to a neurosurgical unit after CT in a district general hospital:***
   - Abnormal CT scan.
   - CT scan normal, but clinical progress unsatisfactory.

   Intracranial abnormalities suggesting need for urgent neurosurgical management:
   - High or mixed density intracranial lesion (size and site).
   - Shift of midline.
   - Obliteration of III ventricle.
   - Relative dilatation of a lateral ventricle(s).

- Obliteration of basal cisterns.
- Intracranial air; or
- Subarachnoid or intraventricular haemorrhage.

Note: Neurosurgical opinion should be sought on clinical information and images transferred electronically to the neurosurgical unit.

6. ***Further investigations include***
   - *Glucose* – to exclude hypoglycaemia.
   - *Arterial blood gases.*
   - *Coagulation studies* – risk of disseminated intravascular coagulopathy in severe head injuries.

ICP monitoring

The normal ICP is 15 mmHg or less, and an elevated ICP is associated with increased mortality. If it rises above 20 mmHg active therapy is advised.

The *Cerebral Perfusion Pressure (CPP)* is calculated using the formula:

$$CPP = MABP - ICP$$

This pressure must be above 70 mmHg to provide adequate oxygen to a severely injured brain.

An ICP monitor should be inserted in a patient who remains in coma despite resuscitation and when CT demonstrates cerebral oedema or diffuse axonal injury.

Management techniques in prevention and treatment of raised ICP

1. Although hyperventilation was previously the cornerstone of treatment for reducing ICP it is now appreciated that aggressive and prolonged hyperventilation produces cerebral ischaemia by causing cerebral vasoconstriction and impaired cerebral perfusion.

   Aim to keep the pCO_2 at 30 mmHg (4 kPa) or above. Levels between 25 and 30 mmHg (3.3–4 kPa) are acceptable in the presence of raised intracranial pressure. Every effort should be made to avoid hyperventilating the patient with a pCO_2 of less than 25 mmHg.

2. ***Fluid control***
   - *Intravenous fluids* should be administered as appropriate. This is particularly important in a patient who is hypovolaemic as this will cause significant deterioration of a head-injured patient.

     Avoid the use of hypotonic fluids. Avoid glucose containing fluids as they may cause hypoglycaemia which is harmful to the damaged brain.

     Hyponatraemia is to be avoided as this results in cerebral oedema.
   - *Mannitol* – its use before a CT in the emergency management of head injury is controversial. It should only be administered with the consent of a neurosurgeon, or to buy time when neurosurgical intervention will be delayed, and the patient is deteriorating. Dose of 0.5–1.0 g/kg is used over a 15–20 min period and may control raised ICP temporarily.

3. Corticosteroids. Their use is currently being evaluated in a multicentre RCT entitled the 'CRASH study'.

4. High-dose barbiturates. Has no role in early treatment of raised ICP.

5. The role of agents to minimize secondary brain damage such as *nimodipine* (calcium channel-blocking agent) and that of other agents that limit the cellular damage caused by the release of free radicals (lipid peroxidase inhibitors and free radical scavengers) are undergoing clinical trials.

6. Hypothermia. A number of small single-centre trials have consistently shown a cerebral protection effect in patients with head injuries. The results of a large multicentre trial are awaited to define its role.

Complications

1. Intracranial haematomas

- *Extradural* – usually related to bleeding from the middle meningeal artery.
- *Intradural*
  - (a) *subdural* – usually due to bleeding from superficial veins ruptured indirectly by shearing forces or by direct impact.
  - (b) *intracerebral.*
- *Subarachnoid.*
- *Mixed.*

Rapidly expanding intracranial haematoma, usually extradural, may be imminently life-threatening. In such circumstances *burr holes* can be considered if a surgeon, properly trained in this procedure, is available and only with the advice and consent of a neurosurgeon. Generally in the UK, patients are transferred to a neurosurgical unit for surgical decompression.

2. Epilepsy. Prolonged or repeated seizures should be treated aggressively as they increase cerebral hypoxia, oedema and raise ICP.

- *Treatment*
  - (a) *Lorazepam/diazepam* – respiratory function must be closely monitored.
  - (b) *Fosphenytoin/phenytoin* – at a rate of 50 mg/min, with continuous ECG monitoring.
  - (c) *Phenobarbitone.*
  - (d) *General anaesthesia* with either propofol or thiopentone.

- *Post-traumatic epilepsy* occurs in about 5% of all patients admitted with closed head injury and in 15% of those with severe head injuries. The following factors are linked with late epilepsy:

(a) Early seizures occurring within the first week.
(b) An intracranial haematoma.
(c) Depressed skull fracture.

Further reading

American College of Surgeons. Advanced Trauma Life Support Instructor Manual 1997.

Gentleman D *et al.* Guidelines for resuscitation and transfer of patients with serious head injury. *British Medical Journal*, 1993; **307:** 547–52.

Maas AIR, Dearden M, Teasdale G M, *et al* (on behalf of the European Brian Injury Consortium). EBIC Guidelines for Management of Severe Head Injury in Adults. *Acta Neurochir (Wein)*, 1997; **139:** 286–94.

Report of the Working Party on the Management of Patients with Head Injuries. 1999, The Royal College of Surgeons of England.

The Society of British Neurological Surgeons. Guidelines for the initial management of head injuries: recommendations from the Society of British Neurological Surgeons. *British Journal of Neurosurgery*, 1998; **14:** 349–52.

Teasdale GM, Murray G, Anderson E, *et al.* Risks of traumatic intracranial haematoma in children and adults, implications for managing head injuries. *British Medical Journal*, 1990; **300:** 363–7.

Working Party of the Neuroanaesthesia Society and Association of Anaesthetists. *Recommendation for the Transfer of Patients with Acute Head Injuries to Neurosurgical Units.* London: Neuroanaesthesia Society of Great Britain and Ireland and the Association of Anaesthetists of Great Britain and Ireland, 1996.

Related topics of interest

Abdominal trauma (p. 4); Interhospital transfer (p. 194); Genitourinary trauma (p. 164); Maxillofacial injury (p. 226); Spine and spinal cord trauma (p. 307); Thoracic trauma (p. 321); Trauma scoring and injury scaling (p. 329)

HEART FAILURE

Morbidity and mortality for all grades of symptomatic chronic heart failure are high, with a 20–30% one-year mortality in mild to moderate heart failure and a greater than 50% one-year mortality in severe heart failure. These prognostic data refer to patients with systolic heart failure, as the natural course of diastolic dysfunction is less well defined.

Severe acute heart failure is a medical emergency requiring effective management. The aims of treatment are improvement of haemodynamic status, relief of pulmonary congestion and improvement of tissue oxygenation. Additionally assessment of the underlying cause is important as timely intervention may improve the prognosis in selected cases, e.g. severe aortic stenosis.

Symptoms and signs in heart failure

1. ***Symptoms***
   - Dyspnoea.
   - Orthopnoea.
   - Paroxysmal nocturnal dyspnoea.
   - Reduced exercise tolerance, lethargy, fatigue.
   - Nocturnal cough.
   - Wheeze.
   - Ankle swelling.
   - Anorexia.

2. ***Signs***
   - Cachexia and muscle wasting.
   - Tachycardia.
   - Pulsus alternans.
   - Elevated jugular venous pressure.
   - Displaced apex beat.
   - Right ventricular heave.
   - Crepitations or wheeze.
   - Third heart sound.
   - Oedema.
   - Hepatomegaly (tender).
   - Ascites.

Precipitating causes of heart failure

- Arrhythmias, especially atrial fibrillation.
- Infectious (especially pneumonia).
- Acute myocardial infarction.
- Angina pectoris or recurrent myocardial ischaemia.
- Anaemia.
- Alcohol excess.

- Iatrogenic cause – for example, post-operative fluid replacement or administration of steroids or non-steroidal anti-inflammatory drugs.
- Poor drug compliance, especially in anti-hypertensive treatment.
- Thyroid disorders – for example, thyrotoxicosis.
- Pulmonary embolism.
- Pregnancy.

European Society of Cardiology's guidelines for diagnosis of heart failure

1. ***Essential features***
   - Symptoms of heart failure (for example, breathlessness, fatigue, ankle swelling) *and*
   - Objective evidence of cardiac dysfunction (at rest).

2. ***Non-essential features***
   - Response to treatment directed towards heart failure (in cases where the diagnosis is in doubt).

Assessment of severity

Clinical and radiographic assessment provides a guide to severity and prognosis – the Killip classification can be used which is as follows:

Class	*Clinical features*	*Hospital mortality (%)*
Class I	No signs of left ventricular dysfunction	6
Class II	S3 gallop with or without mild to moderate pulmonary congestion	30
Class III	Acute severe pulmonary oedema	40
Class IV	Shock syndrome	80–90

Complications of heart failure

1. Arrhythmias. Atrial fibrillation; ventricular arrhythmias (ventricular tachycardia, ventricular fibrillation); bradyarrhythmias.

2. Thromboembolism. Stroke; peripheral embolism; deep venous thrombosis; pulmonary embolism.

3. Gastrointestinal. Hepatic congestion and hepatic dysfunction; malabsorption.

4. Musculoskeletal. Muscle wasting.

5. Respiratory. Pulmonary congestion; respiratory muscle weakness; pulmonary hypertension (rare).

Treatment

- Sit the patient in an upright position and initiate high-flow oxygen via a face mask.
- Monitor the patient in a high-dependency area.
- Arterial blood gas analysis provides information regarding oxygenation and acid–base balance. The base excess is a guide to tissue perfusion: a worsening

base excess indicates lactic acidosis and is a poor prognostic feature. Correction of hypoperfusion will correct the metabolic acidosis. Bicarbonate infusion should only be reserved for refractory cases.

1. ***Initial drug treatment***
   - Loop diuretics – These provide a transient venodilatation and lead to symptomatic improvement prior to diuresis.
   - Parenteral opiates (morphine or diamorphine) relieve anxiety, pain and distress and reduce myocardial oxygen demand. They also induce transient venodilatation, thus reducing preload, cardiac filling pressures and pulmonary congestion.
   - Nitrates (sublingually, buccal or intravenous) – Reduce preload and cardiac filling pressures and are particularly valuable in patients with angina.

2. ***Second line drug treatment***
   - Sodium nitroprusside is a potent directly acting vasodilator which is reserved for refractory cases of acute heart failure.
   - Inotropes (dopamine and dobutamine) – These may assist haemodynamic status and peripheral perfusion by increasing myocardial contractility.
   - Phosphodiesterase inhibitors e.g. enoximone, are occasionally used and work by increasing myocardial contractility and venodilatation.
   - Intravenous aminophylline is rarely used for its weak inotropic effect, diuretic effect as well as bronchodilating properties.

3. ***Advanced management***
   - Assisted ventilation may be warranted in severe cases and helps reduce myocardial oxygen demand and improves alveolar ventilation.
   - Circulatory assist devices (intra-aortic balloon pumping and left ventricular assist devices) may temporarily improve haemodynamic status and peripheral perfusion by providing mechanical support.

Further reading

The Task Force on Heart Failure of the European Society of Cardiology. Guidelines for the diagnosis of heart failure. *European Heart Journal,* 1995; **16:** 741–51.

The CONSENSUS Trial Study Group. Effects of enalapril on mortality in severe congestive heart failure: results of the cooperative north Scandinavian enalapril survival study (CONSENSUS). *New England Journal Medicine,* 1987; **316:** 1429–35.

HEAT ILLNESS

Heat stroke

Heat stroke describes the syndrome produced by over-heating of the body core. It is an uncommon but severe form of heat illness that may be rapidly fatal. The rectal temperature is >40.5°C and sweating may stop. There is often severe metabolic upset with increase in metabolic rate and oxygen consumption. The mortality is high (10%) and may result from shock, arrhythmias, myocardial ischaemia, renal failure and neurological dysfunction. Complication and death are more related to the underlying disease than to the actual temperature.

Aetiology

1. ***Exertional heat stroke.*** Commonly a young, healthy individual takes excessive exercise. The armed forces and long distance runners are most at risk. Predisposing factors include lack of acclimation, lack of cardiovascular conditioning, dehydration, the wearing of heavy clothes and excessive exercise.

2. ***Classic heat stroke*** is most common in the elderly. The underlying defect may involve impaired heat dissipation. Underlying diseases include cardiovascular disease, neurological disorders, obesity, the use of anticholinergic or diuretic drugs, dehydration and the elderly or very young.

3. ***Neuroleptic malignant syndrome*** occurs in 0.2% of those on neuroleptics, usually within a month of starting. Haloperidol is the most common agent. An idiosyncratic reaction with symptoms of muscle rigidity, extrapyramidal abnormalities, and autonomic dysfunction. Tends to develop insidiously over 1–3 days, either after initiation of treatment or when the dose is increased. The mortality is significant and associated with respiratory complications.

4. ***Malignant hyperthermia of anaesthesia*** is a rare autosomal dominant disease e.g. suxamethonium and halothane.

5. ***Drug induced.*** Anti-cholinergic drugs, alcohol abuse and withdrawal, salicylate overdose and drug abuse (cocaine and amphetamines).

6. ***Hormonal hyperthermia.*** e.g. thyrotoxicosis and phaeochromocytoma.

7. ***Hypothalamic hyperthermia*** is rare, except in association with cerebrovascular accidents.

History

The presenting feature is likely to be of *acute onset*, with a core temperature *above 40 °C*. Confusion or coma is present. The patient is flushed, the skin is dry, the pulse rapid and hypotensive. If a young fit patient presents collapsed after exercise it is vital that the rectal temperature is recorded.

Complications

1. ***Cardiac***
   - Myocardial ischaemia.
   - Arrhythmias.
   - Hypotension.
   - Congestive heart failure.

2. ***Neurologic***
   - Seizures.
   - Confusion.
   - Delerium.
   - Coma.
   - Persistent peripheral neuropathies.

3. ***Metabolic***
   - Hypoxia.
   - Hypoglycaemia.
   - Electrolyte disturbances.
   - Acid–base disturbances.

4. ***Haematological***
   - Leucocytosis and thrombocytosis.
   - Disseminated intravascular coagulopathy.

5. ***Renal failure.***

6. ***Myoglobinuria and rhabdomyolysis.***

Treatment

The most important step is to diagnose and treat the underlying disorder. Physical cooling is essential. The rapidity of treatment is more important than the precise method of cooling.

These patients require admission and if unconscious or temperature raised for some hours admit to an ICU/HDU.

1. ***High flow oxygen.***
2. ***Secure venous access.***
3. ***Remove all clothing.***

4. ***Immersion in ice water*** is ideal for the true hyperthermic emergency, but is not usually feasible. Other treatments may include intravenous, peritoneal lavage, gastric lavage or enemas with ice water, and even extracorporeal circulation. Soak sheets in water at 20°C and have fans blow room air over the patient. An alternative is to wrap ice in sheets and place in the axillae, groins and behind the neck. Stop cooling when rectal temperature reaches 38°C.

5. ***Check blood glucose*** urea and electrolytes, CPK, calcium, phosphate, full blood count and clotting screen. *Monitor* – continuously monitor pulse, blood pressure, respiratory rate, ECG, GCS and rectal temperature.

6. ***Monitor urinary*** output and check for myoglobin.

7. ***Commence i.v. fluids.*** 1 litre normal saline (room temperature) over the first 30 minutes and continue as guided by clinical examination, electrolyte disturbance and urinary output.

8. ***Check arterial blood gases.***

9. ***Diazepam*** if fits occur.

10. ***Consider Dantrolene*** for the treatment of malignant hyperthermia and neuroleptic malignant syndrome.

Heat exhaustion

A common but usually benign condition. The rectal temperature is <40.5°C. It is a metabolic/vascular upset due to water and salt depletion or imbalance.

Water depletion

Water depletion results from deprivation of water in hot environments. The patient complains of thirst, is clinically dehydrated with an elevated serum sodium and chloride, but normal haematocrit.

1. ***Treatment.*** Consists of oral rehydration of water or intravenous infusion of 5% glucose, if the patient is unable to swallow. Death occurs when the weight loss is 15–25% of body weight, due to excess salt in the body fluids.

Salt depletion

Salt depletion develops gradually over a few hours or days in people working in hot environments, particularly if unacclimatized. Early features include malaise, headaches and fatigue. There may be sudden collapse with confusion and vomiting. Muscle cramps which are very painful develop if there is associated muscular exercise. Dehydration, associated with a normal serum sodium and chloride but raised haematocrit.

1. ***Treatment.*** Oral treatment with 25 g sodium chloride in 5 litres of water by mouth is often adequate, and then ensure adequate daily salt intake. In severe cases or if associated with vomiting intravenous isotonic saline is required. Most patients recover within a few hours.

Further reading

Simon, HB. Hyperthermia. *New England Journal of Medicine*, 1993; **329:** 483–7.

INFECTIOUS GASTROENTERITIS

Criteria for the diagnosis of infectious gastroenteritis include the co-existence of acute diarrhoea (three or more unformed stools per day) plus one or more of the following signs and symptoms:

- Abdominal pain.
- Nausea.
- Vomiting.
- Fever.
- Passage of bloody stools.
- Faecal urgency, or tenesmus.

Traveller's diarrhoea is defined as acute diarrhoea occurring after crossing national boundaries.

There should be a careful assessment of the current medical status of all cases to identify co-existing disease that may exacerbate the illness. The potential for significant fluid loss must be recognized. Fluid replacement should initially be with oral rehydration solutions. Anti-diarrhoeal medications are generally of little value and should be specifically avoided in cases of dysenteric illness.

All patients admitted to hospital should be ideally assessed in single room accommodation. Investigations should be appropriate to the symptoms but take special care to consider specific complications, e.g. haemolytic uraemic syndrome.

Anti-microbial therapy is generally not recommended. Empirical treatment with a quinolone such as Ciprofloxacin should be reserved for high-risk patients.

Statutory requirements for notification to Public Health Authorities must be adhered to. The following cases should be notified:

- Cholera.
- Dysentery.
- Food poisoning or suspected food poisoning.
- Typhoid or paratyphoid fever.

In England and Wales notify the Consultant in Communicable Disease Control (CCDC), and in Scotland the Consultant in Public Health Medicine (CPHM). The initial communication should be by telephone and should not await laboratory identification of a cause. Written notification on a standard certificate should follow as soon as possible.

Assessment of severity of illness

The following features suggest a more severe illness and indicate a lower threshold for hospitalization and the administration of antibiotic therapy:

- Fever.
- Shock.
- Blood in the stool.

- Pre-existing medical conditions; immunodeficiency, inflammatory bowel disease, diabetes mellitus, renal impairment, heart disease, gastric hypochlorhydria.
- Drug therapy; immunosuppressive or systemic steroid therapy, protein pump inhibitors/H_2 receptor blockers.
- Increasing number of stools per 24 hours.
- Age greater than 60.

Infection control

The potential for spread of gastroenteritis pathogens is greatest when the individual has diarrhoea. Some small round viral pathogens can be spread by the aerosol route, especially if the index case is vomiting.

All patients must be cared for in suitable single cubicles. Staff must observe strict infection control procedures to prevent the spread of faecal–oral pathogens. This includes the use of gloves and protective clothing (apron) and a strict regime of hand washing.

Assessment of hydration

Most of the clinical features of dehydration result from combined water and salt losses. The major losses in salt and potassium occur in early stages of the illness.

Adults in the UK will rarely exhibit anything more than mild losses. The fluid loss varies according to the pathogen and the length of symptoms. The losses from toxin mediated food poisoning may be quite rapid and profound with prostration and the development of severe dehydration over a few hours.

Fluid replacement

The basic principle of fluid replacement is to estimate the deficit and replace this over the first 12–24 hours. Also replace the daily requirement for fluid/electrolytes, plus an additional volume for ongoing losses.

Oral hydration should be used across the age range from paediatrics to geriatrics. Two litres of oral rehydration solution (ORS) should be used as sole fluid intake in the first 24 hours, thereafter ORS should be administered at a rate of 200 ml per loose stool with no other dietary or fluid restriction.

In cases of moderate to severe dehydration, especially if there is persistent vomiting, then intravenous therapy is required. If the individual is passing urine this requires use of isotonic saline with potassium replacement. If the patient can take oral fluids, then proportional amounts can be given as ORS.

In severe dehydration progressive acidosis will ensue because 20% of body sodium is coupled with bicarbonate. In this situation 20% of replacement fluids should be in the form of sodium bicarbonate (isotonic 1.26% solution).

Management of gastroenteritis

	Degree of dehydration		
	Mild	*Moderate*	*Severe*
Typical causes	24 h diarrhoea 24 h vomiting	48 h diarrhoea Diabetic keto-acidosis Vomiting of pyloric stenosis Salt losing chronic renal failure	Fulminating diarrhoea > 10 stools/day, > 48 h explosive, toxin-mediated diarrhoea
Average water loss	1.0 – 2.0 litres ECF	2.0–4.5 litres ECF	4.5–8.5 litres ECF
Average sodium loss	2.5–5.0 mmol/kg	5–10 mmol/kg	10–20 mmol/kg
Common symptoms	Lassitude Anorexia/nausea Light headedness Postural hypotension	Apathy/tiredness Giddiness Nausea/headache Muscular cramps	Profound apathy/weakness Convulsion leading to coma
Common signs	Nil of note	Pinched face Dry tongue/sunken eyes Reduced skin elasticity Postural hypotension (systolic >90 mmHg) Tachycardia Oliguria	Oligaemia/shock Tachycardia Marked peripheral vasoconstriction Systolic BP < 90 mmHg Uraemia/olig/anuria
Other features		If water has been taken as fluid replacement, hyponatraemia will develop	Patients may be moribund and if depletion continues without replacement then death can occur within a few hours

Anti-diarrhoeal agents

Anti-motility agents, e.g. opiates, Loperamide, Diphenoxylate. These agents are commonly used to some effect in non-infection. However, they have been shown to be dangerous in shigellosis and should be avoided in any patient with dysenteric symptoms including *E. coli* 0157H infection and *Cl. difficile* colitis.

Bismuth subsalicylate – Bismuth salts reduce the number of stools, but do not have a significant effect on stool water losses.

Absorbency – e.g. kaolin, charcoal. Although theoretically they may bind exotoxins, studies have shown there to be no effect in cholera or infantile gastroenteritis.

Microbiological investigations

In hospital, stool specimens should be obtained from all patients fulfilling the diagnostic definition of infective gastroenteritis. Microbiological investigations are essential if an outbreak of gastroenteritis or food poisoning is suspected in which case the Public Health authorities must be informed. In cases of suspected food poisoning detail the nature of the suspect food and the approximate incubation period.

Other indications for stool samples include:

- Fever.
- Blood in stool (request dysenteric pathogens and *E. coli* 0157H).
- Weight loss (request microscopy and culture).
- Recent anti-microbial use (request *Clostridium difficile* culture/toxin detection).
- Recent travel (request examination for ova, cysts and parasites, and culture).
- Severe dehydration.
- High-risk patients.
- Immunodeficiency (request *Isospora* and *Cryptosporidia*).

Multiple specimens are usually unnecessary, except for the microscopic diagnosis of giardiasis when a maximum of three are usually sent.

Hospital in-patient management

Factors influencing hospital admission include:

1. ***Personal***
   - Recent foreign travel.
   - Elderly patients.
   - Poor home/social circumstances.
2. ***Clinical***
   - Fever.
   - Bloody diarrhoea.
   - Abdominal pain and tenderness.
   - Tenesmus.
   - Severe dehydration, requiring Iv. rehydration.
   - Faecal incontinence.
   - Vomiting.
   - Shock.
   - Protracted diarrhoea greater than 10 days.
   - High-risk patients.

Patients admitted to hospital require blood cultures for those who are febrile or 'high risk'. Patients who have blood in the stools need exclusion of bacterial or amoebic dysentery, haemolytic uraemic syndrome and other illnesses such as inflammatory bowel disease and gastrointestinal malignancy.

Haemolytic-uraemic syndrome (HUS)

There has been a recent rise in the notification of *E. coli* 0157H which carries an associated risk of HUS. The development of HUS is insidious and occurs on average five to seven days after the acute episode. In all cases of bloody stools a baseline full blood count and biochemistry profile (urea and electrolytes, creatinine, lactate dehydrogenase and bilirubin) are required. The haematology laboratory should be asked to look at the blood film for fragmented red blood cells. These examinations should be repeated during the illness, especially when renal impairment or anaemia are expected and again 10–14 days after the start of diarrhoeal symptoms.

Anti-microbial therapy

Anti-microbials such as Erythromycin, Tetracycline and Cotrimoxazole are of no benefit. Quinolones have been shown to modify illness and to curtail faecal excretion of gut pathogens.

Empirical therapy cannot generally be recommended. However, the following algorithm is suggested:

Your adult patient has diarrhoea

⬇ *Yes*

Diarrhoea: 3 or more unformed stools/day
+ one of the following signs or symptoms:
– abdominal pain
– nausea, vomiting, fever, blood in stool, tenesmus

⬇ *Yes*

Infective gastroenteritis likely

Yes ⬇
HIGH-RISK PATIENT
⬇
Age >60
Other risk factors
Yes ⬇

Yes ⬇
DYSENTERIC SYMPTOMS
Fever, bloody diarrhoea
Abdominal pain
Yes ⬇

Obtain stool sample for culture if possible

⬇

Consider Ciprofloxacin 500 mg bd orally for 5 days

REVIEW PROGRESS

Management of gastroenteritis

	Commonly used oral treatment regimes
Shigellosis	Ciprofloxacin 500 mg bd 5 days
Uncomplicated Salmonellosis	Ciprofloxacin 500 mg bd 5 days
Campylobacteriosis	Ciprofloxacin 500 mg bd 5 days
Cholera	Tetracycline 500 mg qds for 5 days Doxycycline 300 mg single dose
Enterotoxigenic *E. coli*	Treatment not usually recommended
Cl. difficile	Metronidazole 400 mg 8 hourly, 7–10 days Vancomycin 125 mg 6 hourly, 7–10 days

Further reading

Farthing M. *et al.* The management of infective gastroenteritis in adults: a consensus statement by an expert panel convened by the British Society for the Study of Infection. *Journal of Infection*, 1996; **33:** 143–52.

INHALATION INJURIES

Sepsis and shock have traditionally been the common causes of death in burn victims. With advances in the management of shock and infection, inhalation injury has become the major cause of death. Factors predisposing to inhalation injury include exposure to fire in an enclosed space and decreased conscious level (e.g. head injury, drugs and alcohol).

Mechanism of injury

Injury occurs by exposure to heat, particulate matter and toxic gases.

- Heat. The degree of heat injury is related to the temperature, duration of exposure and the humidity. Steam has a high specific heat capacity and therefore transfers more heat energy to the exposed tissues of the airway than gases.
- Particulate matter. This is produced as a result of incomplete combustion of organic matter. Smoke particles are generally less than 0.5 μm in diameter. They are small enough to reach the terminal bronchioles where they cause an inflammatory reaction leading to bronchospasm and oedema.
- Toxic gases. These cause injury by one of three mechanisms: interference with oxidative phosphorylation leading to tissue hypoxia (carbon monoxide and hydrogen cyanide); pulmonary irritation leading to bronchospasm and oedema (e.g. oxides of sulphur, nitrogen and chlorine) and systemic toxicity (e.g. ammonia).

Diagnosis

The diagnosis may not be immediately evident but is suggested by the presence of one or more of the following:

- exposure to fire in an enclosed space, particularly if smoke is present;
- history of explosion;
- decreased conscious level or confusion;
- respiratory symptoms or signs (e.g. hoarseness, loss of voice, wheeze or stridor);
- signs of oropharyngeal burn (including burnt eyebrows or nasal hairs and the presence of soot particles in the nose, mouth or pharynx);
- presence of carbonaceous sputum.

Investigations

In many cases the initial investigations will be normal and serve as a baseline to monitor progress. Routine investigations include:

- arterial blood gases;
- chest X-ray;
- carboxyhaemoglobin levels.

Fibre-optic bronchoscopy may be useful in confirming the diagnosis of inhalation injury by demonstrating the presence of soot particle and oedema of the upper airways.

Management

- One hundred percent oxygen is administered via a humidifier.
- Oedema of the upper airways may occur early and may make orotracheal intubation difficult or impossible. Therefore early intubation should be considered in all cases of upper airway burn or if inhalation injury is suspected.
- Patients are usually observed for a minimum of 24 hours as late onset bronchospasm may develop.

Further reading

Manfo W. Initial management of burns. *New England Journal of Medicine*, 1996; **335:** 1581.

Settle JAD. *Burns: the first five days.* London: Smith & Nephew, 1986.

Related topics of interest

Airway (p. 28); Burns (p. 74); Carbon monoxide poisoning (p. 80)

INTERHOSPITAL TRANSFER

Ideally all patients will be triaged to the hospital appropriate to the patients needs, realistically however, patients may require definitive care at another hospital and thus require secondary transfer.

In 1988, a survey by the Clinical Shock Study Group in Glasgow, estimated that 10 000 patients with life-threatening illness are transferred between hospitals annually in the UK.

Delays in transfer may result in avoidable mortality in view of the association between increasing duration of illness before transfer. Life-threatening injuries that can be stabilized, operatively or non-operatively, at the initial hospital must be treated prior to transfer as inadequate resuscitation (untreated hypoxia, hypotension etc) prior to transfer will jeopardize the patient's outcome.

The *referring physician* should complete the primary and secondary surveys, and institute appropriate resuscitation to *stabilize* the patient. The referring and *receiving physicians* should communicate directly to decide:

- the method of transportation;
- the transfer personnel who must be adequately skilled, appropriately equipped to monitor the patient and able to administer treatment en route as required.

Transfer protocol

The American College of Surgeons guidelines are:

1. ***Referring physician.*** Should speak directly to the receiving physician and provide the following details:
   - the patient's identity;
   - brief history, including pre-hospital details;
   - details of the clinical finding in the department and treatment administered.
2. ***Transferring personnel.*** Knowledge of the patients condition and requirements during transfer including:
   - airway control;
   - fluid replacement;
   - special procedures that may be necessary;
   - revised trauma score;
   - resuscitation procedures;
   - potential complications to be anticipated en route.
3. ***Documentation.*** A written record of events will accompany the patient and include:
   - patients details;
   - history of injury/illness;
   - pre-hospital and hospital vital signs;
   - treatment record;
   - fluids given by type and volume;
   - investigations performed with results;

- diagnosis;
- time of transfer;
- details of referring and receiving physician.

4. ***Priorities pre-transfer.*** Resuscitation and stabilization of the patient based on this suggested outline.

   - *Respiratory*
     (a) Insert an airway or endotracheal tube as necessary.
     (b) Determine rate and method of administration of oxygen.
     (c) Provide suction.
     (d) Provide mechanical ventilation when needed.
     (e) Insert a chest tube as needed.
     (f) Insert a nasogastric tube to prevent aspiration.

   - *Cardiovascular*
     (a) Control external haemorrhage.
     (b) Establish 2 large-bore IV lines and infuse appropriate fluids.
     (c) Restore blood volume loss and continue replacement during transfer.
     (d) Insert an indwelling catheter to monitor urinary output.
     (e) ECG monitoring.

   - *Central nervous system*
     (a) Assist ventilation for head-injured patients.
     (b) Administer mannitol after neurosurgical consultation.
     (c) Immobilize the spine.

   - *Investigations*
     (a) Radiographs of the cervical, spine, chest, pelvis, and extremities if indicated.
     (b) Haemoglobin, haematocrit, type and crossmatch, pregnancy test on all females of childbearing age and arterial blood gases.
     (c) ECG.
     (d) Urinalysis.
     (e) Blood alcohol and/or drugs as indicated.

   - *Wounds*
     (a) Clean and dress open wounds after haemorrhage control.
     (b) Tetanus prophylaxis as necessary.
     (c) Antibiotics as necessary.

   - *Fractures.* Splintage and traction.

5. ***Management***
   - Continued monitoring of vital signs including pulse oximetry.
   - Continued support of the cardiorespiratory system.
   - Continued blood volume replacement.
   - Appropriate medication to maintain the patients clinical state.
   - Communication with the receiving hospital.
   - Continuing written record of events during transfer.

Further reading

American College of Surgeons. *ATLS Student Course Manual*, 1997. Chapter 12: Transfer to Definitive Care, pp. 325–335.

Related topic of interest

Trauma Scoring and Injury Scaling (p. 329)

INTRAOSSEOUS INFUSION

Since the 1830s fluids have been administered intravenously. An alternative route is by intraosseous infusion. This was first carried out by Tocantins and O'Neill in 1936 on experiments with rabbits. The first clinical trial of its use was published by them in 1940.

Intraosseous infusion is commonly used in paediatrics and recommended for children 6 years of age or younger who require vascular access that cannot be achieved in a timely manner via another route. It has also been used in adults.

It is a reliable, safe procedure with a less than 1% complication rate. It is useful in emergencies when rapid vascular accesses by other methods are unsuccessful in conditions such as:

- Cardiopulmonary arrest.
- Shock.
- Major trauma.
- Extensive burns.
- Status epilepticus.
- Overwhelming sepsis.

Anatomy

Fluid or drugs infused via the intraosseous route rarely diffuse more than a short distance before entering the network of venous sinusoids within the medullary cavity. These sinusoids drain into central venous channels and exit bone via nutrient or emissary veins to enter the circulation.

The use of bone marrow of long bones as a route for infusion is generally limited to young children. Red marrow is gradually replaced by less vascular yellow marrow after about the fifth year of life. This change begins in the distal part of the limbs and progresses proximally.

Physiology

Animal studies have demonstrated the successful rapid infusion of crystalloid and blood in a fluid bolus of 20 ml/kg in less than 10 minutes.

Comparisons after injection of adrenaline have demonstrated that intraosseous and central venous injection result in similar blood levels during cardiopulmonary resuscitation.

Method

- The technique of intraosseous infusion is suitable for use in and out of hospital, paramedics having demonstrated success rates of 80–94% correct siting of intraosseous needles.
- Needle insertion can be practised on a variety of models, from chicken legs to mannikins.
- Various needles have been used, including spinal needles (gauge 18–20) and bone marrow biopsy needles (gauge 12–18) but specifically designed intraosseous needles are available. They vary in gauge (14–18), length and trocar

tip and have a positioning mark to indicate probable depth for ideal placement into the bone marrow. The trocar includes a handle to allow controlled pressure during insertion. The newer needles are a threaded screw-tip design to allow atraumatic stabilization at the access site to help prevent leakage.

Site of insertion

- The antero-medial surface of the *proximal tibia* is the preferred site of insertion. The tibial tuberosity is palpated and the needle inserted on the subcutaneous surface, 1–3 cm distal to the tuberosity, thus avoiding damage to the epiphyseal growth plate. This is an ideal site since it is easily located with only a layer of skin covering bone and is free from any significant neurovascular structures or major muscle groups. Use of this site is limited to children up to the age of six.
- The *distal tibia* – the needle is inserted proximal to the medial malleolus where it will not endanger the epiphyseal plate or saphenous vein. The cortex of the bone and the overlying tissues are both thin.
- The *distal femur* is an alternative site (although bony landmarks are often difficult to palpate) as are the *sternum* and *ileum*.

Contraindications

This procedure is only recommended in life-threatening conditions where vascular access is vital and thus there are few contraindications.

- Needle placement through an area of cellulitis or an infected burn increases the risk of *infection* and should be avoided if possible.
- Ipsilateral *fractures, vascular injuries* and *multiple unsuccessful attempts* preclude reliable venous outflow.
- *Osteogenesis imperfecta* and *osteopetrosis* increase the risk of iatrogenic fractures.

Drug administration

- Emergency drugs (adrenaline, atropine, bicarbonate, calcium, glucose, lignocaine, naloxone) and fluids (crystalloids and colloids including blood) can be administered intraosseously at essentially the same dosages and rates as when given intravenously.
- Strong alkaline and hypertonic solutions should be diluted.
- Saline boluses administered after each drug will hasten delivery to the systemic circulation.
- When rapid fluid replacement is required fluid should be infused under pressure and bilateral infusions may be necessary.

Complications

Major complications are infrequent and the majority of difficulties are technical. To minimize complications it is recommended that correct placement be verified prior to infusion and signs of extravasation checked for. The intraosseous needle should be removed promptly once venous access is obtained.

- Failure to enter the marrow cavity or incorrect placements have been reported in 0–18% of attempts. This may lead to extravasation of fluid or subperiosteal infiltration.
- *Osteomyelitis* is a rare complication (0.66%). Increased incidence is associated with prolonged needle placement, pre-existing bacteraemia and the use of hypertonic fluid infusions.
- Localized cellulitis, abscess formation and skin necrosis are reported.
- Pain.
- Compartment syndrome.
- Fractures.
- Fat and bone marrow micro-emboli.
- Though epiphyseal growth plate could be at risk from incorrect needle placement no cases have been reported.

Further reading

Fisher DH. Intraosseous infusion. *New England Journal of Medicine*, 1990; **322:** 1579–81.

Related topic of interest

Intravenous fluids (p. 200)

INTRAVENOUS FLUIDS

Intravenous fluids are used for volume replacement in shock or for normal daily maintenance when the patient cannot take fluids and electrolytes orally. There are three broad groups, crystalloids, colloids and blood.

Crystalloids

These consist of a solution of electrolytes and/or dextrose in water. They may be isotonic with plasma or hypertonic. Those containing dextrose have a very low calorific value, the purpose of the dextrose being to make them isotonic.

Composition of standard isotonic crystalloids

Saline 0.9% (N/saline)	Sodium	150 mmol/l
	Chloride	150 mmol/l
	Energy (kcal/l)	0
Saline 0.45%	Sodium	75 mmol/l
Dextrose 2.5%	Chloride	75 mmol/l
	Energy (kcal/l)	100
Saline 0.18%	Sodium	30 mmol/l
Dextrose 4%	Chloride	30 mmol/l
	Energy (kcal/l)	160
These solutions may have potassium added at a concentration of 20 mmol/l		
Dextrose 5%	Energy (kcal/l)	200
Hartmanns solution	Sodium	131 mmol/l
(Ringer's Lactate)	Chloride	111 mmol/l
	Potassium	5 mmol/l
	Lactate	
	Energy (kcal/l)	0

Although Hartmanns solution is more physiological in composition that N/saline, there is no obvious additional benefit in using it. Ringer's solution has the same composition as Hartmanns without the addition of lactate.

Isotonic crystalloid solutions are the first choice for fluid replacement in shock. In Grade I and Grade II shock they may be all that is required. In Grade III and Grade IV shock colloid and blood are usually required, although crystalloids are usually used in the early stages of resuscitation. As a rule of thumb, crystalloid resuscitation equires replacement of the estimated circulating volume loss with three times that volume of crystalloid. It is important when using crystalloids for resuscitation to use solutions containing electrolytes only (N/saline or Hartmanns solution).

Isotonic crystalloids are also used for replacement of water and electrolytes, for maintenance (e.g. postoperatively) and/or for replacing pre-existing losses (e.g. in diarrhoea and vomiting).

Isotonic dextrose (dextrose 5%) is used to replace water loss. It has no significant calorific value (200 kcal/l). In routine practice it is used in combination with normal saline to provide maintenance therapy. Average daily requirements of fluid and electrolytes for a 70 kg man are 150 mmol sodium chloride, 3 litres of water and 60–80 mmol potassium. This can be given as 1 litre N/saline and 2 litres dextrose 5%, with the addition of 20 mmol potassium per bag.

Colloids

These are solutions of macromolecules which tend to stay in the circulation. They have a greater effect on intravascular volume per unit volume than crystalloids and that effect is longer lasting. They consist of four groups of solutions, one, albumin, from blood, and three which are synthetic, the gelatins, starches and dextrans.

1. Albumin (human albumin solution). This consists of a solution of isotonic 4.5% albumin. It contains no blood group factors and therefore does not require crossmatching. There is no evidence to suggest that there is any benefit to be had from the use of albumin over the synthetic colloids. There has been some debate recently as to whether the use of albumin rather than crystalloid in resuscitation increases mortality. At present this hypothesis remains unproven.

2. Gelatins. There are two synthetic gelatins currently available, polygeline (Haemaccel®) and succinylated gelatin (Gelofusine®). These are similar in composition being modified gelatin solutions. The only significant differences are that polygeline contains potassium (5 mmol/l) and calcium (12.5 mmol/l). This means that polygeline should not be given in the same giving set as blood as the calcium may lead to clotting of the set. Neither solution interferes with crossmatching of blood unless given in large volumes.

3. Starches. There are two hydrolysed starch preparations available, Hetastarch (Hespan®) and Pentastarch (Pentaspan®). They have a longer half life in the circulation than the gelatins and have a measurable effect on haemodynamic status for up to 24 hours. There is research to suggest that they are more effective in preventing capillary leak than the gelatins. Because of their long half life they probably should not be used as first line agents in resuscitation.

4. Dextrans. These are used less than they used to be because they interfere with haemostasis and crossmatching, a disadvantage which the other colloids do not share. They consist of glucose polymers of various lengths in solution. Dextran 70 is the most common one used. It is hypertonic and has a greater effect on volume expansion per unit volume than any of the other colloids.

Crystalloid versus colloid

As mentioned above there is debate as to the use of albumin in resuscitation, although there is little good evidence to support or refute its use. There is still controversy as to the relative benefits of colloids versus crystalloids in the management of traumatic hypovolaemic shock.

1. ***Crystalloid pros***
   - Crystalloids move rapidly out of the vascular space (this is the reason that such large volumes are required to replace blood loss) and therefore correct extravascular fluid deficits as well as intravascular.
   - They have no significant side effects.
   - They are cheap.

2. ***Crystalloid cons***
   - For a given volume of blood loss it takes three times that volume of crystalloid to make good the loss.
   - Crystalloids dilute plasma so reducing its osmotic pressure. This is thought to increase the incidence of adult respiratory distress syndrome.

3. ***Colloid pros***
   - Replace blood on a volume for volume basis.

4. ***Colloid cons***
   - May increase the incidence of adult respiratory distress syndrome if capillary leak is present.
   - May cause anaphylaxis.
   - May inhibit reticuloendothelial function.
   - Considerably more expensive than crystalloids.

5. ***Blood and blood products.*** Blood is fractionated to produce blood products. The practice now is wherever possible to replace only that component that is required. This means that whole blood is now rarely available. In trauma resuscitation blood transfusion is used to replace lost red blood cells, other fluids are used to replace plasma volume lost.

Blood is supplied at a temperature of 4°C. If more than one or two units are to be transfused it should be warmed in a blood warmer either before transfusion of during transfusion.

Blood can be supplied in three states of readiness.

Group O Rhesus negative. This blood is commonly known as 'universal donor' blood. It is used in cases of exsanguinating haemorrhage. It is usually stored in a blood fridge in the A&E department.

Type specific blood. This can be ready to transfuse within 15 minutes of the laboratory receiving the patients blood. Transport times of samples to the lab and transfer of blood from the lab may add to this ideal time. The blood is ABO and Rhesus compatible, but has not been fully matched. It is uncommon to have significant reactions against such blood.

Fully cross-matched blood. This may take up to one hour to match from the time the patients blood sample has arrived in the lab.

In practice few patients require O negative blood. The laboratory may be requested to carry out a full crossmatch but with the possibility that the blood may be required before that full match has been completed.

Fluid replacement in children

- *Maintenance*

  The standard formula is:

Weight	Daily requirement	Hourly requirement
First 10 kg	100 ml/kg	4 ml/kg
Second 10 kg	50 ml/kg	2 ml/kg
Each subsequent kg	20 ml/kg	1 ml/kg

- *Resuscitation*
  (a) Crystalloid or colloid, 20 ml/kg as a bolus, followed by repeated boluses of 20 ml/kg as required.
  (b) Blood, 10 ml/kg aliquots.

Further reading

The Advanced Paediatric Life Support Group. *Advanced Paediatric Life Support.* BMJ Publishing Group, 1997.

Lawrance RJ. Blood transfusion: indications and hazards. *Recent Advances in Surgery*, 1992; **15:** 119–35.

Pflederer TA. Emergency fluid management for hypovolaemia. *Postgraduate Medicine*, 1996; **100**(3): 243–4, 247–8.

Trentz O, Friedl HP. Fluid resuscitation in acute trauma and multiple injuries. *Current Opinion in Anaesthesiology*, 1992; **5:** 255–7.

Related topic of interest

Shock (p. 291)

LIMPING CHILD

Limping or the inability to weight bear is a common reason for children to present to the A&E department. A careful history and examination combined with selective use of X-rays and blood tests usually allows a diagnosis to be made. Indiscriminate use of whole limb X-rays should not be seen to be an acceptable substitute for careful clinical examination.

Conditions that may occur at any age

- Fracture.
- Soft tissue injury.
- Foreign body.
- Septic arthritis
- Osteomyelitis.
- Malignancy.
- Abdominal pathology (e.g. acute appendicitis).
- Groin/genitalia pathology (e.g. hernias, testicular torsion).

Conditions that occur in specific age groups

1. Congenital dislocation of the hip. Congenital dislocation of the hip occurs in 1–2 babies per thousand births. It is now usually detected during neonatal screening. Occasional cases present later between the ages of 0–3 years when the child begins to walk. The male to female ration is 1:5. The child will present with an abnormal gait, either a limp, waddling gait or Trendelenburg gait. AP and frog lateral view of the hip will usually reveal a shallow acetabulum and dislocated head of femur. Referral for orthopaedic management is required.

2. Irritable hip (transient synovitis). This is the most common cause of hip pain and limp in childhood. The condition usually occurs between the ages of 1–6 years. It is more common in boys than girls. The condition is often associated with an upper respiratory tract infection. The child presents with a limp and may complain of pain in the hip or knee. The diagnosis is essentially one of exclusion. More serious conditions such as septic arthritis are excluded on clinical grounds and where necessary by use of laboratory tests such as white cell count, ESR and C reactive protein. An ultrasound examination of the hip will reveal an effusion. X-ray is not indicated as the first line imaging technique unless the child is in the age range for slipped upper femoral epiphysis. Once the diagnosis is made the management in most cases is conservative. Rest is advised and analgesia prescribed. The child is reviewed in 24–48 hours to exclude the development of septic arthritis. The condition usually resolves spontaneously within 2–3 days although some cases may persist for up to 10 days. Cases persisting for longer than this may warrant admission for bed rest.

3. Perthes disease (osteochondritis of the femoral head). Perthes disease occurs in about 1 in 2000 children. The initial presentation is usually a limp associated with pain and restricted movement. The condition usually presents between the ages of 4–7 years but may occur as early as 3 years of age and as late as 10 years. Boys are affected five times more commonly than girls. The age of the child should alert to the possibility of the diagnosis. The initial X-ray may be normal. Only about 5% of children with irritable hip develop Perthes disease. Over a period of 1–2 years segmental necrosis of the femoral head occurs leading to fragmentation and collapse. Healing then occurs over a period of 2–3 years. Mild cases are treated conservatively. More severe cases require intervention to maintain the shape of the femoral head within the acetabulum whilst healing occurs. On occasion the child at first presentation may have advanced disease. Referral for orthopaedic management is required.

4. Slipped upper femoral epiphysis (coxa vara). Slipped upper femoral epiphysis is less common than either Perthes or congenital dislocation of the hip. It occurs most commonly in the 10–14-year age group in girls and the 12–16-year age group in boys. Boys are more commonly affected than girls. It is bilateral in 20% of cases. The child is usually obese and tall with gonadal immaturity. They present with pain in the hip, thigh or knee. AP and lateral views of the hip reveal the slip of the epiphysis downwards and backwards.

5. Toddlers fracture. This is an undisplaced fracture of the tibia occurring in toddlers. It presents as a limp. Careful examination will identify the tibia as the site of maximal tenderness. In minor fracture tenderness will be minimal and may be difficult to elicit. Gentle rotational stress of the tibia will reveal the fracture. Initial X-ray is normal.

6. General management plan. A history is taken to elicit the type and duration of symptoms and any associated factors (e.g. intercurrent infection). Care should be taken in attributing the limpto a recently sustained injury. Many children have minor accidents on a regular basis.

When approaching the child with a limp care must be taken to maintain the confidence of the child during the examination and not to inflict unnecessary pain. Watching the child walk will indicate the side of the limp. Examination starts on the normal side. Each joint and bone is observed for evidence of trauma and inflammation. The whole length of the limb is palpated for tenderness and skin temperature. Each joint is examined for effusion and range of movement. This examination should reveal the side and likely site of pathology.

If an injury is suspected X-rays of the relevant bone or joint only should be requested. If hip pathology is suspected an ultrasound is the investigation of choice, except in the case of slipped upper femoral epiphysis when an AP and lateral hip views should be obtained.

Protocols vary on how to manage the well child with a clinical diagnosis of irritable hip. Some units advocate admitting all such cases. The following management plan allows the vast majority of such cases to be managed as out-patients. You should however consult and follow your local procedures.

If the clinical diagnosis of irritable hip is made out-of-hours and the child is well and apyrexial, ultrasound investigations and blood tests can be deferred until the next working day. The child should rest and be given simple analgesia as required. The parents are advised to bring the child back earlier if the symptoms get worse or if the child develops a temperature or becomes unwell.

If the diagnosis is of a toddler's fracture, the child is treated in an above knee plaster for ten days and reviewed. At review the plaster is removed. If the child is pain free and without a limp they are discharged. If the child complains of pain or has a limp the tibia is re-X-rayed. If a fracture is present the periosteal reaction will be seen. The above knee plaster is re-applied and the child referred to the fracture clinic.

Further reading

Danby KW, Lipton G. Evaluation of limp in children. *Current Opinion in Paediatrics*, 1995; 7(1): 88–94.

Related topics of interest

Ankle sprain (p. 43); Anterior knee pain (p. 48); Back pain (p. 62); Fractures – principles of treatment (p. 155); Septic arthritis (p. 289)

LOCAL ANAESTHESIA

Elizabeth Jones

Local anaesthetic agents reversibly block the conduction of nerves by impairing the propagation of action potentials. They exist in two forms: a base (fat soluble) and a cation (water soluble). The base form is able to diffuse into the axon where it dissociates, enabling the cationic form to block the sodium channel. The equilibrium of the two forms is determined by the pKa of the local anaesthetic and the pH of the surrounding tissues. The susceptibility of nerves depends on several factors including nerve size and myelination, thus small nerve fibres (C and Aδ fibres) tend to be more easily blocked with higher doses being required to block other sensory modalities and motor fibres.

Classification

Broadly into two groups: according to the intermediate chain within the structure.

1. ***Amides***
   - Lignocaine.
   - Prilocaine.
   - Bupivacaine.
   - Levo-bupivacaine.
   - Ropivacaine.

2. ***Esters***
   - Cocaine.
   - Amethocaine.
   - Benzocaine.
   - Procaine.

Metabolism

Local anaesthetics are metabolized in the liver, with additional hydrolysis of esters occurring in the plasma (plasma cholinesterase).

Vasoconstrictors

Most local anaesthetics cause vasodilatation (except cocaine) therefore vasoconstrictors are used, e.g. adrenaline, felypressin.

1. ***Effects***
   - Increase the duration of the anaesthetic.
   - Reduce blood loss.
   - Reduce absorption and systemic toxicity.

Vasoconstrictors should not, however, be used for digits, the nose, ears or penis because of the risk of ischaemic necrosis.

Maximum recommended dose of adrenaline for use in local anaesthetics = 500 mcg.

Choice and dose

Choice and doses of local anaesthetic depends on:

- The route of administration (local infiltration and nerve blocks, haematoma blocks, intravenous regional anaesthesia, surface anaesthesia).
- The duration of anaesthesia required.
- Patient's age, weight and general health. (Note: in obese patients the ideal weight should be used to avoid overdosage; reduce doses in the elderly).

Guide to maximum doses (local infiltration)

			Total
Lignocaine	Plain	3 mg/kg	200 mg
		e.g. 20 ml of 1% lignocaine for a 70 kg adult	
	With adrenaline	7 mg/kg	500 mg
Bupivacaine		2 mg/kg	150 mg
	(same maximum with or without a vasoconstrictor)		
Prilocaine	Plain	6 mg/kg	400 mg
	With adrenaline	9 mg/kg	600 mg

Adverse

1. ***Local***

- Hypersensitivity. True allergic reactions are reported with ester local anaesthet-ics but are extremely rare with amides. Preservative hypersensitivity problems, however, have been reported with amides.
- Injury to adjacent structures. Good knowledge of applied anatomy is essential.
- Spread of infection. Local infiltration should be avoided in inflamed or infected tissues because of the risk of spreading infection. Other good reasons to avoid the use of local anaesthetics in this situation are that it is painful; there is poor efficacy due to the acidic pH of the tissues; and there is increased risk of systemic toxicity due to the vasodilatation.

2. ***Systemic.*** Usually related to the absorption of large doses in vascular areas (e.g. head and neck, intercostal blocks) or to an inadvertent intravascular injection.

- Central nervous system: local anaesthetics also have a membrane stabilizing effect on central neurones. In overdose, inhibitory neurones are affected first thus excitatory manifestations are seen: dizziness, tremor, restlessness, anxiety, peroral paraesthesia, tinnitus, grand mal seizures. Larger doses cause depression of the vital centres in the pons and medulla with respiratory depression and loss of consciousness. (Note: the adverse effects may not progress in the orderly fashion listed above; convulsions may be the first sign of overdosage, especially in the event of an inadvertent intravenous injection).
- Cardiovascular system: local anaesthetics in overdose reduce myocardial excitability, cause peripheral vasodilatation (except cocaine) and block autonomic ganglia, thus may produce hypotension and arrhythmias, including

ventricular fibrillation. (Note: ventricular arrhythmias may occur with bupivacaine without any CNS warning signs of toxicity.)

Management of local anaesthetic overdose

Stop procedure and give high-flow oxygen. The airway and breathing will need to be supported as necessary. Convulsions are treated using intravenous benzodiazepines. Hypotension is treated with intravenous fluids and adrenaline. Prolonged cardiopulmonary resuscitation may be necessary because of the refractory nature of cardiac arrhythmias caused by local anaesthetic overdose. Bretylium and amiodarone have been used for bupivacaine arrhythmias.

Lignocaine

- Local anaesthetic with rapid onset and adequate duration of 30–90 minutes (plain – with adrenaline).
- Used for local infiltration, nerve blocks, surface anaesthesia.
- EMLA (Eutectic Mixture of Local Anaesthetics) (Lignocaine 2.5%, prilocaine 2.5%). It needs to be applied one hour before painless venepuncture is attempted.
- Lignocaine gels and spray: Used for mucous membrane anaesthesia.

Prilocaine

- Local anaesthetic with many characteristics in common with lignocaine.
- Less potent than lignocaine but less toxic at correct doses.
- Available plain and with felypressin as vasoconstrictor.
- Felypression is an analogue of vasopressin. It exhibitis fewer myocardial side effects than adrenaline.
- Used for local infiltration, nerve and epidural blocks, surface anaesthesia and is the only drug recommended for intravenous regional anaesthesia.
- Large doses (>600 mg) cause methaemaglobinaemia due to the metabolite o-toluidine. This may need treatment with 1% methylene blue, 1 mg/kg i.v. (See contraindications for Bier's block).

Bupivacaine

- Slower onset of action (up to 30 minutes) but longer duration of action (up to 8 hours for a nerve block).
- Used for local infiltration, peripheral nerve blocks and epidural block. Toxicity limits dose and use. It is contraindicated for intravenous regional anaesthesia (Bier's block) because of the risk of cardiac arrest, which is resistant to treatment, if bupivacaine is inadvertently released into the systemic circulation.

Levobupivacine

- Most of the toxic side effects of racemic bupivacaine arise from the R-enantiomer of bupivacaine. Levobupivacine has been developed in the hope that it is safer. It would appear that it has less toxic effects on the heart and CNS.
- Current indications for use in adults include major and minor nerve blocks during surgery, post-operative pain management and obstetrics.

Ropivacaine

- Local anaesthetic in the pure S-enantiomer. Developed in the search for a safer, long acting LA to replace bupivacaine. Claims for ropivacaine include reduced myocardial, CNS toxicity and reduced motor nerve blockade.
- Therapeutic indications include management of surgical pain e.g. epidural blocks, field blocks and acute pain management in obstetric practice.

Cocaine

- Alkaloid derived from the leaves of *Erythroxylum coca* tree.
- High toxicity limits its use to specific topical applications where its rapid absorption through mucous membranes and potent vasoconstrictor actions result in excellent surface anaesthesia.

Amethocaine

- Use limited to surface anaesthesia because of significant systemic toxicity. Hypersensitivity has been reported.
- Anaesthesia of the cornea is rapidly obtained using a 0.5 or 1% solution.
- Ametop: Topical gel containing amethocaine. Indicated for surface anaesthesia of intact skin. Painless venepuncture is possible after 30 minutes of application and intravenous cannulation after 45 minutes. The gel should be removed after 45 minutes. Skin anaesthesia persists for up to 6 hours. It should only be used on intact and non-inflamed skin to avoid the problems of rapid absorption and systemic toxicity.

Local anaesthetic procedures

1. Local infiltration. Subcutaneous injection of local anaesthetic in close proximity to the site of surgery. Pain produced by infiltration may be reduced by using warmed local anaesthetic solution, a narrow-bored needle and providing counter-stimulation, e.g. rubbing, in close proximity to the injection site. (Note: contraindications to local infiltration.) Useful for wound exploration, debridement, removal of foreign bodies and suturing.

2. Peripheral nerve block. Injection of local anaesthetic in the proximity of a peripheral nerve to provide anaesthesia in the dermatome supplied by that nerve.

3. Digital nerve block. 1% lignocaine plain and a 25 G needle on a 5 ml syringe is used to anaesthetize the palmar digital branches of the median and/or ulnar nerves by injecting 1.5–2 ml either side of the base of the relevant digit. The palmar digital branches supply the dorsum of the digits to a variable degree, therefore it is often necessary to infiltrate over the proximal part of the dorsum of the digit to anaesthetize the dorsal branches of the radial nerve. Up to 15 minutes should be allowed for the local anaesthetic to take effect.

4. Femoral nerve block. Femoral nerve (L2–L4)

Used to provide analgesia for a fractured shaft of femur.

Contraindications: Local sepsis, coagulopathy, lack of co-operation. The femoral nerve supplies motor fibres to quadriceps and sensory fibres to the anterior thigh and medial aspect of the knee and calf. Above the inguinal ligament, the nerve lies on iliacus muscle, deep to the fascia lata drawing a fascial sheath around them. The femoral nerve lies outside this sheath: behind and lateral to the artery, separated from the artery by a fibrous septum from fascia iliaca. Below the inguinal ligament the vein, artery and nerve are covered by fascia lata.

Difficulties with the block may result from anatomical variations: the nerve may branch before passing into the legs and its exact relationship to the artery is variable.

Method: Lignocaine 1%, bupivacaine 0.5% alone or combined are used. (Note: if used 50:50 the maximum dose of each will be reduced by 50% because the toxicity is additive.) The femoral artery is palpated at the mid-inguinal point (half-way between the anterior superior iliac spine and the pubic symphysis). 21 G needle on a 20 ml syringe is inserted 1 cm lateral to the artery until 2 'pops' or loss of resistance are felt as the needle penetrates the fascia lata and fascia iliaca. Local anaesthetic is injected with repeated aspirations at 5 ml intervals.

Complications:

- Haematoma.
- Intravascular injection.
- Failed block.
- Damage to the femoral nerve.

5. *Nerve plexus block.* Large volumes of low concentration local anaesthetics are injected in the proximity of a nerve plexus. The onset is slow (30–45 minutes for an axillary brachial plexus block) but longer duration may be achieved. Contralateral venous access and full monitoring and resuscitation equipment must be available.

6. *Haematoma block.* A Colles fracture may be manipulated following injection of 1% lignocaine (plain) into the haematoma around the fracture site. Location of the correct site on the dorsal aspect of the radius is achieved by aspiration of fracture haematoma into the syringe containing local anaesthetic. A tangential light source across the syringe will demonstrate fat globules from the fracture site before 10 ml of local anaesthetic is injected. 3–5 ml can be injected around the ulnar styloid.

Complications: In converting a closed fracture into an open one by injecting into the fracture site there is a theoretical risk of sepsis. In practice when strict aseptic techniques are used, this risk is small.

7. *Intravenous regional anaesthesia: Bier's block.* Described by Bier in 1908. Indicated for surgery below the elbow, and fracture manipulation, e.g. Colles fracture.

Complications:

- Local anaesthetic toxicity.
- Methaemaglobinaemia.

Contraindications:

- Limb infection.
- Coagulopathy.
- Peripheral vascular disease.

- Sickle cell disease.
- Ischaemic risk – crush injury.
- Neurological disease.
- Uncontrolled hypertension.
- Epilepsy.

Staff and equipment: Deaths have occurred due to inadvertent release of local anaesthetic causing systemic toxicity of local anaesthetic especially in the past when bupivacaine was used. Bupivacaine is not licensed for a Bier's block.

There are still risks: large doses of 0.5% prilocaine are used and therefore steps must be taken to minimize inadvertent systemic toxicity. Equipment must be regularly checked and maintained; trained staff (two doctors and a nurse) must be present during the procedure, with easy access to resuscitation equipment; patient must be consented, starved and monitored.

Procedure: Insert a 20 G intravenous cannula in the dorsum of the hand on the side to be manipulated. A second cannula is placed in the opposite arm for use in an emergency. Exsanguinate the limb by elevating the arm whilst compressing on the brachial artery for a period of about three minutes. Whilst still elevated, inflate the special 15 cm wide tourniquet cuff to 100 mmHg above systolic BP (maximum 300 mmHg). Lower the arm and check the tourniquet is not leaking. A trained person should monitor the tourniquet time and cuff pressure throughout the whole procedure. Warn the patient about warmth, skin discolouration and altered sensation. Slowly inject the 0.5% prilocaine (1–3 mg per kg, e.g. 40 ml for 70 kg adult, 30 ml for an elderly or frail adult). Regional anaesthesia is achieved in five minutes. The operator is now committed to keeping the cuff inflated for at least 20 minutes to prevent a large bolus of local anaesthetic being released on early deflation of the cuff. Manipulations, application of POP and X-rays must be completed within the maximum tourniquet time of one hour. Deflate the cuff slowly, watching for signs of toxicity. Normal sensation returns within two to five minutes. The patient should be observed for one hour because of the risk of delayed toxicity. In addition, the circulation in the limb should be checked prior to discharge.

Further reading

Knudsen K, Beckman-Suurkula M, Blomberg S, Sjovall J, Evardsson N. Central nervous system and cardiovascular effects of i.v. infusions of ropivacaine, vupivacaine and placebo in volunteers. *British Journal of Anaesthesia*, 1997; **78:** 507–4.

Markham A, Faulds D. Ropivacaine: a review of its pharmacology and therapeutic use in regional anaesthesia. *Drugs*, 1996; **52**(3): 429–49.

McClellan KJ, Spencer C. Levobupivacaine. *Drugs*, 1998; **56**(3): 355–62.

Peutrell JM, Mather SJ. *Regional Anaesthesia in Babies and Children.* Oxford University Press, 1997.

Vickers MD, Morgan M, Spencer PSJ, Read MS. *Drugs in Anaesthetic and Intensive Care Practice.* Butterworth Heinemann. Eighth edition, 1999.

Wildsmith JAW, Armitage EN. *Principles and Practice of Regional Anaesthesia.* 2nd edition Churchill and Livingstone, 1993.

MAJOR INCIDENT PLANNING

Mark Poulden

A health service major incident exists when the number of live casualties are such that special arrangements are necessary to deal with them or an occurrence presents a serious threat to the health of the community or the health service is disrupted.

It can further be classified by the cause – natural (earthquake) or man-made (transport accident); by whether the incident exceeds the capacity of the service (including special arrangements) to cope – compensated or uncompensated; by whether the infrastructure (roads etc) is intact or disrupted – simple or compound.

Major incident phases

- Standby and declaration;
- the initial response;
- establishing command and control;
- ensuring safety of self, scene and survivors;
- establish communication links;
- scene assessment;
- carry out triage sieve and sort;
- begin emergency treatment at scene and in casualty clearing station;
- establishing a temporary mortuary;
- transportation to receiving hospitals;
- stand down;
- debriefing.

A successful plan

Each hospital that is able to receive casualties 24 hours a day is required to have a major incident plan. For success it must:

1. Establish plans for all potential disaster sites in your area (e.g. football stadia, industrial sites), including potential special incidents e.g. radioactive leaks;
2. Develop an all hazard approach such that it is easily adaptable whatever the incident;
3. All staff involved should have action cards detailing their role and responsibilities. Safety, training and equipment of staff is paramount;
4. Link with the plans of other agencies, both pre-hospital and in-hospital;
5. Identify a medical incident officer to oversee medical resources at scene, and a mobile medical team for emergency on-scene treatment. These staff must be easily identifiable, equipped and trained for their role. Thought must be given for these staff not coming from the main receiving hospital;
6. Be practised and assessed regularly. This may be table-top paper exercises or full combined service response with simulated patients. Accurate evaluation and action to update and improve the plan follows;
7. Establish and test communication links (communications failure is the most often cited reason for problems). Accurate information from the scene is

essential for the developing response but also to provide information to relatives, police and the media;

8. Have unique, accurate documentation of casualties location, condition, treatments and response. Likewise a log of all events and decisions;
9. Teach major incident triage and treatment principles. These aim to do the most for the most. This means the seriously injured being managed on their likelihood of survival based on condition, accessibility and resources available at the time. Treatment addresses the ABCs, remembering analgesia;
10. Have procedures in place to deal with the uninjured survivors, relatives and the dead;
11. Consider use of other agencies e.g. WRVS – food and support, St Johns – transport of the walking wounded etc.
12. Establish principles for media liaison;
13. Include a debrief with availability of social and psychological support not just for victims and relatives, but also rescue workers. Psychological trauma is an important cause of morbidity;
14. Aid the police in forensic activity.

Further reading

Dealing With Disaster: Homeoffice.gov.uk/epd/dwd.htm (ISBN 185 893 9208)
Department of Health: doh.gov.uk/epcu/epcu/index.htm
Major Incident Medical Management and Support: Course and Manual; ALSG.
Planning for Major Incidents, The Health Service Guidance; HSC 1998/197.

MAJOR INJURIES – INITIAL MANAGEMENT

The standard adopted for the initial management of major trauma in the UK is that set by the Committee on Trauma of the American College of Surgeons. This is taught using the methodology laid down in the Advanced Trauma Life Support manual and taught on ATLS courses in the UK under the direction of the ATLS Steering Committee of the Royal College of Surgeons of England. This manual and the associated courses teach one system of management.

The system is based upon the concept of a primary survey with simultaneous resuscitation, a secondary survey to map out all of the patients injuries and definitive management.

During the course of the primary and secondary survey further information should be sought to aid management. This must not detract from the immediate priority to identify immediately life-threatening injuries and resuscitate them.

The essential features of the history may be recalled by the use of the acronym **AMPLE.**

Allergies.
Medications past and current.
Past illnesses/pregnancy.
Last meal.
Events/environment related to the injury.

Primary survey and resuscitation

The aim of the primary survey and resuscitation phase is to identify immediately life-threatening problems in a systematic order (primary survey) and address those problems as they are met (resuscitation). Note the survey and resuscitation are carried out concurrently not consecutively. The order of priority follows the same order as with other resuscitation scenarios, with appropriate modifications for the unique features of trauma:

Airway with cervical spine control.
Breathing.
Circulation.
Disability (neurological function).
Exposure and environment factors.

Airway

On the basis that obstruction to the airway will result in severe neurological damage leading to death within a few minutes, management of the airway is of the highest priority. However the control of the airway must be undertaken with due consideration to the possibility of a cervical spine or cord lesion. Although not an immediately life-threatening problem failure to adequately control the cervical spine may lead to significant morbidity and mortality in the trauma victim.

The patient without adequate cervical spine immobilization should be approached from the head end of the trolley and the neck immobilized with both hands. This is sufficient until adequate mechanical immobilization can be applied (semi-rigid collar, sand bags and tape).

The airway is inspected for foreign bodies and obvious trauma. If the patient is able to speak they are unlikely to have an immediately life-threatening airway problem.

High-flow oxygen is applied via a face mask with a reservoir bag attached.

If a life-threatening airway problem is present it must be addressed before moving on to an assessment of breathing.

Management of the airway

The principle underlying the management of an acute airway problem is that the least invasive manoeuvre required to secure the airway should be used. This is achieved by moving progressively from basic to advanced techniques in a stepwise fashion until the airway is secured.

Basic airway manoeuvres

Full flow oxygen should be administered as outlined above. Such a system should allow a 90–95% concentration of oxygen to be delivered to the patient. If a foreign body or fluid is the cause of the problem it should be removed manually or with suction (blind sweeps of the airway should not be undertaken in children). The next step in the sequence is to use manual airway manoeuvres such as a jaw thrust (ensuring that the cervical spine is not moved) and/or chin lift. If these techniques do not work an airway adjunct such as an oropharyngeal or nasopharygeal airway should be inserted. In the majority of cases these simple procedures will ensure a clear airway.

Advanced airway manoeuvres

If the basic manoeuvres do not work then an advanced technique should be considered. The first stage in advanced airway management is tracheal intubation by either the oral or nasal route. Nasotracheal intubation is more likely to move the cervical spine than the oral route. If tracheal intubation does not succeed then a surgical airway must be established. There are two methods, needle cricothyroidotomy and surgical cricothyroidotomy.

Needle cricothyroidotomy

This technique is applicable in all age groups. A needle is introduced into the cricoid membrane and oxygen is jet insufflated. This technique provides only a temporary respite as it does not provide adequate ventilation and carbon dioxide levels will rise to unacceptable levels over a 30–40 minute period.

Surgical cricothyroidotomy

This is via the same route as needle cricothyroidotomy but because it is an open technique a tracheostomy tube may be inserted which ensures adequate ventilation as well as oxygenation.

Breathing

The neck is examined for distended veins and for evidence of tracheal shift. The chest is exposed. The sequence of observe, palpate, percuss and auscultate is followed. The respiratory rate and work of breathing are assessed. Four immediately life-threatening conditions are specifically sought:

- Tension pneumothorax.
- Open pneumothorax/'sucking chest wound'.
- Flail chest.
- Massive haemothorax.

If any of the above mentioned immediately life-threatening injuries is identified they should be addressed before moving on to circulation.

Management of immediately life-threatening breathing problem

1. ***Tension pneumothorax*** is treated by immediate needle decompression (insertion of a chest tube is deferred until the patient is stable during the secondary survey).

2. ***Open pneumothorax*** is treated by covering with an impermeable square of material taped down on three sides to allow air to escape.

3. ***Flail chest and massive haemothorax*** will usually be evident at this stage but will not in general require intervention until further along the primary survey.

Circulation

The circulation is assessed using the pulse rate, volume and quality, peripheral perfusion (capillary refill and colour). Blood pressure is measured when convenient.

Management of circulatory problems

Exsanguinating haemorrhage should be controlled by applying direct pressure. Tourniquets should not be used.

All victims of major trauma require venous access with at the minimum two large bore, short, peripheral lines. If it is not possible to insert peripheral venous lines the sequence to follow is:

- Percutaneous venous cut down (usually at the saphenous vein on the medial aspect of the ankle). In children under 6 years the intraosseous route is the route of choice.
- Femoral or saphenous vein cannulation.
- Central venous lines are not required in the primary survey. Their function is to monitor response to the fluid replacement, not as a route for fluid replacement.

Disability (neurological function)

A detailed neurological examination is not required at this stage. All pertinent information relating to immediately life-threatening neurological problems can be obtained by assessing pupillary size and reaction and conscious level. Unequal pupils suggest the possibility of an intracranial bleed with midline shift. Decreased conscious level indicates amongst other things threat to the airway.

Exposure and environmental factors

The patient should be completely uncovered in preparation for the secondary survey. The environment should be kept warm and draught-free to avoid hypothermia, which may develop rapidly in the traumatized patient even within the resuscitation room.

Secondary survey

Only when the primary survey is complete and the patient fully resuscitated and stable should the secondary survey be commenced. The purpose of the secondary survey is to carry out a complete head-to-toe examination of the patient looking for any additional injuries. This includes the following:

- Head and skull.
- Maxillofacial.
- Neck.
- Chest.
- Abdomen.
- Perineum/rectum/vagina.
- Musculoskeletal.
- Complete neurological examination.
- 'Tubes and fingers in every orifice'.

If at any stage of the secondary survey the patients state deteriorates, the survey should be stopped and the patient reassessed from the beginning of the primary survey sequence.

1. Routine investigations

- FBC
- U&E
- Glucose
- Pregnancy test
- 12 lead ECG
- Chest and pelvis X-ray

2. Monitoring

- Arterial blood gas analysis and ventilatory rate
- End-tidal carbon dioxide
- ECG
- Pulse oximetry
- Blood pressure

Cross-table lateral C-spine X-ray has been considered mandatory in the past as part of the primary/secondary survey. It is now recognized that although it may provide useful information if it shows a lesion, that a normal X-ray does not exclude a fracture or cord lesion. Therefore irrespective of the result of the cross-table films the patient must be treated as if they have a cervical spine lesion until this is definitively excluded.

Specialized diagnostic procedures to confirm suspect injuries should only be performed after that patient's life-threatening injuries have been identified and appropriately managed. These include:

- Computerized tomography.
- Contrast studies.
- Extremity X-ray.
- Endoscopy and ultrasonography.

Definitive care

After identification of the patient's injuries, management of life-threatening problems and obtaining special studies, definitive care begins.

Transfer

If the patient's injuries exceed the hospital's immediate treatment capabilities, the patient will require a timely and safe transfer to an appropriate facility.

Further reading

Amercian College of Surgeons Committee on Trauma. *Advanced Life Support Course for Doctors.* Chicago, 1997.

Details of course dates and locations may be obtained from the Royal College of Surgeons of England.

Related topics of interest

Abdominal trauma (p. 4); Airway (p. 28); Burns (p. 74)

MANAGEMENT OF ACUTE POISONING

Acute poisoning is responsible for approximately 100 000 hospital admissions per year in England and Wales. The fact that in-patient mortality remains less than 1% is due in part to systemic management strategies. Provision of information by the network of Poisons Centres throughout the British Isles plays an important role in the implementation of these strategies. However, initial advice on specific issues can be obtained from the internet on TOXBASE on http://www.spib.axl.co.uk.

General points

The management of most acute poisonings is supportive. The main priority is cardio-respiratory support.

1. ***Airway***

- Level of consciousness should be assessed using either the Edinburgh or Glasgow Coma Scale (GCS).
- In patients with grade 2 Edinburgh Coma Scale or above the oropharynx should be cleared of obstruction (including dentures).

2. ***Breathing***

- Adequacy of breathing should be assessed and supplemental oxygen given as necessary.
- Loss of cough or gag reflex demands endotracheal intubation with a cuffed tube.
- Arterial blood gas estimation will confirm the need for assisted ventilation if breathing remains inadequate.
- Insertion of an oro- or nasopharyngeal airway and placement in the left lateral position should secure the airway.
- If spinal injury is a possibility a hard collar is mandatory prior to manipulation of the airway.

3. ***Circulation***

- The most frequent manifestation of circulatory disturbance is hypotension. Most cases respond to elevation of the foot of the bed, if this fails measurement of central venous pressure and urine output should be employed.
- If central venous pressure is low, crystalloid or colloid volume expansion is indicated.
- On occasion, enhancing the elimination of a known cardiodepressant drug may be effective.
- Rhythm disturbances often settle with normalization of oxygen tension, acid–base and electrolyte status.

4. ***Disability***

- Use Glasgow Coma Scale or Edinburgh Coma Scale.
- Control of convulsions: occur in poisoned patients for several reasons:

(a) as a convulsant effect of the poison; tricyclic anti-depressants are the commonest cause;
(b) after cerebral hypoxia from respiratory or cardiovascular depression;
(c) from hypoglycaemia;
(d) as severe muscle spasms due to spinal or peripheral effects on the mechanisms controlling muscle tone;
(e) owing to withdrawal in physically dependent subjects; the agents usually responsible are alcohol, opioids, barbiturates, and benzodiazepines;
(f) occasionally anticonvulsant poisoning can be associated with worsening of seizures in patients with epilepsy.

5. Common patterns of poisoning ('Toxidromes') include

- Coma, hypotension, flaccidity. Benzodiazepines; barbiturates; ethanol; opioids, beta-blocking drugs and many others. It is rare for poisoned patients to show no improvement in conscious level by 12 h after admission. Consider other pathology in these circumstances.
- Coma, hyper-reflexia, tachycardia, dilated pupils. Tricyclic antidepressants; (sometimes extensor plantar responses), anticholinergic agents; phenothiazines.
- Malaise, restlessness, nausea, weakness. Carbon monoxide; addictive states and withdrawal; solvents; insecticides; lead, mercury; arsenic.
- Restlessness, hypertonia, hyper-reflexia, pyrexia. Monoamine oxidase inhibitors; anticholinergic agents; strychnine; phencyclidine; amphetamine.
- Behavioural disturbances. Psychotropic drugs; anticholinergic drugs, adverse effects of prescribed or self-administered agents, e.g. corticosteroids, pseudoephedrine; addictive states and withdrawal; solvent abuse; psilocybe ('magic') mushrooms.
- Burns in mouth, dysphagia, abdominal pain, distension. Corrosives; caustics; paraquat.
- Renal failure. Paracetamol; inorganic mercurial compounds; acids (phosphoric, formic, oxalic); phenols (disinfectants, wood preservers); secondary to rhabdomyolysis or shock; arsine, lead.
  - Jaundice, hepatic failure. Paracetamol, carbon tetrachloride, amanita phalloides, phosphorus; organic lead.
  - Convulsions may be associated with: tricyclic antidepressants; phenothiazines; carbon monoxide; monoamine oxidase inhibitors; mefenamic acid; ethylene glycol; opioids; theophylline; isoniazid; hypoglycaemic agents; organo-phosphate insecticides; salicylates; lithium; amphetamines; strychnine; lead, cyanide; withdrawal states.

The laboratory testing and measurement of drugs in acute poisoning

Samples of blood, urine, gastric aspirate or contaminated items should be collected for analysis as follows:

1. Blood collection heparinized tubes for specific drug measurement.

2. Urine or gastric contents 20 ml in a clean container with no preservatives for a drug screen. Note that drug screens are best carried out on urine samples.

Analysis of these samples should be requested according to these guidelines:

- If the patient is seriously ill (or deteriorating) then a drug screen may be necessary at once.
- If a specific drug is suspected, will the knowledge of the actual concentration affect the immediate therapy?
- Particular problems should be discussed with your local consultant biochemist or a Clinical Toxicologist (call the National Poisons Information Service).

Gut decontamination

Evidence of benefit to the vast majority of poisoned patients from some of the older techniques of gut decontamination is lacking. This has led to recent changes in recommendations from Poisons Centres in the USA and Europe.

1. Syrup of ipecachuana and other emetics. The use of emetics is no longer generally recommended. No study exists to demonstrate a significant reduction in drug absorption or toxicity following ipecachuana administration. Indeed it may, by forcing gastric contents beyond the pylorus, increase poison absorption. Vomiting and other effects (e.g. drowsiness) induced by the syrup can mask the true diagnosis, increase morbidity and rarely fatalities have been reported in association with its use.

2. Gastric lavage. As a means of drug recovery, gastric lavage is poor and probably contributes little to the course of most poisonings. As with syrup of ipecachuana, absorption may be increased and a small risk exists of respiratory, cardiovascular, biochemical and mechanical complications. Lavage is now generally only recommended up to an hour after poison ingestion if a potentially life-threatening amount of poison has been ingested. Patients for whom the time of ingestion is uncertain or severely symptomatic patients may benefit from gastric lavage. This should be discussed with a senior colleague or with a poisons centre.

Lavage should always be performed by staff experienced in the technique, as protection of the airway is vital. It is contraindicated when the airway cannot be protected, after ingestion of petroleum distillates (e.g. white spirit) or corrosive substances, where there is increased risk of bleeding or perforation, or if the patient refuses the procedure. If in doubt, check with the poisons centre.

3. Whole bowel irrigation (WBI). In this technique a polyethylene glycol electrolyte lavage solution is instilled via a nasogastric tube at a rate of 2 litres per hour in an adult. This is continued until 10 litres of solution have been used or the rectal effluent becomes clear although the validity of these end points has been questioned. WBI may rarely be considered in poisonings where other methods of decontamination (in particular activated charcoal) are ineffective, e.g. with iron, lithium and other metals and in cocaine body packers. In practice it is seldom required. It should not be continued for more than 8 hours as there is a risk of systemic absorption of the irrigation fluid. ***A physician considering using WBI is strongly advised to consult with a poisons centre.***

4. Activated charcoal. Many poisons are adsorbed by activated charcoal and as a means of gut decontamin-ation it compares favourably with gastric emptying techniques. Some important toxins poorly absorbed by charcoal are listed below:

Cyanide	Lead salts	Acids
DDT	Lithium preparations	Alkalis
Ethanol	Mercury salts	
Ethylene glycol	Methanol	
Ferrous salts	Organic solvents	
Fluorides	Potassium salts	

Single dose charcoal at a dose of 50–100 g for adults and 1g per kg body weight for children can be given by mouth or via nasogastric tube (if vomiting or any doubt about the airway) up to an hour post-poison ingestion. There are insufficient data to support or exclude the benefit of single dose activated charcoal after this period. The exception to this time limit is following ingestion of agents for which the administration of repeated doses of charcoal is recommended.

Repeated dose charcoal is useful in preventing absorption of some sustained release preparations even when they present over 1 hour post ingestion. This is continued until the stools turn black or lack of symptoms suggests that the ingested dose is unlikely to be of harm. In multiple dose form charcoal also increases the elimination of certain toxins (see below). This technique acts by adsorbing drugs that are secreted in bile as well as those drugs that pass from the circulation into the gut, either passively or by active secretion (*'gastrointestinal dialysis'*).

Dosage for adults is 50 g stat followed by 12.5 g hourly or 25 g every 2 hours, and for children an initial dose of 1 g per kg followed by 1 g per kg every 4 hours. To prevent constipation a **single dose** of sorbitol (50 ml of 70% solution for adults) is sometimes given. Charcoal is continued until either there is sustained clinical improvement or a significant reduction in plasma concentration of the poison where appropriate. Complications are unusual but include vomiting and charcoal aspiration, bowel obstruction, electrolyte and acid–base disturbances. Vomiting, if problematical, may respond to high dose intravenous metoclopramide or if necessary, intravenous ondansetron. It is important to avoid using multiple dose charcoal in patients with absent bowel sounds or who may be at risk of bowel obstruction. Caution is advocated in using this technique in young infants, and in drowsy or unconscious patients, the airway must be protected.

Eliminating poisons

Drugs which may require gastrointestinal dialysis, peritoneal dialysis, haemodialysis or haemoperfusion if there is severe intoxication, clinical deterioration, or high drug concentrations, include the following (discuss with Poisons Unit).

1. Gastrointestinal dialysis. Some drugs for which repeat-dose activated charcoal is sometimes indicated:

- carbamazepine;
- phenobarbital;
- theophylline;
- dapsone;
- quinine.

Some modified and sustained release preparations.

2. ***Haemodialysis.*** Salicylates; phenobarbitone; barbitone (but not short acting barbiturates); methanol/ethanol; ethylene glycol; lithium; isopropanol; salt poisoning (following attempts at emesis).

3. ***Haemoperfusion.*** Salicylates; short and medium acting barbiturates; disopyramide; theophylline; phenytoin; carbamazepine, chloroquine.

Detaining a patient under the Mental Health Act 1983

An in-patient may be detained in hospital against his/her will under the provision of Section 5(2) of the Mental Health Act.

An 'application' is made by one doctor in respect of the patient on the grounds that:

- '*he is suffering from mental disorder of a nature or degree which warrants the detention of the patient in hospital for assessment..... for at least a limited period*'

and

- '*he ought to be so detained in the interests of his own health or safety or with a view to the protection of other persons*'

A brief report is made on a prescribed form (Mental Health Act – Form 12). These forms are available from the Medical Records Officer. The report must be 'received by the managers' if possible within 1 hour of Form 12 being signed and for this the on-call manager shouldbe contacted. The patient may then be detained for a period of up to 72 hours. A psychiatric opinion would usually be required as soon as possible (see below) to advise on management and to consider whether a 28 day assessment order and/or transfer to a psychiatric ward would be appropriate.

A patient can only be transferred between hospitals on a Section 5(2) if these hospitals are directly managed units within the same district. In all other circumstances a Section 2 or 3 would be required, and a psychiatrist should be called.

A patient may not be admitted to hospital from a Casualty Department or an out-patient department under a Section 5(2).

Advice and consultation

At all times there is a duty psychiatrist on call to advise on the telephone.

Consent to treatment and Common Law

'*A patient has the right under common law to give or withhold consent prior to examination or treatment.*' (NHS Management Executive. A guide to consent for examination and treatment. London: Department of Health 1990, HC(90) 22).

There are clearly occasions when examination or treatment proceeds without a patient's consent; for example, where an unconscious patient cannot indicate his or her wishes. In such cases a doctor acts under Common Law. Where there are problems with consent, consultation with relatives may be appropriate and clear records should be kept of such consultations and of any action taken.

It should not be assumed that refusal to give consent indicates a mental disorder, although there are times when a psychiatric opinion may be helpful. The Mental

Health Act (1983) only deals with issues relating to mental illness. There are no such statutory provisions for the treatment of physical illness in the absence of informed consent.

Common Law

Common Law is based on judicial precedent and custom as distinct from statute law. In many cases, it will not only be lawful for doctors to give essential treatment to patients unable to give their consent, it will also be their common law duty to do so. Actions taken without a patient's consent under Common Law may be said to be taken '*in accordance with a responsible body of relevant professional opinion*' e.g. a patient who is confused, disorientated and paranoid may appropriately be physically restrained from discharging him/herself and given sedation (IM if necessary) under Common Law without use of the Mental Health Act. Rigid guidelines in such circumstances are hard to give. Common sense and '*acting in good faith*' should cover most such problems.

MAXILLOFACIAL INJURY

D Burke

The incidence of serious maxillofacial injury has fallen significantly since the introduction of legislation in the mid 1980s making the wearing of seatbelts compulsory. Such injuries may be of only cosmetic significance. Some may be life threatening due to airway obstruction. If the maxillofacial injury occurs as part of multiple trauma then it is treated according to the standard priorities.

Orbital blow-out fracture

These are caused by a blow to the eyeball causing a fracture to the floor of the orbit and prolapse of orbital contents into the maxillary antrum.

*1. **Clinical signs***
- Peri-orbital haematoma.
- Diplopia.
- Enophthalmos.

*2. **Diagnosis.*** The suspicion of a fracture rests upon eliciting a history of the mechanism and examining for diplopia and enophthalmos. Enophthalmos is best seen by standing above the patient and looking down at both eyes. The affected globe will be seen to have retracted into the orbit.

Radiographically the fracture is best seen on the AP orbital view when the characteristic 'tear drop' sign can be seen. This is opacity in the roof of the maxillary antrum of the affected side, best appreciated by comparison with the normal side.

Zygomatic arch fracture

Usually caused by a direct blow to the zygoma in a fist fight. Two types of fracture are recognized:

- Tripod fracture: This occurs through the zygomaticotemporal and zygomatico-frontal sutures and the infraorbital foramen.
- Zygomatic arch fracture: An isolated fracture of the arch.

*1. **Clinical signs.*** The tripod fracture is associated with:
- Bruising and swelling over the cheek.
- Flattening of the cheek contour.
- Infraorbital nerve paraesthesia.
- Diplopia.
- Subconjunctival haemorrhage.

The isolated zygomatic arch fracture is associated with:

- Bruising and swelling over the zygoma.
- Flattening of the cheek contour (unless minimally displaced).

*2. **Diagnosis.*** The history of a blow to the cheek suggests that a zygoma fracture may exist. The patient is examined looking for diplopia, infraorbital nerve paraesthesia and flattening of the cheek contour. Flattening of the cheek contour is best appreciated by viewing both cheeks from above. Comparison of both sides will show a depression of the affected side. If the fracture presents late, then soft tissue swelling may obscure the depression, X-rays will reveal the deformity. Failure to X-ray and diagnose the depression can lead to significant cosmetic deformity. In the case of the isolated arch fracture bony tenderness may be the only clinical sign.

Radiographically the tripod fracture requires in addition to the standard AP and lateral skull views, a 10–15° occipitomental view to show vertical displacement and 30° occipitomental view to show horizontal displacement. The arch fracture may require a shoot down view to demonstrate depression.

Nasal fracture

These occur as a result of a blow to the nose.

*1. **Clinical signs***

- Localized bleeding from the nostril.
- Deformity (depression or lateral displacement).
- Swelling.
- Septal deviation.
- Septal haematoma (uncommon).

*2. **Diagnosis.*** The diagnosis that an injury has occurred is usually evident. It is not always possible to determine whether there is a fracture present or not due to the often considerable swelling that has occurred by the time the patient has presented.

There is no need to X-ray as a routine as nasal fractures are only treated if they cause cosmetic deformity or obstruction to breathing. There is often blood occluding the affected side of the nose. It can therefore be difficult to determine whether obstructed breathing is due to the presence of blood or because of septal deviation.

The patient is instructed to return in 5–7 days if there is cosmetic deformity or obstruction to breathing for an ENT review. Bleeding from a fractured nose almost always stops spontaneously.

The only condition requiring urgent intervention is the presence of a *septal haematoma.* This has the appearance of a blueberry attached to the septum. Urgent drainage is required to prevent necrosis of the septum with subsequent collapse of the bridge of the nose.

Maxillary fracture

These fractures occur as a result of a frontal impact, usually of considerable force. Originally classified by LeFort, detailed knowledge of this classification is not required for their management in the A&E department.

*1. **Clinical signs***

- Bilateral facial swelling.
- Bilateral peri-orbital haematoma.
- Malocclusion of the teeth.
- Mobile maxilla.

- Infraorbital and superior dental nerve paraesthesia.
- Dish face appearance (due to backwards displacement of the maxilla).
- Soft palate haematoma.
- CSF rhinorrhoea.

2. ***Diagnosis.*** The mechanism of injury and swelling over the cheeks will suggest the diagnosis. Not all clinical signs will be present. The array and severity of signs will depend on the type of fracture, e.g. dish face deformity only occurs when the maxilla slips backwards.

Maxillary mobility may be assessed by grasping the teeth between the index finger and thumb and rocking it gently backwards and forwards. Only one side may be mobile.

Malocclusion can be observed by inserting a tongue depressor between the cheek and gums to observe occlusion. The patient, if conscious, will be able to tell if the teeth fit together normally (it may need to be explained that the term 'normal' means normal for them, many people 'normally' have malocclusion).

These fractures pose a real threat to the airway both as a result of the bleeding associated with them and as a result of the maxilla migrating posteriorly and causing obstruction. Manually elevating the fracture can relieve airway obstruction and reduce bleeding. There are usually associated injuries.

Standard radiography usually needs to be supplemented with CT scans to fully define the fracture.

Mandibular fracture

This occurs as the result of a blow to the jaw. Multiple fractures are common (50%) and often occur at sites distant from the impact. Forty percent involve the condyle, 20% the angle and 20% the body. They may be compound within the mouth.

1. ***Clinical signs***
   - Malocclusion.
   - Step deformity along the lower border of the jaw.
   - Mobile fragments.
   - Sublingual haematoma.
   - Inferior dental nerve paraesthesia.

2. ***Diagnosis.*** The mechanism of injury in combination with localized pain, swelling and malocclusion suggest the diagnosis. Care should be taken to examine the whole of the jaw to exclude second fractures.

Most A&E departments can obtain orthopantomographs (OPG) which reveal the majority of fractures. If the OPG is normal but the patient complains of malocclusion, condylar views may be required to exclude a condylar fracture.

Temporomandibular dislocation

Commonly occurs spontaneously when the patient yawns, it may also be the result of trauma. The patient presents with inability to close the mouth. The dislocation rarely requires sedation or anaesthesia to reduce.

Dental trauma

In all instances when a tooth is fractured be it an isolated injury or as part of a more complex maxillofacial injury, the possibility that a fragment has been inhaled must be considered. If the whole tooth or all of the component parts cannot be identified then chest radiography is required to look for the fragments. The fragment itself may not be seen, but inspiratory and expiratory films may show air trapping. If an inhaled fragment is missed the patient may present at a later date with signs of chest infection and radiographic signs of segmental collapse.

1. *Classification of tooth fractures*

- *Grade I.* Fracture involving the enamel.
- *Grade II.* Fracture involving the enamel and dentine.
- *Grade III.* Fracture involving the enamel, dentine and pulp (the pulp is visible as a red dot at the centre of the fracture).
- *Grade IV.* Fracture involving the root.

Management

Fractures that only involve the enamel are generally painless and do not require immediate management. The patient is advised to make an appointment with their own dentist. Fractures involving the dentine, pulp or root are exquisitely tender to hot, cold and air. They require early referral to a dentist for coating which relieves pain and reduces the risk of infection.

Displaced teeth

The main risk with displaced primary teeth is that they may be inhaled. They should be referred to a dentist for assessment and possible extraction because the roots are shallow and provide little anchorage.

Displaced permanent teeth should where possible be preserved for cosmetic reasons. The patient should be referred to a dentist for reduction and splintage.

Avulsed teeth

Avulsed primary teeth should be discarded as the roots are too shallow to anchor the tooth in place.

Avulsed permanent teeth should be retained and an attempt made to re-implant them early. Up to 50% of re-implanted permanent teeth take. The tooth should be kept moist whilst awaiting re-implantation. It should not be wiped. It can be kept in normal saline or milk, or in the case of an adult gently placed back in the socket and held in place pending splintage.

Further reading

Hawkesford J, Banks JG. *Maxillofacial and dental emergencies.* Oxford Handbooks in Emergency Medicine – 7. Oxford: Oxford University Press, 1994.

Related topic of interest

Cervical spine – acute neck sprain (p. 190)

MENINGITIS

In 1990 there were 2572 notifications of meningitis is England and Wales. The majority of cases were *meningococcal* (1138), *haemophilus influenzae* (431), *viral* (353), and *pneumococcal* (156).

Bacterial meningitis can be a fulminant, rapidly fatal illness requiring immediate recognition, diagnosis and therapy. Meningitis may occur in acute and chronic forms but presentation of the chronic form is rare.

The key to preventing morbidity of these patients is early diagnosis and treatment with the appropriate antibiotic. The causes of death include septic shock, cerebral oedema and brain coning.

Susceptibility is determined by predisposing factors such as:

- Immunocompromised patients;
- Post splenectomy;
- Sickle cell;
- Alcoholism;
- Hypogammaglobulinaemia;
- Cirrhosis;
- Diabetes.

The mortality varies with the organism – *Neisseria meningitidis* (7–14%), *Haemophilus influenzae* (3–10%), *Streptococcus pneumoniae* (15–60%) and *Listeria monocytogenes* (20%). Mortality is highest in the very young and old and those patients with underlying disease.

Permanent neurological sequelae include:

- Mental retardation;
- Deafness;
- Cranial nerve palsies;
- Hydrocephalus;
- Subdural effusion;
- Cerebral venous thrombosis;
- Epilepsy.

Organisms

1. Bacterial. *Haemophilus influenzae, Neisseria meningitides* and *Streptococcus pneumoniae* cause approximately 90% of all cases of proven bacterial meningitis. Less common pathogens include Gram-negative bacilli, *Listeria* and *Staphylococcus aureus.* Age is the most important variable in considering which organism is most likely to be the pathogen.

- Birth–3 months: Group B streptococci; *Escherichia coli*; *Listeria monocytogenes*
- 4 months–5 years: *Haemophilus influenzae*; *Neisseria meningitides*

- 6–65 years — *N. meningitides*, *S. pneumoniae*
- Over 65 years — *S. pneumoniae*, Gram negative bacilli, *Listeria monocytogenes*

2. ***Viral.*** Is probably three to four times more common and most often occurs in the summer in patients under the age of 40. The most common virus is the enterovirus with flavivirus, mumps and Herpes simplex following.

Pathophysiology

Colonization of the pathogen, usually in the nasophyarynx, is followed by systemic invasion and intravascular replication. Systemic invasion is more likely in the predisposed, that includes those with cellular and immunologic deficiency. Additionally there is a HLA B12 association with *Haemophilus* infection in children. The next step is blood–brain penetration, once this occurs replication within the CSF is facilitated by the lack of adequate immune defence systems in the CSF. Pathogens are usually limited to the subarachnoid space. Altered membrane permeability at the blood–brain barrier is one of the possible mechanisms for the cerebral oedema and the subsequent risk from herniation and death.

Clinical features

Unfortunately the classic triad of fever, neck stiffness and impaired consciousness is present in only 50% of cases.

1. ***The presentation is either***:
   - *The acute form* (10%) – symptoms develop within 24 hours, progress rapidly to altered states of consciousness, and have a mortality of 50% in bacterial cases.
   - The other 90% are *sub acute* with symptoms developing over 1–7 days. They are precedent viral type illness followed by a relatively rapid onset of fever, vomiting and stiff neck.

2. ***Tuberculous meningitis*** may present with an abrupt onset of meningeal signs but more commonly presents as a slow onset of vague illness with fever, headache and mental state changes. Tuberculous disease may be also located outside the CNS, usually pulmonary or miliary.

3. Only 20% of cases with bacterial meningitis present in a completely alert and orientated manner and 10% are in coma. Deteriorating level of consciousness correlates with worsening prognosis. An abnormal mental state may be the only sign in the elderly.

4. ***Rash*** can be identified in 50% of cases with meningococcal infection, but often begins as a maculopapular rash before the characteristic petechial rash develops.

5. ***Seizures*** occur in about 10% of cases and are significantly more common in pneumococcal than meningococcal meningitis.

6. ***Fundoscopic abnormalities*** are unusual (4%).
   Papilloedema takes 24–48 hours to develop and is rarely seen early on.

7. ***Cranial nerve palsies*** (notably III, IV, VI and VII) and focal neurological signs occur in 10–30% of cases. They may be an early sign in *Listeria monocytogenes* meningitis.

8. Other associated findings include *otitis media, sinusitis* and *pneumonia* that are most common with *S. pneumoniae* but can occur with *H. influenzae.*

Paediatric

1. Child under 3 years. Bacterial meningitis is most common in this age group but the diagnosis is more difficult. The classical signs of neck rigidity, photophobia, headache and vomiting are often absent. The signs and symptoms in this age group are mainly related to the raised intracranial pressure that is usual in children with bacterial meningitis.

- Drowsiness.
- Irritability.
- Poor feeding.
- Unexplained pyrexia.
- Convulsions with fever.
- Apnoea or cyanotic attacks.
- Purpuric rash.

2. Child aged 4 and over. More likely to present with the more classical signs of headache, vomiting, pyrexia, neck stiffness and photophobia. The presence of an ill child and purpuric rash is almost pathognomic of meningococcal infection and warrants immediate treatment.

As raised ICP is the rule in the child with bacterial meningitis the concern is the formation of coning, which is the direct cause of death in as many as 30% of deaths. If contraindications to lumbar puncture exist then *blood and throat cultures* are taken before prompt treatment with intravenous antibiotics. Blood cultures will identify the organism in 90% of cases within 24–48 hours with Haemophilus or pneumococcal meningitis but only 50% of cases of meningococcal meningitis.

There is no place for routine computed tomography before or after lumbar puncture in the child with clinically uncomplicated acute bacterial meningitis. Once stabilized a *CT scan* should be arranged.

Relative contraindications to lumbar puncture include:

- papilloedema;
- coma;
- hypertension;
- bradycardia;
- bradypnoea or irregular respirations;

- fixed dilated or irregular pupils;
- impaired doll's eye movements;
- recent or prolonged convulsive seizures;
- focal seizures;
- decerebrate or decorticate posture;
- focal neurological signs;
- septic shock;
- coagulation disorder.

Treatment

Attention to the patient's airway, breathing and circulation then:

1. On arrival in hospital the admitting doctor should without delay take blood for culture and a coagulation screen. If bacterial meningitis is suspected antibiotic treatment should be started immediately.

Afterwards take:

- throat swab, which should be plated as soon as practicable by a microbiologist;
- disrupt and swab, or aspirate any petechial or purpuric skin lesions for microscopy and culture.

2. An EDTA specimen should be taken at the time of first blood sample so that they may be sent for polymerase chain reaction studies if needed.

A baseline clotted blood sample for serological blood testing should be collected within 24 hours.

The Working Party recommend a **lumbar puncture** in all adult patients with suspected meningitis except when a clear contraindication exists or if there is a confident clinical diagnosis of meningococcal infection with a typical meningococcal rash. Antibiotics should be given first.

3. Antibiotic therapy. The consensus statement produced by the British Infection Society recommends the following:

- meningitis with a typical meningococcal rash be given 2.4 g benzylpenicillin intravenously 4-hourly or 2 g ampicillin intravenously 4-hourly;
- For adults aged 18–50 years without a typical meningococcal rash 2 g ceftri azone intravenously 12-hourly or 2 g cefotaxime intravenously 6-hourly;
- if lumbar puncture has to be delayed in patients without a typical meningococcal rash **OR** if the patient comes from an area of the world (Spain for example) where penicillin resistant pneumococci are common, then add vancomycin intravenously 500 mg 6-hourly or 1 g 12-hourly (or 600 mg rifampicin intravenously 12-hourly). For adults aged over 50 years without a typical meningococcal rash consider addition of 2 g ampicillin intravenously 4-hourly to ceftriaxone or cefotaxime as above;
- if there is a clear history of anaphylaxis to beta-lactams give chloramphenicol intravenously 25 mg/kg 6-hourly or 1 g 12-hourly. Vancomycin is given because of the possibility of penicillin-resistant pneumococci and the likely failure of chloramphenicol in this group. Additional co-trimoxazole should

be given in those over 50 years old. Neither chloramphenicol nor vancomycin is effective *in vivo* against *Listeria monocytogenes* meningitis, and co-trimoxazole alone has been used successfully for this infection.

4. Septic shock and adult respiratory distress syndrome. May necessitate ventilation and intensive care support.

5. Convulsions. With intravenous diazepam or phenytoin.

6. Hyperpyrexia. With paracetamol in the first instance.

7. Headache. May require treatment with codeine phosphate.

8. Fluid administration. Patients should be kept euvolaemic and not be fluid restricted in an attempt to reduce cerebral oedema. Hyponatraemia in children with bacterial meningitis is most induced by fluid volume depletion.

9. Inappropriate antidiuretic hormone secretion. Restriction of fluids and monitoring of the serum sodium.

10. Steroids. The Working Party consider the administration of steroids is appropriate in adults with meningitis but not with septicaemia. They suggest administering Dexamethasone 4–6 mg 6-hourly on admission, either shortly before or simultaneously with antibiotics to adults with an impaired conscious level, focal or lateralized neurological signs, markedly raised opening pressure at lumbar puncture or evidence of cerebral oedema on brain scanning. The evidence is supported for *Haemophilus influenzae* and pneumococcal meningitis.

11. Tuberculous meningitis. It is recommended that Prednisolone should be given in those with abnormal mental states or focal neurological signs.

12. Mannitol. Mannitol should be considered in patients with impaired conscious levels, lateralized neurological signs, markedly raised opening pressure at lumbar puncture or evidence of cerebral oedema on brain scanning.

13. Immunotherapy. The current status of immunotherapy and adjunctive therapy are uncertain.

14. Intensive care. Intensivists should be involved early. The Working Party recommend that the following patients require intensive care unit facilities and expertise:

- those with cardiovascular instability with hypotension not responding promptly to fluid challenges, oliguria persisting for more than 2–3 hours, or increasing metabolic acidosis;
- those with respiratory instability with an unprotected airway, dyspnoea/tachypnoea or hypoxaemia;
- those with neurological impairment and/or seizures;
- those with central nervous system depression sufficient to prejudice the airway and its protective reflexes.

Prevention of secondary cases of meningitis

- It is important to consider prophylaxis for close contacts of patients with meningitis.
- Report to the CCDC who will instigate chemo prophylaxis and vaccination.
- Contact tracing of tuberculous meningitis should also follow standard procedure.

Differential diagnosis

1. ***Differential diagnosis includes:***

   - posterior fossa tumours;
   - acute hydrocephalus;
   - cerebral abscess;
   - subdural haematoma;
   - bleeding from an arteriovenous malformation;
   - meningoencephalitis;
   - herpes simplex encephalitis;
   - Reye's syndrome;
   - intracerebral haemorrhage.

Further reading

Begg N. *et al.* Consensus Statement on Diagnosis, Investigation, Treatment and Prevention of Acute Bacterial Meningitis in Immunocompetent Adults. *Journal of Infection* 1999; **39:** 1–15.

Mellor DH. The place of computed tomography and lumbar puncture in suspected bacterial meningitis. *Archives of Disease in Childhood* 1992; 1417–1419.

Related topics of interest

Antibiotics (p. 50); Coma (p. 97)

MENINGOCOCCAL DISEASE

Meningococcal disease may present either as meningococcal meningitis or meningococcal septicaemia. There are in the region of 3000 cases per annum. The disease is seasonal, being more prevalent in winter months.

Two age groups are at particular risk, namely children under the age of two in whom group B predominates and young people aged 15–24 in whom group C strains are more common (this may occur in clusters). Mortality from meningococcal septicaemia ranges from 20–40%.

The prompt recognition and treatment of meningococcal disease is essential.

Management

Upon recognition of meningococcal disease (purpuric or petechial rash, or signs of meningitis/septicaemia) call for senior Accident & Emergency staff, anaesthetic or intensive care and paediatric input as appropriate.

Clinically shocked

Look for signs of early compensated shock:

- Tachycardia.
- Cold peripheries/pallor.
- Increased capillary refill time (>4 seconds).
- Decreased urine output (<1 ml/kg/hr).
- Tachypnoea/pulse oximetry <95%.
- Hypoxia on arterial blood gas.
- Base deficit (<–5 mmol/l).
- Confusion/drowsiness/decreased conscious level.
- Hypotension (late sign).

Observations and investigations

1. ***Observe:***

- Heart rate.
- Respiratory rate.
- Blood pressure.
- Perfusion.
- Conscious level.
- ECG monitoring.
- Pulse oximetry.

2. ***Take blood for:***

- Full blood count.
- Glucose.
- Clotting.
- Urea and electrolytes.
- Calcium.

- Magnesium.
- Phosphate.
- Blood gases.
- Cross match.

Treatment

Patient should be treated in the resuscitation room. Early involvement of senior staff including A&E, paediatrics, anaesthetists or ITU staff is essential.

- ABC and oxygen (10 l/min).
- Perform bedside glucose analysis. If hypoglycaemia present (glucose <3 mmol/l) treat with 5 ml/kg 10% dextrose bolus i.v. and then dextrose infusion at 80% of maintenance requirements over 24 hours.
- Insert 2 large i.v. cannulae or intraosseous needles.
- Give i.v. Cefotaxime (80 mg/kg) or Ceftriaxone (80 mg/kg).
- Aggressive volume resuscitation – use 20 ml/kg colloid as a bolus and repeat. Use 4.5% human albumin solution or fresh frozen plasma (FFP) or Haemaccel/Gelofusine.
- Observe closely for response/deterioration.
- Do not lumbar puncture.

If the patient is still shocked after 40 ml/kg volume replacement, call the anaesthetist and contact PICU.

- Continue boluses of 10–20 ml/kg of colloid.
- Consider peripheral inotropes (Dopamine, Dobutamine).
- Nasogastric tube.
- Urinary catheter.
- Consider cuffed ET tube and chest X-ray.
- Anticipate pulmonary oedema (consider PEEP).
- Central venous access.
- Consider adrenaline infusion (central) if poor response to volume resuscitation and peripheral inotropes.

Intubation

Atropine 20 mcg/kg (maximum 600 mcg) and Thiopentone 3–5 mg/kg and Suxamethonium 2 mg/kg (caution high potassium). Then morphine (100 mcg/kg) and Midazolam (100 mcg/kg) every 30 minutes.

Anticipate and correct:

- Hypoglycaemia.
- Acidosis. Correct metabolic acidosis if pH <7.2. Use 1 mmol/kg of sodium bicarbonate intravenously over 20 minutes. This is equivalent to 1 ml/kg of 8.4% sodium bicarbonate. In neonates give 2 mmol/kg 4.2% sodium bicarbonate.
- Hypokalaemia. If potassium is <3.5 mmol/l. Give 0.25 mmol/kg over 30 minutes intravenously with ECG monitoring. Caution if anuric.

- Hypocalcaemia. If total calcium is <2 mmol/l or ionized calcium <1 mmol/l. Give 0.1 ml/kg 10% calcium chloride over 30 minutes intravenously (max 10 ml), or 0.3 ml/kg 10% calcium gluconate over 30 minutes (max 20 ml).
- Hypomagnesaemia. Treat if magnesium <0.75 mmol/l. Give 0.2 ml/kg of 50% magnesium sulphate over 30 minutes intravenously (max 10 ml).
- Anaemia.
- Coagulopathy (fresh frozen plasma 10 ml/kg).
- Central venous access required CXR and urinary catheter.
- Consider adrenaline infusion if poor response to volume replacement and Dopamine/Dobutamine infusion.
- Transfer to ITU.
- Raised intracranial pressure.

Raised ICP

1. ***Look for signs of raised intracranial pressure such as:***

- Decreasing or fluctuating level of consciousness.
- Hypertension and relative bradycardia.
- Unequal, dilated or poorly responsive pupils.
- Focal neurological signs.
- Seizures.
- Abnormal posturing.
- Papilloedema (late sign).

2. ***If present treat:***

- ABC and oxygen (10 l/min).
- Bedside glucose.
- Steroids (Dexamethasone 0. 4 mg/kg bd for 2 days).
- Cefotaxime or Ceftriaxone 80 mg/kg.
- Treat shock if present.
- Do not lumbar puncture.
- Give Mannitol 0.25 g/kg as a bolus followed by Frusemide 1 mg/kg.
- Intubate and ventilate to control $PaCO_2$ (4–4.5 kPa).
- Sedate (and muscle relaxation) for transport.
- NG tube.
- 20° head-up position, midline and avoid neck lines.
- Phenytoin 18 mg/kg over 30 minutes for seizures (ECG monitoring).
- Urinary catheter (especially after Mannitol/Frusemide).
- Transfer to ITU.

Features of meningitis only

If clinical features of meningitis:

- Dexamethasone 0.4 mg/kg bd for 2 days.
- Cefotaxime/Ceftriaxone 80 mg/kg.
- Close observation and repeat review.

Diagnosis

Diagnosis is made using the following tests:

- Blood cultures.
- Throat swab.
- Skin aspiration/scrapings from skin showing haemorrhagic rash.
- Rapid antigen screen.
- EDTA specimen for PCR.
- Convalescent serology.

Prophylaxis of contacts

- Inform Public Health Department.
- Give Rifampicin (bd for 2 days)
  < 1 years 5 mg/kg
  1–12 years10 mg/kg
  > 12 years 600 mg.
- Or Ceftriaxone (single i.m. dose)
  < 12 years 125 mg
  > 12 years 250 mg.
- Or Ciprofloxacin as single 500 mg dose (adults only).

Further reading

Pollard AJ, Nadel S, Habibi P, Faust SN, Maconochi I , Mehta N, Britto J, Levin M. Early Management of Meningococcal Disease. Department of Paediatrics, Imperial College School of Medicine, St Mary's Hospital, London W2. *Archives of Disease in Childhood*, 1999; **80:** 290–6.

MISSILE INJURIES

The incidence of gunshot wounds is increasing in the UK. However they are still sufficiently rare that few doctors in civilian practice will encounter more than a few cases. The lessons learnt and relearnt in every major conflict is that antibiotics are no substitute for aggressive, early management of the initial wound.

Ballistics

The tissue damage caused by a missile is a consequence of the energy imparted to the tissue by the missile and the properties of that tissue. The velocity of the missile is the most significant determinant of its wounding potential and is demonstrated by the formula: kinetic energy = (mass × velocity^2).

A missile which passes through a tissue will impart only a fraction of its potential energy to the tissue. One that is stopped by the tissue will impart all of its energy. Fragmentation or deformity of the missile will lead to greater energy transfer to the tissues. In general high-velocity missiles cause more damage than low-velocity missiles.

Types of bullet

1. ***Military ammunition.*** These are clad in metal jackets which act to reduce deformation (a requirement under the Hague Convention).

2. ***Civilian and police ammunition.*** This ammunition is not clad in metal. The intention is to promote deformation, thus maximizing tissue destruction and reducing the chance that the missile will exit the victim's body. This reduces the probability that a missile exiting the victim's body will hit an innocent bystander.

Mechanism of tissue damage

Tissue damage occurs by one of three mechanisms.

1. ***Laceration and crushing.*** This is injury caused directly in the track of the missile. It is characteristic of low-velocity weapons such as hand guns and submachine guns. Unless the missile fragments or deforms on its journey through the tissue there will be little damage outside the missile track.

2. ***Shock waves.*** High-velocity missiles produce a shock wave travelling at up to 1500 m/s as a result of tissue compression in front of the missile. This shock wave may only last a few milliseconds, but generates a pressure of up to 100 atmospheres causing damage at a distance from the track. The shock wave propagates along blood vessels and may cause significant damage to solid organs.

3. ***Temporary cavitation.*** High-velocity missiles may produce a cavity in front of the missile path as tissues expand away from them. The cavity may be 30–40 times the diameter of the track. The pressure within the cavity is subatmospheric. As the cavity collapses debris and bacteria are drawn in leading to contamination of the

already damaged and devitalized tissues. The final cavity will be considerably smaller that the original cavity understating the degree of tissue damage caused.

Factors influencing tissue damage

1. *Mass and velocity.* As mentioned above the energy of a missile is proportional to its mass and the square of its velocity. Therefore a doubling of the velocity of a missile will lead to a quadrupling of its energy. This explains why high-velocity missiles generally cause more damage than low-velocity missiles.

2. *Instability in flight.* A missile which is aerodynamically unstable in flight will tumble when it enters a tissue. This will increase the energy transfer to the tissue and increase destruction.

3. *Fragmentation.* Fragmentation is more likely to occur with a high-velocity missile than a low-velocity one. Some missiles are designed to fragment by making the casing weak. The fragments produce multiple tracks in the tissues. Because fragments are lighter than the original missile they are more likely to be stopped by the tissues, this maximizes energy transfer to the tissues.

4. *The nature of the tissue.* The more dense and unyielding a tissue is, the more energy is transferred to it. Bone and solid organs are more susceptible to damage that gas-filled organs.

5. *Entrance/exit wounds.* The wound as the point of impact is determined by:

- The shape of the missile.
- The relation of the missile and its position relative to the impact site.
- Fragmentation/shotgun, bullet fragments, special bullet.

If there is only one wound, it logically must be the entrance wound.

Commonly the wound is round or oval with a surrounding 10^2 mm blackened area of burn or abrasion. The injection of gas into the subcutaneous tissue from close-range may produce crepitus around the entrance wound. Powder burns or tattooing of the wound edges may be present. Exit wounds are usually ragged, irregular or stellate. Do not assume that the trajectory of a bullet follows a linear path between an entrance and exit wound.

6. *Management.* As in all significant injuries the priorities for treatment are the ABCs.

The tissue damage should be assumed to be more extensive than the external injury suggests and surgical exploration and debridement carried out. All devitalized tissue should be excised and the wound left open to drain. Delayed primary closure may be indicated several days postoperatively.

The major complications are gas gangrene and tetanus caused by the clostridial organisms, *Cl. tetani* and *Cl. perfringens.*

Further reading

Owen-Smith MS. *High Velocity Missile Wounds.* London, Edward Arnold, 1992.
Ryan J, Rich N (eds). *Ballistic Trauma: Clinical Relevance in Peace and War.* London, Edward Arnold, 1995.

Related topics of interest

Antibiotics (p. 50); Major injuries – initial management (p. 215); Tetanus (p. 317)

MONITORING – PULSE OXIMETRY AND END-TIDAL CARBON DIOXIDE

Whilst there is no substitute for good clinical observation monitoring devices are essential to A&E management. Monitoring in the pre-hospital setting is simple and non-invasive but in the Accident and Emergency Department more complex monitoring is available.

The traditional indices include temperature, pulse rate, blood pressure, electrocardiogram (ECG), respiratory rate and forced expiratory volume (FEV_1). Additional non-invasive monitoring includes non-invasive automated blood pressure (NIBP), pulse oximetry, capnography, transcutaneous oxygen and carbon dioxide detection, and conjunctival oxygen and carbon dioxide detection. Invasive monitoring includes arterial, central venous, Swan Ganz and intracranial pressure monitors.

Pulse oximetry

The early detection of hypoxia clinically is difficult. Pulse oximetry allows for a continuous, reliable, non-invasive estimation of the PaO_2 and has been heralded as 'a fifth vital sign'. The value of pulse oximetry in the prehospital setting requires further evaluation, although its use as a non-invasive monitor in the A&E department is well established.

The potential errors of pulse oximetry must be understood by those interpreting the oxygen saturation. Pulse oximetry is based upon differences in the optical transmission spectrum of oxygenated and deoxygenated haemoglobin measuring the absorbance of light at two wavelengths, 660 nM (where there is a maximum difference in absorbance between oxygenated and deoxygenated blood), and the control wavelength of 940 nM. The probe is fixed to a finger, toe, nose, ear-lobe or forehead and contains an emitter and a detector for light at the two wavelengths. The relative amount of haemoglobin present in solution and its degree of oxygenation can be determined.

Studies have shown a close correlation between pulse oximeter saturation and arterial haemoglobin saturation in conscious volunteers during anaesthesia and in critically ill patients.

1. Uses

- To aid in detection of hypoxaemia.
- During apparent tonic–clonic seizures may help to identify patients with low arterial oxygen tension who need immediate intervention.
- During patient transfer in the hospital setting, in the pre-hospital setting where pulse oximetry was found to be of benefit in detecting and monitoring hypoxia in patients with airway obstruction, depressed respiration due to head injury, and in closed chest injuries.
- The monitoring of procedures carried out under sedation such as the manipulation of fractures and dislocations.
- For accurate monitoring of the systolic blood pressure.
- As a non-invasive assessment of peripheral arterial occlusive disease.
- For assessment of collateral blood flow to the hand.

- To monitor pregnant patients and their infants at delivery and on the neonatal intensive care unit on the fetus before and during labour.

2. ***Limitations of use include:***
- It will not reveal the patient with hypoventilation when being delivered high-flow oxygen.
- Poor perfusion – shock, hypothermia.
- Movement artefact.
- Severe anaemia.
- Methaemoglobin, carboxyhaemoglobin.
- Electrical interference.
- Optical interference e.g. nail polish.

3. ***Complications*** are rare but burns and skin necrosis have been reported.

End-tidal CO_2 detection

Capnography is a valuable tool to assess ventilatory failure. In conditions of cardiovascular stability, the end-tidal CO_2 concentration bears a constant relationship to $PaCO_2$. If the alveoli from all areas of the lung are emptying synchronously, end-tidal CO_2 will be synonymous with alveolar PCO_2.

1. ***Uses***
- End-tidal monitoring identifies inadvertent misplacement of an endotracheal tube in the oesophagus.
- To detect sudden changes in the breathing circuit (disconnection, leaks, obstruction, twisting of tubes, or ventilator or valve malfunction).
- To aid blind nasal intubation.
- To monitor cardiopulmonary resuscitation (return of spontaneous circulation precedes a palpable pulse). The measurement of end-tidal CO_2 as a guide to the probability of survival needs further evaluation.

FEFtm end-tidal CO_2 detector – this small, disposable monitor uses a colormetrically controlled reaction to allow estimation of the end-tidal CO_2. In the non-arrested patient it allows verification of tracheal location of the endotracheal tube, although careful attention to ensure the correct placement is still appropriate. In the arrested patient interpretation requires caution. It may indicate an absence of cellular metabolism, inadequate CPR or incorrect tube placement.

Further reading

Phillips GD, Runciman WB, Ilsley H. Monitoring in Emergency Medicine. *Resuscitation*, 1989; **18:** S21–S35.
Tremper KK, Barker SJ. Pulse oximetry. *Anaesthesiology*, 1989; **70:** 98–108.
Zorab JSM. Who needs pulse oximetry? *British Medical Journal*, 1988; **296:** 658–9.

Related topic of interest

Interhospital transfer (p. 194)

MYOCARDIAL INFARCTION

Liam Penny

In the UK there are estimated to be 200 000 admissions each year for myocardial infarction. Acute myocardial infarction most commonly results from thrombosis within an epicardial coronary artery, triggered by fissuring or rupture of an atheromatous plaque. Platelet aggregation and fibrin deposit on the plaque leading to clot formation and occlusion of the artery.

Approximately 50% of deaths occur within one hour of onset of symptoms usually due to an arrhythmia. The in-hospital mortality is age dependent, with a mortality of less than 5% for patients less than 55 years and 12% for patients greater than 65 years.

The diagnosis is based on two out of three findings:

- A classical history.
- Typical ECG changes (which may include including evolving Q waves, ST elevation).
- A diagnostic rise in serum cardiac enzymes (e.g. CK, CKMB, myoglobin, Troponin T).

Symptoms

The commonest presentation is central chest discomfort with characteristic features:

- Characteristically a constriction, compression or pressure.
- Radiation to the neck, jaw, arms and back.
- Angina is precipitated by exercise. However, an MI occurs at rest or limited exertion, etc.
- Associated with sweating, shortness of breath, nausea and vomiting.

The patient presents typically with pain that lasts longer than 30 minutes unrelieved by GTN. However the presentation may be atypical or detected incidentally. May or may not occur in someone with antecedent history of angina.

Management

Physical examination is rarely helpful but complications such as heart failure, heart valve lesions, and arrhythmias and risk factors such as hypertension, evidence of peripheral vascular disease, diabetes and hypercholesterolaemia may be detected. This should not delay prompt treatment.

1. Oxygen. Via a mask or nasal cannulae at a flow rate of 4–6 l/min.

2. Intravenous access. A large bore i.v. line should be sited and blood taken for serum potassium, cardiac enzymes, blood glucose.

3. ECG monitoring. Because of the high incidence of arrhythmias, especially VT/VF, during the early hours of infarction.

4. 12 lead ECG. Repeat every 15–30 minutes if not diagnostic of acute MI.

5. Analgesia. This is a high priority as the release of catecholamines potentiate arrhythmias and may extend the infarct.

- Make the patient comfortable.
- Entonox useful in the pre-hospital setting and nalbuphine has been used.
- Sublingual nitrate initially, unless the patient is hypotensive (systolic BP < 90 mmHg).
- If unsuccessful or pain severe, small (2.5–5 mg) intravenous doses of diamorphine should be titrated to the patients needs. This should be accompanied by an anti-emetic such as metoclopromide (10 mg).

6. Beta-blockers. The ISIS-1 trial showed that intravenous atenolol (15 mg in aliquots of 5 mg), followed by oral atenolol limits infarct size and reduces the incidence of ventricular rupture. Contraindications include heart failure, hypotension and patients with asthma (*ISIS-1*).

7. Aspirin. All patients should receive aspirin (300 mg chewed or soluble) as soon as possible because it reduces mortality and reinfarction rates (*ISIS-2*).

8. Heparin. If rtPA is used an intravenous heparin bolus (5000 units), followed by 1000 units/h adjusted to maintain the APTT twice normal. Heparin is not required with streptokinase.

Consider subcutaneous heparin if high risk of DVT or cardiac thrombus (large anterior MI).

9. Magnesium sulphate. The *LIMIT-2* trial showed that Magnesium sulphate reduces mortality after acute MI. However, data from ISIS-4 suggests no benefit. Magnesium should be considered for ventricular arrhythmias.

10. Angiotensin converting enzyme inhibitors. Long-term survival and quality of life are improved if angiotensin converting enzyme inhibitors are administered to patients with significantly impaired left ventricular function (SAVE). These are usually started when the patient is haemodynamically stable after 24 hours.

Thrombolytic therapy

The early administration of thrombolytic therapy reduces morbidity (left ventricular function, coronary patency) and mortality in patients with ST elevation MIs.

Thrombolytic therapy has limitations because normal coronary flow is achieved in only 30–55% of cases. Additionally 5–10% of patients who are successfully treated experience coronary re-occlusion exposing them to the hazard of re-infarction.

The time window for benefit, up to 12 hours from onset of continuous symptoms, with ST elevation or new left bundle branch block is unequivocal. Its use in patients with MI or after 12 hours is not likely to benefit ST depression.

Maximum benefit is attained if thrombolysis is given as soon as possible after onset of symptoms (*minutes = muscle*). Every 30 minutes of time saved results, on average, in one additional year of life for patients.

1. Streptokinase is the cheapest drug, but is antigenic and may cause a pseudo-allergic reaction. Streptokinase should not be re-administered. Neutralizing antibodies develop within days and may persist for years.

2. Alteplase *(rtPA)* is the drug of choice in patients with systolic blood pressure <90 mmHg and it is non-antigenic, and used in those patients previously exposed to streptokinase. It should be considered in those in whom possible urgent surgical intervention is required (e.g. pacing, angioplasty, CABG).

3. ***Newer thrombolytics.*** Molecules of tpA are becoming available.

   (a) Reteplase – this can be administered as a double bolus.
   (b) TNK – tpA – this can be administered as a single bolus.

Half dose tpA and gp iib/iiia receptor antagonist may lead to faster and more stable reperfusion.

4. ***The inclusion criteria for thrombolysis are:***

Basic criteria

- Cardiac pain >30 minutes within 12 hours of onset, unresponsive to GTN.
- ECG criteria either:
  ST elevation >2 mm in two contiguous chest leads
  or ST elevation >1 mm in two inferior leads
  or new bundle branch block.

5. ***Active contraindications to streptokinase thrombolysis include:***

- Active internal bleeding (melaena, haematemesis, acute SAH, CVA).
- CVA or SAH in last six months.
- Major trauma or surgery in last 10 days (includes liver or renal biopsies).
- Evidence of head injury.
- Full cardiac resuscitation in last 10 days.
- Suspected aortic dissection.
- Brain tumour.
- Acute pancreatitis.
- Oesophageal varices.
- Cavitating pulmonary disease (TB, aspergilloma, bronchiectasis etc.).
- Previous streptokinase.
- Persistent systolic BP <90 mmHg.
- Possible emergency surgery required (including internal pacing, angioplasty or CABG).
- Peptic ulceration within six months and not already on effective treatment.
- Bleeding disorder.
- Arterial or subclavian/internal jugular venous puncture within ten days.
- Diastolic or systolic hypertension >200/110.
- Pregnancy (caution during menstruation).
- Proliferative diabetic retinopathy.
- Infective endocarditis.
- History of severe renal or hepatic dysfunction.
- Established gut or lung tumour.

6. ***Adverse reactions include:***

- Pyrexia, allergic reactions.
- Rarely anaphylaxis.
- Transient hypotension.

- Reperfusion arrhythmias – especially idioventricular rhythm.
- Haemorrhage, including CVA.

7. ***Reversal of thrombolysis:***

- Give fresh frozen plasma.
- Give tranexamic acid (10 mg/kg by slow i.v. injection) and aprotinin.

Coronary angioplasty

In specialist centres acute primary angioplasty can be more successful than thrombolysis at recanulating occluded coronary arteries. It should also be considered in those patients with:

- Contraindications to thrombolytic therapy.
- Patients who re-infarct after successful thrombolysis.
- Patients in whom thrombolysis has failed.

Recently the benefits of primary angioplasty in acute myocardial infarction have been shown to be further enhanced by stenting which produces lower rates of re-stenosis after six months.

Further reading

ISIS-3. A randomised comparison of streptokinase vs. tissue plasminogen activator vs. anistreplase and of aspirin plus heparin vs. aspirin alone among 41 299 cases of suspected acute myocardial infarction. *The Lancet*, 1992; **339:** 753–70.

ISIS-2 (Second International Study of Infarct Survival) Collaborative Group. Randomised trial of intravenous streptokinase, oral aspirin, both, or neither among 17 187 cases of suspected acute myocardial infarction: ISIS-2. *The Lancet*, 1988; **ii:** 349–60.

OBSTETRIC EMERGENCIES

The Confidential Enquiries into Maternal Deaths in the United Kingdom 1994–1996 showed that 376 women died in this period giving a maternal mortality rate of 12.2 per 100 000 maternities. There were 134 direct deaths, 134 indirect deaths, 36 fortuitous deaths and 72 late deaths.

The causes of direct deaths (134) are as follows:

- Thromboembolism (48).
- Pregnancy induced hypertension (20).
- Amniotic fluid embolism (19).
- Early pregnancy complications (15) (12 ectopic pregnancies).
- Sepsis (14).
- Haemorrhage (12).
- Uterine rupture (13).
- Fatty liver of pregnancy (2).
- Anaesthesia (1).

The commonest causes of indirect deaths (134) are as follows:

- Cardiac disease (39).
- Epilepsy (19).
- Psychiatric causes (9).

In the UK the majority of Accident and Emergency departments are sited in District General Hospitals with on-site obstetric facilities. The majority of pregnant women with problems related to their pregnancy will usually be referred or will self-refer directly to such units. Instances when such direct referral does not occur include the pregnant patient who has been a victim of trauma, the patient who is unaware that she is pregnant or has concealed the pregnancy or when obstetric facilities are not on site. The pregnant patient presenting to A&E will usually present with vaginal bleeding, abdominal pain, trauma, precipitous delivery or with cardiovascular collapse. When managing any woman of child-bearing age it is wise to consider the possibility that the patient is pregnant until that possibility has been excluded by a negative pregnancy test.

In all cases where the possibility of feto–maternal transfer of blood exists (abortion, antepartum haemorrhage, ectopic pregnancy or trauma) the patient's Rhesus D status must be established to determine whether anti-D immunoglobulin administration is required. Anti-D immunoglobulin must be administered within 72 hours. Standard doses of anti-D are 250 IU where gestation is less than 20 weeks and 500 IU where gestation is over 20 weeks. Where gestation is over 20 weeks, a Kleihauer test should be performed to assess the degree of transplacental haemorrhage. If significant transfer has occurred higher doses of anti-D will be required.

Vaginal bleeding

Bleeding in pregnancy can be divided into bleeding where gestation is less than 20 weeks and bleeding where gestation is more than 20 weeks.

1. ***Causes of vaginal bleeding where gestation is less than 20 weeks:***

- Abortion (the birth of a non-viable fetus, generally less than 24 weeks gestation).
- Ectopic pregnancy (implantation of the ovum in a site other than in the uterine body).

2. ***Causes of bleeding where gestation is more than 20 weeks:***

- Placenta praevia (a placenta located partly or wholly below the lower uterine segment).
- Abruptio placentae (separation of a normally located placenta after 20 weeks gestation).

3. ***Other causes which may present at any stage of pregnancy:***

- Cervical erosions.
- Cervical polyps.
- Infection.
- Labour.
- Uterine rupture.

4. ***Investigations***

- Pregnancy test (ß HCG).
- Full blood count.
- Group and save (or crossmatch).
- Clotting studies.
- Rhesus D status.
- Kleihauer test.
- Pelvic ultrasound.

5. ***Management.*** Because vaginal examination may precipitate torrential bleeding in both ectopic pregnancy (gestation less than 20 weeks) and placenta praevia (gestation more than 20 weeks), vaginal examination should never be performed in cases of ante-partum haemorrhage before an ultrasound examination has been performed. In practice in the majority of A&E departments in the UK this means that the pregnant patient with vaginal bleeding is routinely referred to the on-call obstetrician for management. Aggressive resuscitation prior to transfer to the obstetric team may be required. Early use of blood (O negative if required) should be considered in cases where there is clinical evidence of shock.

Abdominal pain

Abdominal pain in pregnancy may be predominantly pelvic or upper abdominal pain. The causes of upper abdominal pain are the same as for the non-pregnant woman of the same age. It should be remembered that the distribution of pain in bowel pathology in late pregnancy may be different to that of the non-pregnant patient due to displacement of the bowel by the uterus. This is especially important in the diagnosis of appendicitis when failure to appreciate the atypical distribution of pain can lead to late diagnosis and increase the risk of perforation. The causes of pelvic pain in pregnancy can be broadly classified as those which are accompanied by vaginal bleeding and those that are not.

1. ***Causes of abdominal pain in pregnancy associated with vaginal bleeding:***
- Abortion.
- Ectopic pregnancy.
- Placenta praevia.
- Abruptio placentae.

2. ***Causes of abdominal pain in pregnancy not associated with vaginal bleeding:***
- Rupture or bleeding into an ovarian cyst.
- Torsion of an ovarian mass.
- Appendicitis.
- Intestinal obstruction.
- Renal colic.

3. ***Investigations***
- Urinalysis.
- Pregnancy test (ß HCG).
- Serum amylase.
- Ultrasound.

Other investigations are undertaken as clinically indicated (e.g. plain abdominal films if obstruction is considered).

4. ***Management.*** The management of abdominal pain in pregnancy depends upon the diagnosis. The majority of obstetric causes can be excluded after ultrasound examination and vaginal and abdominal examination.

Trauma in pregnancy

Even relatively trivial trauma in pregnancy may lead to significant intra-abdominal or intra-pelvic injury. All pregnant women suffering trauma warrant an obstetric review. Ultrasound examination of the abdomen and pelvis and fetal monitoring are routinely performed in most units. Rupture of the spleen, bladder and small bowel are all more common in the pregnant women after abdominal trauma than in the non-pregnant patient. Specific injuries associated with pregnancy include abruptio placentae and uterine rupture.

The prognosis for the fetus is intimately related to the management of the mother, maternal hypotension being associated with a fetal mortality of 80%. Because of the physiological changes accompanying pregnancy (50% increase in blood volume, 25% increase in cardiac output) the pregnant patient may lose up to 35% of her circulating volume before the classical signs of shock are evident. This difficulty in assessing the degree of shock in pregnancy is exacerbated because blood loss is often occult, being confined to the uterus, pelvis or abdomen. Administration of high-flow oxygen and aggressive fluid resuscitation are indicated.

Collapse in pregnancy

Specific causes of cardiovascular collapse in pregnancy include:

- Amniotic fluid embolism.
- Hypovolaemia.

- Myocardial infarction.
- Pulmonary embolism.

1. Resuscitation. The priorities for resuscitation in pregnancy are the same as in the non-pregnant patient. Modifications to the standard approach for the pregnant patient include:

2. Decompression of the inferior vena cava. The pregnant uterus may compress the inferior vena cava resulting in a reduction in venous return and cardiac output (supine hypotension). This may exacerbate existing hypovolaemia and may lead to cardiac arrest. The uterus can be shifted off the inferior vena cava either by manually displacing the uterus to the left or by rolling the patient onto the left-hand side or elevating the right buttock.

3. Aggressive fluid resuscitation. As noted above the classical signs of shock appear later in the pregnant patient than in the non-pregnant patient. Therefore aggressive fluid administration (including early use of blood) combined with decompression of the inferior vena cava early in resuscitation can improve outcome in arrest due to hypovolaemia.

4. Emergency caesarian section. In some instances of cardiac arrest prompt delivery of the fetus by caesarian section can be life saving for the patient. It is recommended that this procedure is considered in any cardiac arrest lasting for more than 5 minutes. It is therefore mandatory to involve an obstetrician early in the resuscitation of any pregnant woman.

Other conditions which may complicate pregnancy

1. Disseminated intravascular coagulation

Causes:

- Abruptio placentae.
- Amniotic fluid embolus.
- Eclampsia.
- Intrauterine death.
- Missed abortion.
- Sepsis.
- Uterine rupture.

2. Pre-eclampsia. This is characterized by hypertension (a blood pressure over 140/90 mmHg or a rise in diastolic pressure of 15 mmHg over pre-pregnancy level), proteinuria and oedema. Routine assessment of the pregnant woman therefore includes assessment of blood pressure, examination for the presence of oedema and dip-stick testing of the urine for protein. Most patients will carry a shared care record card which will usually include a record of previous measurements and will allow an assessment as to whether the patient requires referral.

3. Eclampsia. This is characterized by seizures in addition to hypertension, oedema and proteinuria. Although it may occur in the absence of preceding pre-eclampsia.

Management of eclamptic fitting:

- i.v. diazepam 10 g repeated as required.
- i.v. Chlormethiazole 0.8% 40–100 ml bolus then 60 ml/h.
- Phenytoin 18 mg/kg given at a rate of 50 mg/minute under ECG control to prevent further fitting.
- Emergency caesarian section to deliver the fetus may be required.

4. DVT and pulmonary embolism. DVT is more common in the pregnant woman than in non-pregnant controls. Embolism to the lungs occurs in 25% of cases. The diagnosis is made by ultrasound examination.

Pulmonary embolus may present as chest pain, shortness of breath, haemoptysis or cardiovascular collapse. Ventilation-perfusion scan will confirm the diagnosis.

In all cases of DVT and PE admission for anticoagulation is required.

5. Amniotic fluid embolism. This is caused by release of amniotic fluid into the maternal circulation. Mortality is 85%. Causes include:

- Abruptio placentae.
- Amniocentesis.
- Labour.
- Trauma.

Further reading

Confidential Enquiries into Maternal Deaths 1994–96. HMSO, London.

Cox C, Grady K. *Managing Obstetric Emergencies.* Oxford, Bios Scientific Publishers Ltd, 1999.

Stevens L, Kenney A. *Emergencies in Obstetrics and Gynaecology.* Oxford: Oxford University Press, 1994.

Related topics of interest

Abdominal pain (p. 1); Gynaecology (p. 168)

OPHTHALMIC EMERGENCIES

The great majority of urgent eye problems can be diagnosed with careful history-taking and with basic examination techniques. A slit-lamp microscope is invaluable, providing illumination and magnification especially for small superficial foreign bodies, penetrating wounds, the track of intraocular foreign bodies, flare in the anterior chamber and small abnormalities of the iris. Use of local anaesthetic drops, and mydriatic drops aid complete examination.

Examination

1. ***Visual acuity***

   - Check the *visual acuity* of each eye separately (other eye completely occluded with a card or palm of the hand). Patients use their own distance glasses (*corrected visual acuity*) or pinhole to correct any refractive error (*pinhole visual acuity*).

     Use a *Snellen chart* at 6 metres (record as 6/6). If this fails then test vision at 3 metres (3/60). Then one metre (1/60), count fingers, detect hand movement, perception of light or no light perception. If there is still no response test whether the patient can:

     (a) Counts fingers (CF).
     (b) Detect hand movement (HM).
     (c) Perceive light (PL).
     (d) Not perceive light (NPL).

     When there is a language problem the Snellen 'E' chart can be used.

     For young children, a single letter of varying size can be used (Sheridan–Gardiner cards). For younger children tests involve identifying pictures or preferential looking. For infants see if they will fix and follow a light such as a pen torch.

2. ***Check the pupil size, shape and regularity of margin.*** Any difference in the pupil size is termed anisocoria. When anisocoria is greater in darkness than in light this indicates a sympathetic paresis. When anisocoria is greater in light than in darkness this indicates a parasympathetic paresis. If the difference in pupil size is the same in both lighting conditions, the diagnosis is *essential anisocoria*, which is of no neurological significance.

   Check the *pupil reactions*. The relative afferent pupillary response (RAPD) is detected using the 'swinging light test'. Only test *accommodation* if the pupils or light reaction are abnormal.

3. ***Test the visual field.*** to confrontation of each eye. Central defects can be detected using the *Amsler grid test* (a 20 × 20 grid of 5 mm squares with a central fixation dot).

4. *Inspect the conjunctiva and sclera*. Look for evidence of inflammation, ulceration, oedema (chemosis), laceration, haemorrhage or focal abnormalities, e.g. pingecula or nodules.

5. *Evert the upper eyelid.* Ask the patient to look down, pull the lashes down and press a cotton bud at the upper border of the tarsal plate to evert the lid. Examine with a bright light and look for:

- A sub-tarsal foreign body which may be removed with a cotton bud.
- Follicles (collections of lymphocytes) prominent in viral infections.
- Papillae – prominent in allergic reactions.

6. *Measure the intraocular pressure.* This is measured using applanation tonometry or pneumotonometry. Normal intraocular pressure is 10–21 mmHg above atmospheric pressure. An estimate of intraocular pressure may be gauged by palpating the eye with two fingers above the upper eyelid when the patient is looking down.

7. *Inspect the cornea.*

8. *Stain with fluoroscein* and use a cobalt blue light to reveal areas of denuded corneal epithelium. Remove contact lenses as they will stain. If small scratches are seen in the upper cornea, evert the upper eyelid as a subtarsal foreign body may be present. Fluoroscein will reveal an abrasion, epithelial defect or dendritic ulcer.

9. *Examine the anterior chamber for:*
- Depth.
- Keratitic precipitus (KP) in iritis – clumps of cells on corneal endothelium.
- Flare and cells – light scatter by protein and particles found in inflammatory conditions.
- Fluid levels of blood (hyphaema) or pus (hypopyon).

10. *Look within the pupil and inspect the iris.* Look for evidence of an iris prolapse.Is the lens damaged, or displaced?

11. *Ophthalmoscopic examination.* A normal *red reflex* may be impaired by a corneal opacity, aqueous turbidity, pupillary exudate, cataract or vitreous haemorrhage.

12. *Retinal examination*. Consider dilatation of the pupil with a short-acting mydriatic e.g. tropicamide 0.5%, but beware of the older patient in whom acute glaucoma may be precipitated, and avoid its use in a head-injured patient. Pupil dilatation is advisable except in the following:

- The anterior chamber is so shallow that a light shone from the side in the plane of the iris throws the nasal part of the iris into shadow (the patient is at risk of angle closure glaucoma).
- The patient is under neurological observation.
- There is a square pupil with an iris-supported lens implant following cataract surgery.

13. *Check the ocular movements.*

Penetrating trauma and intraocular foreign bodies (IOFB)

*1. **These cause damage by:***

- Disruption of ocular tissues.
- Introduction of infection.
- Scar tissue formation.
- Reaction to a retained foreign body, e.g. iron which disperses gradually into the surrounding tissues including retina. Intraocular copper provokes an immediate and severe inflammatory reaction.

2. History. It is essential to maintain a high index of suspicion. High-risk injuries include hammering and chiselling injuries and those involving glass. Remember an IOFB caused by hammering metal may only cause slight pain on entry and no immediate loss of vision.

3. Examination. If a major penetrating injury is self-evident on gross visual inspection it is not necessary to perform a more detailed examination. Pressure on the globe, either directly or indirectly may result in prolapse of intraocular contents. Similarly, foreign bodies or blood clots must not be removed. Plain radiographs are essential if there is any suggestion of a metallic foreign body. Ultrasound scan or CT is required for non-metallic foreign body.

4. Signs and symptoms

- Loss of vision.
- Pain suggests an associated *endophthalmitis* or an inflammatory reaction to the foreign body.
- Corneal perforations always leave a full thickness scar.
- Limbal or scleral perforation may leave a subconjunctival haemorrhage, which, in this situation must never be ignored.
- A small hole in the iris is best seen by retro illumination.
- Always dilate the pupil to look for matching localized lens opacity, or focal retinal haemorrhages. Gonioscopy and three mirror examination of the posterior segment are essential when searching for an IOFB. If in doubt refer to the ophthalmologists.

Penetrating injury with an ocular laceration

It is essential to differentiate between partial and full thickness corneal lacerations because the full thickness may be complicated by endophthalmitis or a retained IOFB. Wounds may self-heal and be difficult to identify. Perform Seidel's test and, if negative, attempt to open the wound by applying pressure on the globe with a glass rod or cotton bud.

Retinal detachment

Separation of the retina from the retinal pigment epithelium usually results from the development of a retinal tear. Commoner in myopic patients.

1. ***Symptoms and signs***
- Progressive loss of visual field.
- Loss of visual acuity.
- Floaters and peripheral flashing lights (photopsia).
- A detached retina appears grey and wrinkled.
- Retinal tears (frequently multiple).

Acanthamoeba keratitis

Uncommon but increasing due to widespread use of soft contact lenses.

1. ***Symptoms and signs***
- Painful red eye – pain is often disproportionate to the size.
- Corneal infiltrates or ulcer.
- Unresponsive to antibiotics.

2. ***Management***
- High index of suspicion.
- Early diagnosis is important.
- Diagnosis is by corneal scraping or biopsy.
- Treatment is with propamide and polyhexamethylene biguanide.

Contact lenses

1. ***Contact lens use results in a number of other complaints:***

- Hypoxia.
- Corneal infiltrates.
- Acanthamoeba keratitis.
- Corneal ulcers/infectious keratitis.
- Giant papillary conjunctivitis.
- Allergy.
- Lost/stuck lenses.
- Contact lens-induced neovascularization.

Acute glaucoma

1. ***Symptoms and signs***
- Usually asymmetrical and present unilaterally; occasionally bilaterally.
- Associated symptoms – headaches, nausea and vomiting.
- Haloes around bright lights.
- Visual acuity reduced.
- Cornea oedematous and cloudy with circumoral infection.
- Pupil is fixed, mid-dilated and oval.
- The anterior chamber is shallow.

Management of acute angle closed glaucoma

Untreated severe visual loss and eventual blindness. Immediate treatment is medical with intravenous acetazolamide 500 mg. Topical pilocarpine 4% breaks the pupil block by inducing miosis. Insert one drop and wait 15 minutes. If no response (miosis) repeat up to four applications. Put pilocarpine 2% into the fellow eye as prophylaxis.

Acute anterior uveitis (iritis)

1. ***Symptoms and signs***

- Usually unilateral, pain.
- Photophobia.
- Redness maximal at limbus/ciliary flush.
- Impaired visual acuity.
- Pupil constricted with adhesions tethering the pupil and the lens (posterior synechiae).
- Keratic precipitants (KPs) on the lower corneal endothelium.
- Anterior chamber cells and flare.
- May be a hypopyon in severe inflammation.

2. ***Associated factors.*** Most causes are idiopathic. Other associations include:

- Infective – Herpes zoster, viral.
- HLA B27.
- Inflammatory bowel disease.
- Ankylosing spondylitis.
- Sarcoidosis.
- Syphilis.
- Tuberculous.
- Reiter's syndrome.

3. ***Treatment.*** Mydriatics such as cyclopentolate or atropine relieve pain and prevent formation of synechiae. Dilate the eye using topicamide and phenylephrine if not contraindicated. Refer to the ophthalmologist who will also prescribe topical steroids.

Chemical burns

The severity of the burn depends on the chemical and how rapidly treatment is initiated.

Alkalis tend to cause more severe injuries than acid because they break down the epithelium and the alkali radical rapidly penetrates deeper. The epithelium provides an effective barrier against weak acids, whereas stronger acids cause protein precipitation which creates a barrier to further tissue penetration.

1. ***Immediate treatment.*** Irrigate and remove any foreign material. Irrigate with copious amounts of physiological saline using an intravenous delivery system. Check pH in the fornices and continue irrigation until pH is neutral.

Topical anaesthesia and a lid speculum are usually required.

Retained material, e.g. plaster, cement must be removed from the fornices. The eyelids should be double everted with a retractor.

Stain with fluorescein and assess epithelial loss.

Mild chemical burns can be treated as corneal abrasions.

Severe chemical burns refer to ophthalmologist for admission.

Further reading

Elagling EM, Roper-Hall MJ. *Eye injuries – an illustrated guide.* Butterworths, London, 1986.
Elkington AR, Khaw PT. ABC of Eyes. *British Medical Journal,* 1990.

Related topic of interest

Maxillofacial injury (p. 226)

ORGAN DONATION

It is uncommon for staff in A&E departments to become directly involved with the issue of organ donation. The majority of tissues and organs that are currently suitable for transplantation must be harvested from heart beating cadaveric donors because they tolerate periods of warm ischaemia poorly. Some tissues may however be harvested from non-heart beating cadaveric donors up to 72 hours after death, e.g. heart valves, skin and bone. In the majority of patients dying in or shortly after admission from the A&E department the Coroner should be consulted before the matter of transplantation is discussed with the relatives.

Exclusion criteria for donation

- Age more than 70 years (60 for heart valves, no upper limit for bone or corneas).
- Hepatitis B surface antigen positive.
- HIV antibody positive.
- Malignant disease (except brain primaries).
- Systemic sepsis.

Transplant co-ordinator

If a patient is considered to be a potential candidate for organ or tissue harvest, the local transplant co-ordinator should be contacted before the matter is discussed with the relatives to ascertain whether the donor is suitable. If a local transplant co-ordinator is not available, the United Kingdom Transplant Support Service Authority (UKTSSA) can be contacted on 0117 975 7575.

The local transplant co-ordinator will provide local protocols to be followed. If no local protocols are available national protocols can be obtained from the United Kingdom Transplant Co-ordinator's Association (UKTCA) on 0191 213 1674.

Criteria for establishing brain stem death

Prior to undertaking formal tests of brain stem function, the following conditions must be satisfied:

- there should be no doubt that the patients condition is due to irremediable brain damage of known aetiology (e.g. post head-injury or intra-cranial bleed);
- there should be no evidence that this state is due to depressant drugs;
- primary hypothermia as the cause of unconsciousness must have been excluded;
- potentially reversible circulatory, metabolic and endocrine disturbances must have been excluded as the cause of the continuation of unconsciousness;
- the patient is being maintained on the ventilator because spontaneous respiration has been inadequate or ceased altogether (the presence of residual effects of neuromuscular blocking agents should be excluded by the elicitation of deep tendon reflexes or by the demonstration of adequate neuromuscular conduction with a conventional nerve stimulator).

Once these preconditions have been met the following tests for diagnosing brain stem death must be carried out by at least two medical practitioners who have been registered for more than 5 years, are competent in this field and are not members of the transplant team. At least one of the doctors should be a consultant. Two sets of tests should be performed. The two practitioners may carry these out separately or together. No time interval between tests is specified, but the interval should be adequate for the reassurance of all those directly concerned. The legal time of death is when the first, not the second set of tests indicate brainstem death.

Tests of brain stem death

- The pupils are fixed and do not respond to sharp changes in the intensity of incident light.
- There is no corneal reflex.
- The vestibulo-ocular reflexes are absent.
- No motor responses are elicited within the cranial nerve distribution by adequate stimulation of any somatic area. There is no limb response to supraorbitial pressure.
- There is no gag reflex or reflex response to bronchial stimulation by suction catheter placed down the trachea.
- No respiratory movements occur when the patient is disconnected from the mechanical ventilator. The $PaCO_2$ should exceed 6.65 kPa, that this value has been attained should be confirmed by direct blood gas measurement.

These criteria apply to children over 2 months of age.

Further reading

Department of Health. *A Code of Practice for the Diagnosis of Brain Stem Death: Including Guidelines for the Identification and Management of Potential Organ and Tissue Donors.* Department of Health, 1998.

OVERUSE INJURY

The term overuse injury refers to a heterogeneous group of conditions with a range of causes.

Pathology

1. Inflammation. Acute overuse leads to inflammation of the tendon sheath, which is characterized by the presence of crepitus. Chronic or recurrent injury leads to thickening and fibrosis of the tendon sheath which is characteristic of the condition tenosynovitis.

2. Ischaemia. Acute ischaemia may affect muscles occupying a tight fascial compartment leading to pain or in extreme cases compartment syndrome. Chronic ischaemia of a tendon may eventually lead to its rupture.

3. Stress fracture. This results from repeated stressing of a bone by a force insufficient to cause an acute fracture.

Specific conditions

1. Inflammation.

2. Paratendinitis crepitans. This is an acute condition associated with intense periods of increased activity, e.g. hammering or digging. There is tenderness, swelling and crepitus over the radial border of the forearm at the wrist.

3. Chronic paratendinitis. This is characterized by pain over the insertion of the Achilles tendon at the heel. The thickened tendon sheath can usually be palpated.

4. Ischaemia.

5. Ruptured extensor pollicis longus tendon. This is usually a late sequel to a Colles' fracture. The condition is probably secondary to ischaemia of the tendon rather than to the tendon rubbing on bone fragments of the original fracture.

6. Stress fracture. The commonest sites for a stress fracture are:

- Tibia (50%).
- Tarsus (25%).
- Metatarsals (10%).

The usual presentation is of localized pain over the fracture site. The pain is worse on weight bearing. X-rays are usually normal initially but re-X-ray after 10–14 days will often reveal the characteristic periosteal reaction around the healing fracture site. Isotope bone scan will show most fractures within 3 days of the injury.

7. ***Other overuse conditions***

- Chondromalacia patellae.
- Patellar tendinitis.
- Repetitive strain injury.
- Rotator cuff syndrome.
- Tennis/golfers elbow.
- Trochanteric bursitis.

Further reading

Wardrope J, English B. *Musculoskeleteal Problems in Emergency Medicine.* Oxford: Oxford University Press, 1998.

Related topics of interest

Anterior knee pain (p. 48); Calf pain-musculoskeletal causes (p. 78); Shoulder problems – soft tissue (p. 299)

PARACETAMOL

Paracetamol ingestion is the commonest toxin or co-ingestant taken in patients presenting to Accident and Emergency Departments. Paracetamol when taken alone accounts for approximately 100 deaths per year.

Hepatocellular necrosis is the major toxic effect and does not present until 72–96 hours after ingestion. A small number of patients will suffer acute renal toxicity which is almost always associated with severe hepatic failure. There are a few cases of renal toxicity in patients with mild or no hepatic damage. Loin pain, haematuria and proteinuria after the first 24 hours strongly suggest renal toxicity. Any patient should be considered at risk of liver damage if they have consumed more than 150 mg Paracetamol per kilogram, or more than 12 g in adults.

The time interval since ingestion is critical in when deciding the treatment. However, remember that patients often give inaccurate histories and if there is any doubt about the timing or the need for treatment it is essential to treat with the antidote. The antidote N-acetylcysteine is maximally effective when administered within the first 8 hours after ingestion.

Any suicidal patient presenting to the Accident and Emergency Department and any patient who deliberately or accidentally overdoses should have a Paracetamol level.

Guidelines for the management of acute Paracetamol overdose have been provided by the National Poisons Information Service 1999. This has been in collaboration with the British Association of Accident and Emergency Medicine at the Royal College of Paediatrics and Child Health. They are only guidance and state that clinical judgment should always prevail. In particular they stress the unreliability of relying on the timing of overdose. They also stress the importance of consideration of other co-ingestions.

Pharmacokinetics

Paracetamol is absorbed rapidly from the gastrointestinal tract with peak plasma concentrations within 30–120 minutes of ingestion. Peak plasma levels almost always occur within 4 hours, hence the importance of awaiting a 4 hour sample as plasma concentrations prior to this cannot be reliably interpreted because of the possibility of continuing absorption and distribution of the drug.

Once absorbed in therapeutic dosage the drug is metabolized in the liver by glucuronidation (60%) and sulphation (30%) and an estimated 4–7% eliminated in the urine. A small amount, approximately 4%, of any dose is metabolized by the hepatic cytochrome P450 system to an active intermediate metabolite N acetyl P benzoquinonemerine (Napqi) and is normally detoxified by conjugation with reduced glutothionine excreted in the urine as merturic acid and cystine conjugates. Unfortunately in overdose when glutothionine is depleted unconjugated toxic metabolites result in hepatocellular necrosis.

Symptoms of overdose

1. In the first 24 hours the patient may be totally asymptomatic, or otherwise complain of nausea, vomiting, anorexia. Hepatic toxicity occurs and there is usually then a latent period of 24–48 h when the patient will feel reasonably asymptomatic. In very severe cases hepatic toxicity may begin in 12–16 h.

2. In the second phase (24–72 h) the patient may complain of right upper quadrant pain. Blood parameters then become abnormal, elevation of liver enzymes and bilirubin, prothrombin time and renal function.

3. In the next phase (72–96 h), the patient develops significant hepatic necrosis with signs and symptoms of acute hepatotoxicity.

Complications include: coagulation defects, jaundice, renal failure, myocardial pathology (rare), hepatic encephalopathy and hypoglycaemia.

If patient survives they will have complete resolution of hepatic function occurring in a time frame of 4 days–2 weeks.

In an extremely large overdose (serum concentration greater than 800 mg/litre) the central nervous system and metabolic abnormalities may occur.

Investigations

1. ***Plasma Paracetamol level.*** This should be drawn at 4 hours.

2. If time of ingestion is unknown, but less than 4 hours may have elapsed, a level should be drawn immediately and repeated in 2–4 hours to show a peak level.

3. If the decision to admit and treat the patient is made additional blood should be drawn – INR, plasma creatinine, ALT, alanine aminotransferase (if unavailable AST aspartate transaminase), bilirubin, electrolytes, glucose, full blood count, platelets.

4. If the Paracetamol is within the toxic range the patient receives antidotal therapy. Liver function tests, bilirubin, prothrombin and creatinine should be checked for normality on completion of the treatment and before discharge. If any is abnormal or the patient is symptomatic further monitoring is required and advice sought from the nearest centre of the NPIS.

Management of adult patients who present within 8 hours of ingestion

1. There is little evidence that gastric lavage will benefit. Although the benefit has not been demonstrated for Paracetamol poisoning administration of activated charcoal may be considered if:
   - more than 150 mg/kg of Paracetamol has been ingested and
   - it can be given within 1 hour of the overdose.

2. Take blood for plasma Paracetamol concentration as soon as 4 hours or more have elapsed since the time of ingestion.

3. Assess whether the patient is at risk of severe liver damage.

4. Treat with antidote N-acetylcysteine according to treatment graph.

5. If NAC is started within 8 hours of the overdose it is reasonable to expect patients to be declared fit for discharge on completion. However, the INR, creatinine and ALT should be checked prior to discharge. Patients are advised to return if abdominal pain or vomiting develops.

Management of all patients who present 8–15 hours after ingestion

1. If a toxic dose of Paracetamol has been ingested start NAC immediately without waiting for the result of plasma Paracetamol concentration.

2. Check plasma Paracetamol concentration and all those treated with NAC measure the INR, creatinine and ALT.

3. Assess risk of severe liver damage and treat according to treatment line.

Management of all patients who present 15–24 hours after ingestion

1. Urgent action is required as the efficacy of NAC is limited more than 15 hours after overdose.

2. Start NAC immediately without waiting for the plasma Paracetamol concentration in patients who have consumed a potentially toxic amount of Paracetamol.

Management of all patients who present more than 24 hours after ingestion

All should have INR, creatinine and ALT and venous blood acid–base balance or bicarbonate measured. Any abnormalities in the tests should be discussed with the NPIS.

Staggered overdose

In patients who have taken several staggered overdoses over a short period of time the plasma Paracetamol concentration will be meaningless. Such patients must be considered at a serious risk and treated with N-acetylcysteine. They can be discharged after treatment or 24 hours from the last Paracetamol dose provided they are asymptomatic and the INR, plasma creatinine and ALT are normal.

High risk patients

Patients who regularly consume alcohol, take enzyme inducing drugs (e.g. Carbamazepine, Phenytoin, Phenobarbitone, Primidone and Rifampicin) and with conditions causing glutothione depletion (e.g. malnutrition and HIV infection) have increased risk of liver damage from Paracetamol poisoning and should be treated using a treatment line which is 50% lower than the standard treatment line.

Antidotes

Cysteine, Methionine and N-acetylcysteine have all been used successfully to prevent hepatotoxicity. Cysteine and Methionine both produce more adverse effects and Methionine is less effective, therefore N-acetylcysteine has emerged as the preferred treatment.

To be most effective N-acetylcysteine should be administered within 8 hours of ingestion.

Recent evidence suggests that when hepatic failure occurs N-acetylcysteine should be administered until the patient recovers or receives a liver transplant.

Dosage for N-acetylcysteine infusion adult

- 150 mg/kg IV infusion in 200 ml 5% dextrose over 15 minutes, then
- 50 mg/kg IV infusion in 500 ml 5% dextrose over 4 hours, then
- 100 mg/kg IV infusion in 1000 ml 5% dextrose over 16 hours.

Dosage for N-acetylcysteine infusion children (<12 years) body weight 20 kg and over

- 150 mg/kg IV infusion in 100 ml 5% dextrose over 15 minutes, then
- 50 mg/kg IV infusion in 250 ml 5% dextrose over 4 hours, then
- 100 mg/kg IV infusion in 500 ml 5% dextrose over 16 hours.

Body weight less than 20 kg: (From the Alder Hey Book of Children's Doses, Sixth Edition 1996)

- 150 mg/kg IV infusion in 3 ml/kg body weight 5% dextrose over 15 minutes, then
- 50 mg/kg IV infusion in 7 ml/kg 5% dextrose over 4 hours, then
- 100 mg/kg IV infusion in 14 ml/kg 5% dextrose over 16 hours.

Adverse reactions

- N-acetylcysteine may cause anaphylactoid reactions after intravenous therapy. They are probably related to high serum N-acetylcysteine levels. Iatrogenic overdose with N-acetylcysteine has resulted in a number of significant adverse effects and a few deaths.
- Local reaction around the infusion site.
- Generalized reaction usually occurs with loading dose within 30 minutes. Symptoms include nausea, flushing, itching, erythematous rash, urticaria, angioedema, bronchospasm and rarely hypotension or hypertension.
- If anaphylactoid reaction present stop N-acetylcysteine. Consider intravenous antihistamine ± steroids. Once the adverse reaction has settled infusing at the rate of 50 mg/kg over 4 hours can usually be resumed without complication.

Action of N-acetylcysteine

N-acetylcysteine is taken up by hepatocytes which act primarily as a precursor for glutothionine replacing reduced glutothionine stores. The maximal effect is best when administered within eight hours of ingestion. Its use is also advocated even after 24 hours and up to 36 hours if toxic levels of Paracetamol or overt toxicity is present. Its use in patients in Paracetamol-induced fulminant hepatic failure has revealed improved survival and reduced morbidity as measured by development of cerebral oedema. In this capacity the N-acetylcysteine works with regard to its antioxidant properties, also helping to decrease neutrophil accumulation and improve microcirculation and tissue oxygen delivery.

Paracetamol in pregnancy

Advice can be sought from the National Teratology Information Service (NTIS). This has prospective follow-up data of 500 pregnancies in which Paracetamol overdose has occurred. This service is funded by the Department of Health and provides a national 24 hour service. Telephone no. 0191-2321524 (office hours) 0191-2325131 (out of hours ask for person on-call for Poisons) Fax 0191-2615733.

Limited evidence (150 cases) suggest that Paracetamol overdose in the first 3 months of pregnancy does not cause an increased incidence of teratogenic effects. Overdose alone is therefore not an indication for termination of pregnancy.

The general principle of management in overdose in pregnancy is that the protection of the mother must take priority over the foetus. She should be assessed and managed as usual.

Further reading

Guidelines for the Management of Acute Paracetamol Overdosage, NPIS guidelines produced and distributed by the Paracetamol Information Centre, 1999. 78 Farquhar Road, London, SE19 1LT
Tel: 020 8670 5577 Fax: 020 8670 5445
Email: *gb@butlers.u-net.com*
Web site: *http://www.pharmweb.net/paracetamol.html.*

PERIPHERAL NERVE INJURY

Peripheral nerves unlike nerves of the central nervous system have the ability to regenerate themselves after injury. The success of this regeneration in terms of functional outcome is determined by the timing of repair and the accuracy of opposition of the cut ends. It is therefore essential that nerve lesions are detected early and referred for expert management.

Mechanism of injury

1. ***Compression.*** This may occur as a result of incorrect application of a plaster cast, e.g. common peroneal nerve compression leading to foot drop as a result of tight application of a below-knee plaster.

2. ***Ischaemia.*** Commonly the result of prolonged application of a surgical tourniquet, e.g. the nerves of the forearm.

3. ***Laceration.*** Usually the result of a penetrating injury due to broken glass, e.g. the median nerve at the wrist.

4. ***Traction.*** Due to a stretching force, e.g. brachial plexus injury following forced abduction of the arm in a motorcycle accident.

Types of injury

Seddon classified peripheral nerve injuries into three types.

1. ***Neuropraxia.*** Caused by blunt trauma to the nerve. The axon is anatomically intact, but there is no nerve conduction. Because the axon is intact there is no Wallerian degeneration. Recovery is spontaneous over a period of time, up to several months.

2. ***Axontomesis.*** Caused by a stretching injury or blunt trauma. The nerve fibres are disrupted inside an intact nerve sheath. There is Wallerian degeneration distal to the lesion. Because the nerve fibres are disrupted recovery is less predictable, but may occur, often with less than full functional recovery.

3. ***Neurotmesis.*** Caused by a penetrating injury or direct incision of the nerve. The axon is paritally or completely divided. Wallerian degeneration occurs distal to the lesion. If the nerve is surgically repaired good functional recovery may be expected in most cases. Recovery of function may again take several months.

Diagnosis

1. ***History.*** If the patient presents with signs and symptoms of a nerve lesion diagnosis presents no problem. Many patients however present with a wound in the region of a nerve which may or may not be associated with a nerve lesion. A high index of suspicion is required in such cases in order that the lesion is not missed. The mechanism of injury will often suggest the possibility of a lesion (e.g. cut with a sharp

object). Clinical examination should reveal that a lesion is present and the nerve involved. The cardinal symptoms are paraesthesia or dysthesia (abnormal sensation) and loss of function.

2. *Examination.* The site of the wound will suggest the likely nerves involved. The motor and sensory (gross and two point discrimination) function should be examined and the presence or absence of sweating of the skin over the territory of the nerve should be sought. If a peripheral penetrating wound is associated with arterial bleeding, particularly in the palm or digit there is almost certainly an associated nerve lesion.

- *Motor.* The motor function of the muscles distal to the lesion should be examined. Comparison of the pattern of motor deficit with the known nerve supply will suggest which nerve is supplied. If there is not complete loss of motor function the reduction in power can be graded thus:

  0 Complete paralysis.
  1 Detectable contracture.
  2 Power but not against gravity.
  4 Power against gravity but reduced from normal.
  5 Normal power.

- *Sensation.* Gross sensation may be assessed using pin prick and fine touch (e.g. cotton wool wisp). Immediately after an injury sensation may be nearly normal, therefore comparision with the normal side should be carried out (the patient should be asked 'is this the same on both sides', merely asking whether they feel the stimulus may elicit a positive response but fail to elicit the information that the sensation is reduced). The area of deficit should be charted out and will give some indication along with the site of the injury of which nerve is affected (there is wide variation in cutaneous distribution of many peripheral nerves).

3. *Two point discrimination.* This is of particular value in assessing peripheral nerve injuries affecting the hand. The normal resolution for two point separation is 3–5 mm. Any increase in this distance is abnormal and suggests a nerve lesion.

4. *Sweating.* Loss of sweating in the cutaneous distribution of a nerve is probably the best early evidence that a nerve lesion is present. A plastic pen is lightly drawn over the digit. If there is no sweat present then the pen glides smoothly over the skin with no apparent resistance. If sweat is present a resistance to movement of the pen is felt. This effect is best appreciated by comparision of the abnormal digit with a normal digit. The absence of sweat on its own should be sufficient evidence to warrant a referral for exploration of the wound.

5. *Management.* Closed injuries are more likely to result in a neuropraxia or axonotemesis. These can be treated conservatively. Such lesions require careful follow up to ensure that function is preserved whilst recovery is taking place.

If a neurotmesis is suspected the patient should be referred for formal exploration. The earlier this is performed, the better the outcome. In children there should be a very low threshold for referring for exploration as exclusion of a lesion by clinical examination may be difficult.

It is generally considered best practice for nerve repairs to be carried out by a surgeon experienced in the use of an operating microscope using either epineural or group fascicular repair.

Contraindications to primary repair:

- The presence of other life-threatening injuries. These should take priority, but document the nerve injury.
- Presence of infection. Delay operation until the infection is cleared.
- Patient unfit for operation.
- Nerve injury due to missile injury. Delayed repair may be feasible.

Factors influencing outcome from nerve repair:

- Timing of repair.
- Age of patient.
- Proximity of lesion.
- Accuracy of axial alignment of the nerve.
- Fascicular apposition.
- Degree of suture line fibrosis.

6. Brachial plexus injuries. The nerve supply to the upper limb is derived from the anterior primary rami of the C5 to T1 nerve roots via the brachial plexus. The roots enter the upper part of the posterior triangle of the neck passing between the scalenus anterior and scalenus medius muscles. The roots combine to form three trunks, upper (C5–6), middle (C7) and lower (C8–T1), which traverse the posterior triangle. Each trunk divides into an anterior and posterior division behind the clavicle which combine in the axilla to form three cords. The cords embrace the axillary artery as they traverse the axilla. Their names describing their relationship to it, lateral, posterior and medial. The lateral cord gives off the musculocutaneous nerve. The medial cord gives off the ulnar nerve and the posterior cord gives off the radial and axillary nerves. The terminations of medical and lateral cords combine to form the median nerve.

Brachial plexus injuries may be broadly classified into supraclavicular lesions (affecting the trunks) or infraclavicular lesions (affecting the individual nerves either singly or in combination).

7. Supraclavicular lesions. Upper trunk injuries (C5–6) cause the Erb–Duchenne lesion characterized by loss of abduction, external rotation and flexion at the shoulder in addition to loss of flexion and supination at the elbow. The arm hangs at the side with the elbow pronated and hand facing backwards (said to resemble the waiters tip position).

Combined upper and middle trunk injuries (C5–7) cause in addition to the features of an upper trunk lesion loss of extension at the elbow, wrist and digits.

Lower trunk injuries (C8–T1) cause loss of flexion of the fingers combined with paralysis of the intrinsic muscles of the hand (Klumpke paralysis). This injury may be associated with a Horner's syndrome due to injury to the cervical sympathetic chain.

8. ***Infraclavicular lesions.*** These are characterized by injury to one or more of the nerves derived from the brachial plexus.

Further reading

Burge P. Peripheral nerve injuries. *Surgery*, 1990; **20:** 59–63.

Related topics of interest

Fractures – principles of treatment (p. 155); Spine and spinal cord trauma (p. 307)

PNEUMOTHORAX – SPONTANEOUS

Pneumothorax describes air within the pleural cavity. Pneumothorax may be spontaneous or secondary to underlying disease such as asthma or emphysema, traumatic or iatrogenic. Spontaneous pneumothorax usually arises from a rupture of a small sub-pleural bleb. After the first spontaneous pneumothorax there is a 10% chance of reoccurrence and after a second pneumothorax this increases to 40%.

A District General Hospital with a catchment population of 200 000 may expect to treat 25 patients with spontaneous pneumothorax annually. Presentation is commonly in the healthy young adult, who tolerates a large air leak well and in the older patient with emphysema, in whom even a small pneumothorax may cause respiratory failure.

The British Thoracic Society have issued guidelines for the management of spontaneous pneumothorax which stress the advantage of *simple aspiration* over *intercostal tube drainage* and the importance of involving the respiratory physician in those cases that are not managed by simple aspiration alone.

Clinical presentation

Patients present with pleuritic pain and/or breathlessness. Rarely they may present with a life threat when the pneumothorax is under tension.

On examination expansion and breath sounds are reduced and the percussion note is hyper-resonant. Tracheal shift away from the affecting side will be present in a tension pneumothorax.

A plain chest radiograph reveals lung collapse and air in the pleural space.

Tension pneumothorax is a clinical diagnosis and should not require radiological investigations for confirmation.

Management

1. ***In chronic lung diseas*** e.g. emphysema, cystic fibrosis, respiratory compromise is commoner, drainage procedures less successful, and referral to a respiratory specialist more likely. This group of patients must be admitted, whether or not they have had aspiration.

2. ***The degree of collapse*** is defined as:
   - *Small* – small rim of air around the lung.
   - *Moderate* – lung collapsed halfway towards heart border.
   - *Complete* – airless lung, separate from diaphragm.
   - *Tension* – any pneumothorax with cardiorespiratory collapse. It requires immediate treatment. It is rare.

3. ***Significant dyspnoea.*** This refers to an obvious deterioration in usual exercise tolerance and necessitates aspiration, whatever the size of pneumothorax.

4. ***Simple aspiration.*** Infiltrate local anaesthetic down to the pleura, in the second intercostal space in the mid-clavicular line (alternatively use the axillary approach). Use a cannula (French gauge 16 or larger), enter the pleural cavity and

withdraw the needle. Connect both the cannula and a 50 ml syringe (Luer lock) to a three-way tap, so aspirated air can be voided.

Discontinue aspiration if resistance is felt or the patient coughs excessively, or more than 2.5 litres is aspirated (i.e. 50 ml removed 50 times).

Repeat chest X-ray in inspiration (an expiration film is unnecessary) and if only a small pneumothorax remains, the procedure is successful.

If the cannula is accidentally withdrawn from the pleural cavity, or becomes kinked, another attempt at aspiration should be considered.

5. Follow up. Arrange for a chest clinic appointment in 7–10 days. The patient must be given a discharge letter and told to attend immediately if any deterior-ation. Air travel or diving are contraindicated until radiographic resolution.

6. Inpatient observation. Observe overnight. If patient stable both clinically and radiographically, discharge with chest clinic follow up.

7. Intercostal tube drainage. Explanation of the procedure to the patient is essential. In the anxious patient premedication with a small dose of midazolam may be necessary.

The site of insertion is the 4th, 5th or 6th intercostal space in the mid-axillary line, on the ipsilateral side (which should be double checked with the chest radiograph).

Position the patient supine with the head of the bed elevated 30° and the patient's arm behind the head, resting away from the chest wall. Mark the site of insertion with a ballpoint or similar pen.

Sterile skin preparation and use of gloves are essential.

Use a 20–24 French gauge (adult) drain and double check by dismantling and reassembling it. Ensure that all the connections fit tightly and that the under-water bottle containing sterile water is ready.

After palpating the intercostal space, raise an intradermal bleb of local anaesthetic and then infiltrate the deeper tissues down to the parietal pleura, particularly around the periosteum on the upper surface of the lower rib (remember that the neurovascular bundle is on the lower surface). At first use a blue, and then green needle with at least 10–20 ml of either 0.5% bupivacaine plus adrenaline or 1% lignocaine. Aspirate intermittently, looking for air in the syringe to confirm that the pleural space has been entered.

When the local anaesthetic has worked, make an incision in the skin and subcutaneous fat; this should be less than 2 cm to ensure a tight fit of the drain. Then insert two horizontal sutures across the incision, leaving them loose for subsequent sealing of the wound on drain removal. Using blunt dissection with forceps or a scalpel, make a wide tract through the intercostal muscles down to and through the parietal pleura.

Remember that the sharp metal point of a trocar does not cut or separate tissue and can be lethal if inserted forcibly.

Once the tube is in the pleural space, withdraw the metal trocar 5 cm and advance the tube in an apical direction. Remove the trocar and connect to the underwater seal, securing it firmly with a suture (one loop through the skin and multiple ties in at least four places on the tube itself). Loop the tube and secure it again with plaster so that it cannot fall out. Ensure that the tube will not kink.

Prescribe adequate oral and intramuscular analgesia.

8. Needle thoracocentesis. A tension pneumothorax should be immediately decompressed by needle thoracocentesis through the second intercostal space in the mid-clavicular line.

Initial management of pneumothorax

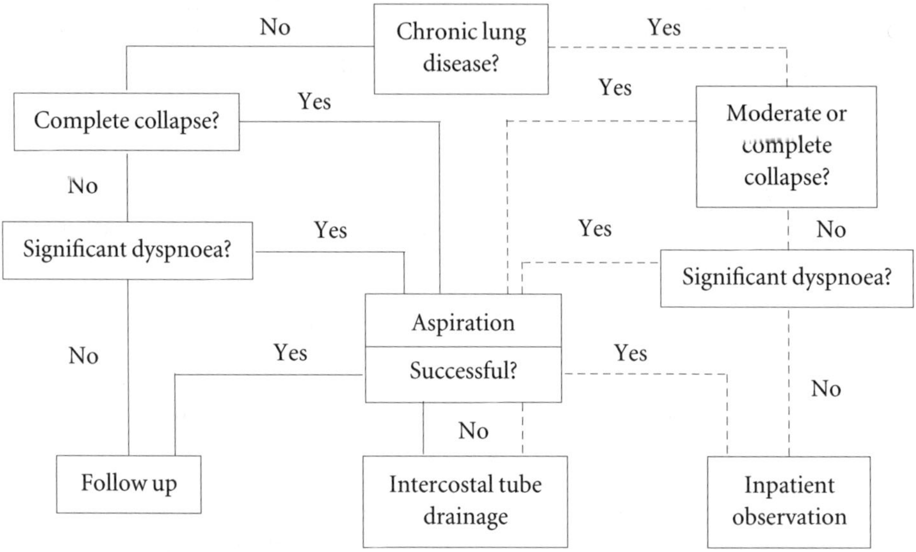

Management of intercostal drains

1. Chest X-ray. Keep the underwater seal below the level of the chest so clamping is unnecessary as it is potentially dangerous. An inspiratory chest X-ray is adequate to confirm positioning of drain.

2. Removal of chest drain. Bubbling should have stopped for at least 24 hours. Before removal consider pre-medication. After removing the suture that holds the drain in place, withdraw the tube while the patient holds his breath in full inspiration. Use the two remaining sutures to seal the wound.

3. Check chest drain. If lung has not re-inflated and there is no bubbling then the tube is blocked or kinked – this should be corrected. Otherwise the tube has become displaced – a replacement should be inserted through a clean incision.

4. Follow up. Arrange for a Chest Clinic appointment in 7–10 days. The patient should be issued a discharge letter with information informing them to return immediately in the event of deterioration. Air travel should be avoided until the radiographic evidence of the pneumothorax has resolved.

Respiratory physician's opinion

Seek advice from the Respiratory Physician for the following:

- Assessing why re-expansion has not occurred (e.g. air leaking around the drain site, tube displaced or blocked, large persistent leak).
- The use of suction to re-expand the lung.
- Whether early thoracic surgery would be appropriate, e.g. failure of conservative measures, need to prevent recurrence.
- Consideration of chemical pleurodesis.
- Management of surgical emphysema.

Management of intercostal drains

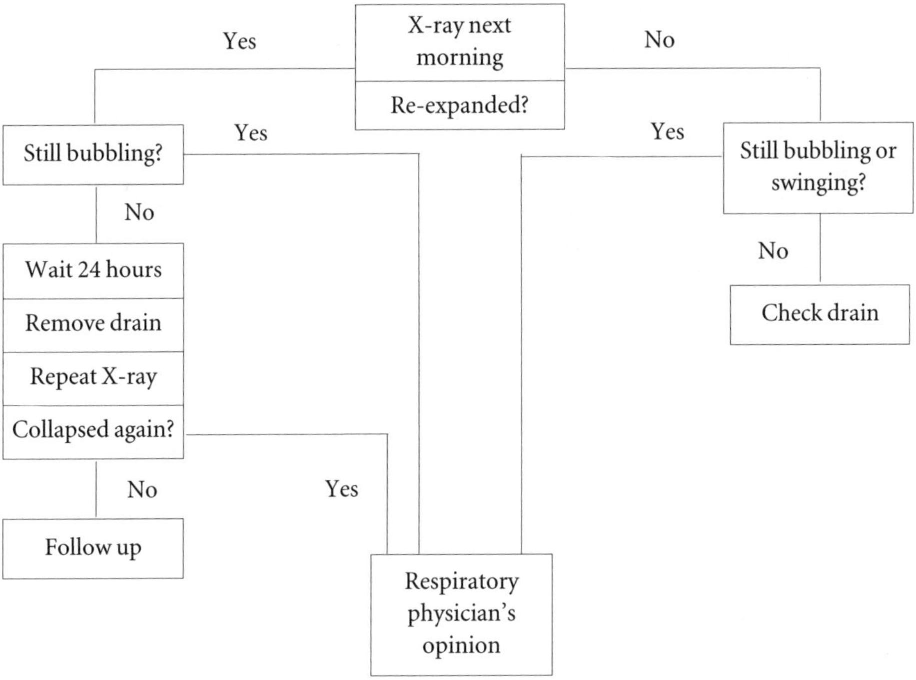

Further reading

Miller AC, Harvey JE on behalf of Standards of Care Committee, British Thoracic Society. Guidelines for the Management of Spontaneous pneumothorax. *British Medical Journal*, 1993; **307:** 114–6.

Peek GJ, Morcos S, Cooper G. The pleural cavity. *British Medical Journal*, 2000, **32:** 1318–21.

POST-TRAUMATIC STRESS DISORDER

Traumatic events are an important source of psychological morbidity. Raphael (1986) concluded that 30–40% of those exposed to a significant disaster showed evidence of significant psychological morbidity one year later. Whereas few now doubt the impact of well publicized mass disasters such as the sinking of the Herald of Free Enterprise, the King's Cross Fire and other disasters, all of which have accumulated their own literature, attention has also turned to the impact of more personal, less publicized trauma such as road traffic accidents or assaults. Mayou et al (1993) reported in adults that one year after a road traffic accident a quarter of those followed up had defined psychiatric disorder, with 11% showing evidence of post-traumatic stress disorder (PTSD). Stallard et al (1998) reported in children that one in three involved in everyday road traffic accidents was found to suffer from PTSD. This was more common in girls but was not altered by the severity of the physical injuries but more the child's perception of the event as life-threatening. The current best estimate of the prevalence of PTSD suggests it has a lifetime prevalence of 5% in males and 10% in females (Kessler 1993).

PTSD is chronic or recurring in a high proportion of patients and is associated with increased mortality, subsequent psychiatric illness, accidental and non-accidental death.

The medical profession and other emergency care staff involved in accident and emergency work are now more fully aware of the psychological aspects of trauma.

Definition

The diagnostic criteria for PTSD initially outlined by the American Psychiatric Association in 1980 and later revised in 1987 are summarized below:

1. The person has experienced an event that is outside the range of usual human experience and which would be markedly distressing to almost anyone, e.g. serious threat to one's life or physical integrity; serious threat or harm to one's children, spouse or other close relatives and friends; sudden destruction of one's home or community; or seeing another person who has recently been or is being seriously injured or killed as the result of an accident or physical violence.

2. The traumatic event is persistently re-experienced in at least one of the following ways.

- Recurrent and intrusive distressing recollections of the event (in young children, repetitive play in which themes or aspects of the trauma are expressed).
- Recurrent distressing dreams of the event.
- Sudden acting or feeling as if the traumatic events were recurring (includes a sense of reliving the experience, illusions, hallucinations, and dissociative (flashback) episodes, even those that occur upon awakening or when intoxicated.
- Intense psychological distress at exposure to events that symbolize or resemble an aspect of the traumatic event including anniversaries of the trauma.

3. Persistent avoidance of stimuli associated with the trauma or numbing of general responsiveness (not present before the trauma) as indicated by at least three of the following:

- Efforts to avoid thoughts or feelings associated with the trauma.
- Efforts to avoid activities or situations that arouse recollections of the trauma.
- Inability to recall an important aspect of the trauma (psychogenic amnesia).
- Markedly diminished interest in significant activities (in young children, loss of recently acquired developmental skills such as toilet training or language skills).
- Feeling of detachment or estrangement from others.
- Restricted range of affect, e.g. unable to have loving feelings.
- Sense of a foreshortened future, e.g. does not expect to have a career, marriage, or children, or a long life.

4. Persistent symptoms of increased arousal (not present before the trauma) as indicated by at least two of the following:

- Difficulty falling or staying asleep.
- Irritability or outbursts of anger.
- Difficulty concentrating.
- Hypervigilance.
- Exaggerated startle response.
- Physiologic reactivity upon exposure to events that symbolize or resemble an aspect of the traumatic event (e.g. a woman who was raped in an elevator breaks out in a sweat when entering any elevator).

5. Duration of the disturbance (symptoms in 2, 3 and 4) of at least one month.

Management

1. ***Debriefing*** involves promoting some form of emotional processing/catharsis or ventilation by encouraging recollection/ventilation/reworking of the traumatic event.

There is no doubt that debriefing is now routinely offered in a number of settings internationally, including the victims of mass disasters, or individuals involved in traumatic incidents in the workplace. Debriefing is usually offered on a voluntary basis, but there are instances, such as debriefing of bank employees in both the UK and Australia, or in some UK police forces, who are victims of trauma, when it can be compulsory. This is in order to reduce the threat of litigation concerning the development of post-traumatic stress disorder. The assumption of such policies is naturally that debriefing can prevent the onset of PTSD.

Debriefing has two principal intentions. The first is to reduce the psychological distress that is found after traumatic incidents. The second, related intention is to prevent the development of psychiatric disorder, usually PTSD.

The effectiveness of debriefing in achieving either of these aims remains unknown. Exponents of debriefing draw attention to its popularity, and claim that it is meeting important needs (e.g. Robinson & Mitchell 1995). Others are more cautious. Recent review (Shalev, 1994; Raphael et al, 1995; Raphael et al, 1996; Rose, 1997) drew attention to the lack of randomized controlled trials.

Single session individual debriefing did not reduce psychological distress nor prevent the onset of post-traumatic stress disorder. Those who received the intervention showed no significant short term (3–5 months) reduction in the risk of PTSD (pooled odds ratio 1.0, 95% CI 0.6–1.8). At one year one trial reported that there was a significantly increased risk of PTSD in those receiving debriefing (odds ration 2.8, 95% CI 1.1–7.5). The pooled odds ration for the two trials with follow ups just included unity (odds ration 2.0, 95% CI 0.9–4.5).

There was also no evidence that debriefing reduced general psychological morbidity, depression or anxiety.

There is no current evidence that psychological debriefing is a useful treatment for the prevention of post-traumatic stress disorder after traumatic incidents. Compulsory debriefing of victims of trauma should cease.

At present the routine use of individual briefing cannot be recommended. It would be more appropriate to focus resources on identifying and treating those with recognizable psychiatric disorders arising from trauma such as acute adjustment disorder, depression and PTSD.

2. The development of programmes such as *group critical incident or stress debriefing*, which is usually provided in groups by mental health professionals and peer support workers needs further evaluation. It has been suggested that planning for this should be incorporated into the Major Incident Plan.

Further reading

Mayou R, Bryant B, Duthie R. Psychiatric consequences of road traffic accidents. *British Medical Journal*, 1993; **307:** 647–51.

Stallard P, Velleman R, Baldwin S. Prospective study of post-traumatic stress disorder in children involved in road traffic accidents. *British Medical Journal*, 1998; **317:** 1619–23.

Wessely S, Rose S, Bisson J. *Brief psychological interventions ("debriefing") for trauma-related symptoms and the revention of post traumatic stress disorder.* The Cochrane Library, December 1998, 1–31.

RAPID SEQUENCE INTUBATION

Emergency airway management is the cornerstone of Emergency Medicine. The National Emergency Airway Management Course has been developed by Dr. Ron M. Walls and his colleagues. This course has recently been introduced in the UK and not only covers rapid sequence intubation (RSI) but also the management of the difficult airway and failed airway.

RSI is the administration of an induction agent followed immediately by a rapidly acting neuromuscular blocking agent to induce unconsciousness and motor paralysis for tracheal intubation.

It is always assumed that the patient is non-fasted and therefore at risk of aspiration.

There are no absolute contraindications and the technique is divided into seven discrete steps – the 7 Ps of RSI:

1. **P**reparation.
2. **P**reoxygenation.
3. **P**retreatment.
4. **P**aralysis with induction.
5. **P**rotection and positioning.
6. **P**lacement with proof.
7. **P**ost-intubation management.

The success rate of RSI approaches 100% in the emergency unit. Complications include unrecognized oesophageal intubation, aspiration of gastric contents, alterations in heart rate and blood pressure and complications as a consequence of the induction agents.

Rapid sequence intubation timing

- Zero–10 min, Preparation:
  1. monitoring (SpO_2, ECG, BP);
  2. laryngoscope and BVM;
  3. endotracheal tube, stylet, syringe;
  4. **all** medications, including long acting maintenance sedation and paralysis;
  5. suction (Yankauer and ET tube suction catheter);
  6. IV (patent);
  7. assess for difficult intubation (the **LEMON** law):
     L – *L*ook externally;
     E – *E*valuate the 3-3-2 rule (3 finger mouth opening, 3 finger mentum-to-hyoid and 2-finger floor-of-mouth to cartilage);
     M – *M*allampati (grade from class I to class IV);
     O – *O*bstruction?;
     N – *N*eck mobility;
  8. immediate access to rescue devices.

- Zero–5 min, Preoxygenation (100% oxygen)
- Zero–3 min, Pretreatment (**LOAD**):
  (a) **L**idocaine. For reactive airway disease or ↑ ICP;

(b) **O**pioid (fentanyl). When sympathetic responses should be blunted (↑ ICP, aortic dissection, ruptured aortic or berry aneurysm, ischaemic heart disease);
(c) **A**tropine. For children ≤ 10 years old;
(d) **D**efasciculation. For ↑ ICP > 5 years/20 kg, penetrating eye injuries.

- Zero, Paralysis + induction.
- Zero + 15 sec, Protection: apply Sellick's manoeuvre and position for laryngoscopy.
- Zero + 45 sec, Placement with Proof: Perform intubation and confirm placement clinically and with $ETCO_2$.
- Zero + 1 min, Post Intubation management:
  (a) monitor haemodynamics and oxygen saturation;
  (b) sedation and long term paralysis if indicated;
  (c) appropriate ventilator settings.

Generic sequence: (for 70 kg adult)

- Zero–5 min, 100% oxygen.
- Zero, etomidate 20 mg; Succinylcholine 100 mg.

Increased ICP

- Zero–5 min, 100% oxygen.
- Zero–3 min, lidocaine 100 mg; vecuronium 1 mg; fentanyl 200 μg.
- Zero, etomidate 20 mg; succinylcholine 100 mg.

Asthma/COPD

- Zero–5 min, 100% oxygen.
- Zero–3 min, lidocaine 100 mg;
- Zero, ketamine 100 mg; succinylcholine 100 mg.

Fatal hyperkalaemia risk: (i.e. burns/crush injuries > 72 h, denervation process)

- Zero–5 min, 100% oxygen; etomidate 20 mg; rapacuronium 100 mg or rocuronium 70 mg.

Further reading

Ron M Walls, Robert C Luten, Michael F Murphy, Robert E Schneider. *Manual of Emergency Airway Management.* Lippincott Williams & Wilkins, 2000.

SCAPHOID FRACTURE

Scaphoid fracture results from a fall onto the outstretched hand or from forced dorsiflexion of the wrist (classically from a kickback from a car starting handle). The fracture is rare in the young and elderly, but does occur. The importance of the injury lies in the risk of non-union, avascular necrosis, and eventually osteoarthritis if the fracture is missed or treated inappropriately. However even optimal treatment of the correctly diagnosed fracture does not guarantee that such complications will not occur. Failure to diagnose or adequately manage such cases leading to complications is a common cause of litigation.

Anatomy

The scaphoid bone is part of the proximal row of carpal bones of the wrist. It articulates with the radius, lunate, capitate, trapezium and trapezoid. The complications of scaphoid fracture are due to anomalies in its blood supply in some individuals. The blood supply to the bone is via small vessels entering the bone along the ligamentous ridge running obliquely along the bone between the two articular surfaces on its proximal and distal surfaces. In most cases these vessels are distributed throughout the ridge. The blood supply to a fractured fragment is maintained. In a proportion of individuals the blood supply to the vessels enters the distal part of the ridge. Fractures involving the waist and proximal pole in such individuals will disrupt the blood supply to the proximal fragment leading to avascular necrosis. Non-union may result from failure to adequately immobilize the fracture or delays in immobilizing the fracture.

Clinical features

There is no pathognomonic test for the presence of a scaphoid fracture. The following should be looked for in any patient (irrespective of age) who presents with pain in the wrist after a fall or forced dorsiflexion:

- Swelling over the anatomical snuffbox.
- Tenderness in the anatomical snuffbox. This is relatively non-specific. When eliciting this sign both wrists should be examined simultaneously. Pressing in the normal snuffbox elicits some tenderness in most individuals!
- Tenderness over the scaphoid tubercle. This is located on the palmar aspect of the wrist underlying the crease line of the wrist.
- Tenderness over the dorsum of the scaphoid.
- Pain on telescoping the thumb (axial compression).
- Pain on forced dorsiflexion of the wrist.
- Weak grip, particularly when pinching the index finger and thumb together.
- Pain on moving the wrist.

When one or more of these signs are elicited in association with the appropriate mechanism of injury and in the absence of another injury to explain the findings then scaphoid fracture should be suspected (scaphoid fracture may co-exist with other injuries).

Differential diagnosis

The signs and symptoms of scaphoid fracture may occur in association with other injuries which include:

- Fracture of the radial styloid.
- Fracture of the base of the first metacarpal.
- Wrist sprain.
- Carpal instability (ligamentous instability of the carpus following an injury).
- Other more complex carpal fractures and/or dislocations.

Radiographic findings

If a scaphoid fracture is suspected then scaphoid views (rather than wrist views) should be requested. Scaphoid views consist of the standard AP and lateral wrist views with two additional oblique views (pronation and supination obliques).

Commonly there will be no fracture visible on the X-ray. This is partly because most patients X-rayed have no fracture and partly because a proportion of scaphoid fractures are not visible on the initial films.

Care should be taken to examine the films for other fractures (see above). Bone cysts, non-union and avascular necrosis from old fractures may also be seen.

Classification

Figures vary from study to study.

- Distal third fracture (20%) including fracture of the tubercle, distal pole and distal third.
- Middle third (70%).
- Proximal third (10%).

Management

If a fracture is seen the wrist is immobilized in a scaphoid plaster and the patient is referred to the next fracture clinic.

The management of the patient with the clinically suspected scaphoid fracture and normal initial X-ray varies. Check and follow your own local protocols. A common method of management is outlined here.

If the initial X-ray shows no fracture there may still be a fracture present. The wrist is immobilized in a tubigrip, scaphoid plaster or Futuro® splint and reviewed at 10–14 days. If clinical examination reveals no tenderness the patient is reassured and discharged without further X-rays. If tenderness is present the wrist is re-X-rayed looking for a fracture. If a fracture is present the wrist is immobilized in a scaphoid plaster and the patient referred to the next fracture clinic. In patients with persistent tenderness and normal second X-rays a bone scan may exclude a fracture and save the patient from prolonged periods of immobilization.

Complications

Non-union occurs in 10% of distal third fractures and 15–20% of proximal third fractures. It may be asymptotic in which case it can be treated conservatively. In symptomatic cases treatment is by bone grafting and screw fixation.

Avascular necrosis of the proximal fragment occurs in 15–40% of proximal third fractures. Treatment is by excision of the avascular component with or without replacement by a silastic spacer. Selective carpal fusion is an alternative but less commonly used treatment.

Further reading

Brondum V, Larsen CF, Skor O. Fracture of the carpal scaphoid: frequency and distribution in a well defined population. *European Journal of Radiology*, 1992; **15**(2): 118–21.

McRae R. Practical Fracture Management. Edinburgh, Churchill Livingstone, 1994.

Tiel-van Buul MM, Roolker W, Broekhuizen AH, Van Beek EJ. The diagnostic management of suspected scaphoid fracture. *Injury*, 1997; **28**(1): 1–8.

Related topics of interest

Fractures – principles of treatment (p. 155); Wrist injury (p. 337)

SEDATION

The purpose of sedation in the A&E department is to reduce anxiety while maintaining the co-operation of the patient, in particular the ability to respond to commands. This is in contrast to the purpose of anaesthesia which is to achieve a state of unconsciousness, analgesia and muscle relaxation. All too often attempts to achieve sedation in the A&E department leave the patient in a state of unconsciousness or near unconsciousness. Sedation is facilitated by the use of techniques to achieve analgesia (local blocks, analgesic drugs or splintage). Sedation implies that the patient can maintain their own airway, anaesthesia implies that they cannot. Therefore while elective anaesthesia requires that the patient be starved for a period pre-procedure (usually 6 hours) sedation does not require pre-procedure starving.

Assessment

The elderly, obese and those with significant pre-existing medical conditions (e.g. cardiac, respiratory, renal or liver disease) are more susceptible to the effects of sedation agents. In such patients the use of sedation is relatively contraindicated. If sedation is used, lower doses may be required.

In children the use of distraction therapy (if available) can be used instead of sedation or as an adjunct.

Equipment

The patient should be placed on a head-down tilting trolley, ensuring that the patient is placed on the trolley such that their head is at the tilting end of the trolley. Oxygen, suction and full resuscitation equipment should be available in the area where the sedation is to be given. All the equipment should be checked to ensure that it is working correctly. An operator trained in the use of this equipment and in resuscitation should be at hand. Supplemental oxygen should be administered at a rate of 2–4 litres/min.

Agents

As mentioned above sedation is facilitated by the concomitant use of agents or techniques to achieve analgesia.

1. Benzodiazepines. In the past diazepam was the agent of choice. However it has a long half life and forms active metabolites. Midazolam is now the preferred option, having a short half life and no active metabolites. In adults it is generally given by the intravenous route where it has a rapid onset of action. The dose is titrated against effect. In children it may be given by the oral route at the dose of 0.5 mg/kg (maximum 15 mg). The onset of action is up to 45 minutes. Approximately 10% of children will exhibit a paradoxical agitation following oral administration. If the first oral dose has not achieved sedation some would recommend a second dose. Midazolam has no analgesic properties, if it is used alone for a painful procedure the sedative effect may be lost.

2. ***Opiates.*** Opiates have predominantly analgesic effects in low doses but as the dose is increased the sedative effect becomes more pronounced. They are best given by the intravenous route rather than by the oral or intramuscular route when their action is less predictable. Morphine or diamorphine is to be preferred to pethidine which has a lower therapeutic index. Opiates can be used in combination with midazolam, but the effects of the two agents are synergistic and cardiac and respiratory depression is more common, particularly in the elderly or those with pre-existing disease. If the combination of an opiate and midazolam is to be used, the opiate should be titrated in first and several minutes allowed to elapse to assess the sedative and analgesic effects before slowly titrating in the midazolam.

3. ***Flumazenil.*** This is a specific benzodiazepine agonist with a relatively short half life.

4. ***Naloxone.*** This is a specific opiate agonist, again with a short half life.

Use of agonists in sedation

Because the specific benzodiazepine and opiate agonists have short half lives, most would use them only to reverse the effects of their respective drugs if problems occur (e.g. the patient becomes unconscious or respiratory depression occurs). The benefit of this approach is that when the patient has fully recovered from sedation the operator can be confident that the effects of the agents have ended. If agonists are routinely administered it is difficult to assess whether recovery is due to the cessation of action of the sedative agent(s) or the effects of the agonist.

Other agents

A variety of other agents including ketamine are used in some areas for sedation, particularly in the pre-hospital environment. It has good analgesic actions and maintains cardiovascular stability.

Monitoring

The mainstay of monitoring during the procedure is the patient's conscious level. The operator should talk to the patient and ensure that they are responsive. Pulse oximetry can be used to monitor oxygen saturation both during and after the procedure. Oxygen saturation should be monitored after supplemental oxygen has been discontinued to ensure that saturation returns to pre-sedation levels or is maintained above 95%. It should be borne in mind that significant respiratory depression can occur in the presence of normal saturation levels when the patient is receiving supplemental oxygen and that CO_2 levels can rise significantly (the pulse oximeter gives no indication of $PaCO_2$). A fall in the patients conscious level may indicate a rising CO_2 level. Alternately a capnograph connected to the outflow of the oxygen mask may be used to give an indication of a rise in end tidal CO_2 level. In most patients end tidal CO_2 correlates with $PaCO_2$. If the oxygen saturation cannot be maintained, the conscious level is falling or end tidal CO_2 is rising the effect of the sedative should be reversed.

The patients BP, pulse and respiratory rate should be monitored both pre- and post-procedure until full recovery is made. Routine ECG monitoring is not required in the fully fit patient.

Discharge

The criteria for discharge are:

- Normal BP, pulse, respiratory rate, oxygen saturation and conscious level.
- Steady gait.
- Toleration of oral fluids.
- Adequate supervision for the next 24 hours.

Patients should be warned not to drive or operate machinery for 24 hours after sedation.

Further reading

Royal College of Surgeons of England. *Guidelines for Sedation by Non-Anaesthetists.* London, Royal College of Surgeons, 1993.

Related topic of interest

Local anaesthesia (p. 207)

SEPTIC ARTHRITIS

Septic arthritis is an acute infection of a joint. Organisms may enter the joint by local spread, e.g. from penetrating wounds, intra-articular injection or secondary to local osteomyelitis where the metaphysis of the affected bone is intracapsular or by haematogeneous spread. Septic arthritis is more common in the extremes of life.

Clinical features

1. ***Children.*** Septic arthritis is commonest in the under-5 age group. The source of the infection is usually a skin lesion or respiratory tract infection. It most frequently affects the large joints of the body. In older children a single joint is usually involved, in the neonatal period multiple joints may be involved. The child will be toxic, unwell with a fever and tachycardia. The joint is swollen, hot, red and exquisitely painful to even the smallest of movements. These signs may not be as florid in the early stages in the younger child or baby.

2. ***Adults.*** In the elderly the clinical signs and symptoms may not be as florid as in the child. They may present initially with confusion and fever. Pain at the site of infection may be minimal.

Investigations

1. ***FBC, WCC, ESR, C reactive protein and blood cultures.*** The white cell count will be raised, as will ESR and CRP. The rise in CRP will occur before that of the ESR, which may be normal or only minimally raised in the early stages. Blood cultures will confirm the organism. Anti-Streptolysin O and anti-staphylococcal titres may be taken to confirm the diagnosis. These will not be available for immediate use but are useful in confirming the organism retrospectively if cultures are negative.

2. ***Aspiration of synovial fluid.*** The joint is aspirated under aseptic conditions. The fluid is sent for immediate microscopy and Gram stain, culture sensitivities and crystals. In the early stages the synovial fluid may show nothing on Gram stain.

3. ***Radiology.*** The early X-rays will usually be normal, although widening of the joint space may indicate an effusion. In neonates osteomyelitis of the adjacent bone may be visible. In the late stages the X-rays will show bone destruction with periosteal new bone formation and loss of joint space. Such changes may not occur if the condition is diagnosed early and treated promptly. Ultrasound examination will reveal an effusion and may be used to guide a needle for aspiration.

Causative organisms

Staphylococcus aureus is the most common infecting organism in all age groups. Other organisms implicated in septic arthritis include the Streptococci, Gonococci, Haemophilus Influenzae, and Salmonella.

Management

The main priority initially is to obtain cultures of both blood and synovial fluid to confirm the diagnosis and guide antibiotic selection. The joint should be surgically drained both to remove infected synovial fluid and to decompress the joint. Antibiotics should be given intravenously. The initial selection will be based upon a knowledge of the likely organisms while awaiting the results of cultures.

In adults the most likely organism is *Staphylococcus aureus*, the drugs of choice are Flucloxacillin and either Clindamycin or Fusidic acid.

Further reading

Esterhui JL Jnr, Gelb I. Adult septic arthritis. *Orthopedic Clinics of North America*, 1991; **22**(3): 503–14.

Shaw DA, Casser JR. Acute septic arthritis in infancy and childhood. *Clinical Orthopaedics and Related Research*, 1990; **257**: 212–5.

Till SH, Snaith ML. Assessment, investigation and management of acute monoarthritis. *Journal of Accident and Emergency Medicine*, 1991; **16**(5): 355–61.

Related topics of interest

Febrile convulsion (p. 153); Limping child (p. 204)

SHOCK

Classification

1. ***Hypovolaemic:*** A reduction in circulating volume due to fluid loss.

- Burns.
- Gastrointestinal fluid loss.
- Haemorrhage.

2. ***Cardiogenic:*** A reduction in cardiac output due to pump failure.

- Arrhythmia.
- Myocardial contusion.
- Myocardial infarction.

3. ***Distributive:*** An increase in the capacity of the circulatory system or leakage of fluid from the circulatory system into the tissues.

- Anaesthesia.
- Anaphylaxis.
- Neurogenic (spinal cord injury).
- Septicaemia.

4. ***Obstructive:*** Obstruction to blood flow.

- Cardiac tamponade.
- Flail chest.
- Pulmonary embolism.
- Tension pneumothorax.

5. ***Dissociative:*** A reduction in tissue oxygen release.

- Anaemia.
- Carbon monoxide poisoning.
- Cyanide poisoning.

Phases of shock

Shock may be divided into two phases based upon clinical features.

1. ***Compensated shock.*** Normal physiological compensatory mechanisms preferentially maintain perfusion and oxygenation to the vital organs at the expense of other organs (e.g. gut and skin). The clinical signs are due to hypoperfusion of these organs and include:

- Cold peripheries.
- Pale skin.
- Reduced capillary return.
- Sweating.
- Tachycardia.
- Tachypnoea.

In compensated shock the patient may become apprehensive or agitated. The blood pressure is maintained within the normal range.

2. Decompensated shock. As the mismatch between circulating volume and metabolic demands increases perfusion of the vital organs is affected. In addition to the clinical features of compensated shock the following signs manifest themselves and progress:

- Decreasing conscious level.
- Fall in urine output.
- Hypotension.
- Kussmal breathing.
- Mottling of the skin.

At this stage recovery may still occur, with or without some residual deficit in vital organ function, if prompt resuscitation is instituted. Failure to institute timely and aggressive treatment for decompensated shock leads eventually to a state of irreversible shock. This phase is characterized by failure to respond to appropriate resuscitative measures and ultimately death. The phase of irreversible shock has no clear boundaries with decompensated shock and is recognized by the failure of resuscitative therapy to produce a response. Therefore all patients who are shocked, irrespective of the apparent degree of shock warrant aggressive resuscitation.

Specific types of shock

1. Hypovolaemic shock. By far the commonest cause of shock. Four clinical categories are recognized based upon the percentage of acute fluid loss. This categorization can only be used to estimate the approximate acute loss of circulating volume as compensatory mechanisms will act to restore some or all of the fluid loss over a period of hours. This classification refers to the young, healthy individual only. The signs of shock will appear earlier in the elderly or those with pre-existing disease as they have less capacity to compensate. Class I and II equate to the compensated phase. Class III and IV equate to the decompensated phase.

- Class I (up to 15% loss of circulating volume). This may be associated with no clinical signs or symptoms. Compensatory mechanisms act to restore the circulating volume within a day.

- Class II (15–30% of circulating volume). This is characterized by mild agitation, tachycardia, tachypnoea and thready pulse. Blood pressure is maintained.

- Class III (30–40% circulating volume). The hallmark of class III shock is hypotension accompanied by confusion, tachycardia and peripheral shut down.

- Class IV (>40% circulating volume). Acute loss of blood of this degree is characterized by profound hypotension, decreased conscious level leading to cardiac arrest due to electro-mechanical dissociation (EMD) now also called pulseless electrical activity (PEA). Immediate aggressive fluid resuscitation may reverse this degree of shock unless fluid loss outstrips the capacity to replace loss (e.g. ruptured aneurysm). Prompt surgical intervention to control bleeding may be indicated.

Treatment. Class I or II shock. Usually only require crystalloid replacement, normal homeostatic mechanisms will replace red cell mass within a few weeks.

Class III and IV shock. This group will require red cell replacement at some stage in their resuscitation. In the initial phase however any fluid which will support the circulation (crystalloid, colloid or blood NOT dextrose) will suffice provided it is given rapidly and in adequate volumes.

Debate currently exists as to the role of hypotensive resuscitation in the management of hypovolaemic shock. There is some debate as to whether aggressive fluid resuscitation may increase mortality in such cases. It is believed that aggressive treatment with intravenous fluids may promote bleeding by washing away established clots, dilute clotting factors and causing relaxation of protective sympathetic vasoconstriction. In the absence of trials to confirm this theory the pragmatic approach would seem to be controlled resuscitation to achieve an acceptable systolic pressure (80–90 mmHg) and early definitive treatment of the underlying cause of fluid loss.

2. Cardiogenic shock. Myocardial infarction is the commonest cause of cardiogenic shock and has a high mortality. Attention should be paid in the first instance to excluding easily treated causes such as tension pneumothorax and cardiac tamponade.

Treatment. Cardiac tamponade is initially treated with pericardiocentesis, tension pneumothorax with needle thoracocentesis. The initial treatment of cardiogenic shock consists of oxygen and reduction of pre-load with intravenous opiates and sublingual or intravenous nitrates. Consideration should be given to the early administration of a thrombolytic agent to reduce the degree of myocardial damage. Ionotropic support is usually required.

3. Septic shock. Increased capillary permeability due to circulating bacterial endotoxins causing complement activation and release of vasoactive substances leads to leakage of fluid from the vascular compartment with a reduction in circulating volume. This is exacerbated by an early fall in peripheral vascular resistance. Initially, cardiac output increases leading to the characteristic early signs of compensated septic shock of warm, pink peripheries. Later, increasing fluid loss combined with myocardial depression produces the classic signs of decompensated shock.

Treatment. The early treatment consists of aggressive fluid resuscitation combined with intravenous antibiotics. Fluid loss may continue at a significant rate when ionotropic support may be required.

4. Anaphylactic shock. This is uncommon although the incidence may be increasing. It is a systemic condition which may manifest itself in its most extreme form as profound cardiovascular collapse. Other manifestations which may be present with or without circulatory collapse include urticarial or other skin rashes, bronchospasm, laryngeal oedema and gastrointestinal symptoms. It usually occurs shortly after exposure to the allergen, although presentation may be delayed. It is recognized that a second episode may occur several hours after the initial episode has subsided. The underlying pathophysiological mechanism of shock is peripheral vasodilatation and increased capillary permeability mediated by vasoactive amines such as histamine.

Treatment. The ABCs are addressed in the conventional order. Adrenaline reverses all of the life-threatening manifestations. It is recommended that it is given i.m. or subcutaneously. In less severe cases i.v. chlorpheniramine and hydrocortisone may suffice. Wherever possible the allergen initiating the process should be removed, often this is not possible.

5. Neurogenic shock. The pathophysiological mechanism is loss of vasomotor tone and dilatation of the vascular bed secondary to interruption of the sympathetic supply to the thoracolumbar outflow. This leads to an increase in volume of the vascular space. The shock may be exacerbated by bradycardia due to interruption of the sympathetic supply to the heart. The diagnosis is often missed in the early stages of trauma resuscitation as hypovolaemic shock is much more common. The associated bradycardia gives a clue, but in the absence of a full history this is often thought to be due to the patient taking beta blockers. The failure to respond to apparently adequate fluid resuscitation often suggests the diagnosis.

Treatment. If neurogenic shock is considered but hypovolaemic shock cannot be excluded then fluid resuscitation should continue. CVP monitoring is invaluable in monitoring response to fluid and indicating when adequate replacement for fluid loss has been achieved. Ionotropes are not usually required.

Further reading

The Advanced Paediatric Life Support Group. *Advanced Paediatric Life Support.* BMJ Publishing Group, 1997.

Amercian College of Surgeons Committee on Trauma. *Advanced Life Support Course for Doctors.* Chicago, 1997.

Dick WR. Controversies in resuscitation: to infuse or not to infuse (1). *Resuscitation*, 1996; **31:** 3–6.

Pepe PE. Controversies in resuscitation: to infuse or not to infuse (2). *Resuscitation*, 1996; **31:** 7–10.

Related topics of interest

Anaphylaxis (p. 38); Intravenous fluids (p. 200)

SHOULDER DISLOCATION

The shoulder is a ball and socket joint. The large humeral head articulates with the relatively small glenoid. This depth of the glenoid is increased by a rim of fibrocartilage, the labrum. The exceptional mobility of the shoulder joint accounts for its being the most commonly dislocated large joint in the body. Over 95% of dislocations are anterior. Most of the rest are posterior with the remaining few being inferior (luxatio erecta) and the extremely rare superior dislocation. Dislocations usually occur in young adults or the elderly.

Anterior dislocation

This results from a fall onto the outstretched hand. This produces external rotation with a consequent anterior dislocation. Occasionally it results from forced internal rotation, e.g. from a tight arm-lock. The force of the injury may cause tearing of the joint capsule and the rotator cuff. The glenoid and/or humeral head or neck may be fractured.

1. Clinical features. The patient complains of pain and is unwilling to move the shoulder. Observation from the front will reveal a prominent acromion (this may be confused with an acromioclavicular dislocation) and loss of the normally rounded contour of the shoulder, more noticeable when compared with the normal side. The humeral head may be palpable, particularly in the axilla. Axillary (circumflex) nerve injury may occur (4%) leading to loss of sensation in the upper outer aspect of the deltoid (the 'regimental badge' region). Axillary nerve injury will also result in weakness in abduction of the shoulder due to paralysis of the central fibres of the deltoid.

2. Diagnosis. An X-ray should always be taken before reduction is attempted, both to confirm the diagnosis and to exclude an associated fracture. Two views of the shoulder should be obtained (although an anterior dislocation is visible on the AP view, a posterior dislocation may be missed), standard AP and a lateral or transaxillary ('shoot down') view. On the AP view the humeral head will be seen to lie below the glenoid. On the lateral or transaxillary view the head will be seen to lie in front of the glenoid. In addition to the dislocation and fracture to the glenoid or humeral neck, a fracture of the posterior articular surface of the humerus may be seen (Hills–Sachs lesion).

3. Management. New dislocations should be reduced as soon as possible, usually in the A&E department. Old dislocations should be referred for reduction under general anaesthetic because of the difficulty of reduction and risk of fracture. Open reduction is frequently required.

Reduction can usually be achieved under analgesia (usually an opiate) or sedation (usually a benzodiazepine). There are several methods described and many variations.

- Kochers manoeuvre. Traction is applied to the arm with the elbow flexed. The shoulder is gradually externally rotated. The arm is then adducted, the elbow moved across the chest and the shoulder internally rotated. Reduction can be sensed as a 'clunking' feeling. Reduction may occur at any time during the manoeuvre.

- Hippocratic method. Traction is applied to the extended arm. The foot is placed in the axilla and the humeral head is eased into place. This method is usually performed under general anaesthesia.
- Gravitational traction. The patient is positioned face down on a trolley with the affected arm hanging over the side. With relaxation (with or without analgesia) the weight of the arm combined with muscular relaxation allows the humeral head to relocate. The patient may be given a weight to hold. This method may take up to an hour to work.
- Milch manoeuvre. The extended arm is gradually abducted from the patients side until it is at 90°. The arm is then gently internally rotated whilst maintaining traction until the humeral head reduces. The moment of reduction may be best appreciated by palpating the humeral head in the axilla. Reduction using this method can often be achieved without analgesia or sedation within 15 minutes.

Once the shoulder is reduced the arm is strapped against the chest. A check X-ray (usually only an AP can be adequately obtained) is taken to confirm the reduction and the function of the axillary nerve is checked and documented. The patient is referred to the next fracture clinic. The immobilization is generally maintained for 3–4 weeks.

4. Complications

- Axillary nerve injury.
- Brachial plexus injury.
- Radial nerve injury.
- Axillary artery injury.
- Fracture of the humeral head or neck.
- Fracture of the glenoid.
- Recurrent dislocation (more than one episode of dislocation).

Posterior dislocation

This may result from a fall onto the outstretched hand followed by internal rotation, as theresult of direct trauma to the shoulder, during an epileptic seizure or secondary to an electric shock.

1. Clinical features. This injury is often missed because it is not considered (e.g. in the post-ictal patient) or because it is associated with more severe injuries (e.g. after an electric shock). The arm will be seen to be held adducted and in internal rotation. It is painful to move.

2. ***Diagnosis.*** Definitive diagnosis is made on X-ray. The standard AP view will reveal a symmet-rical appearing humeral head, the 'light bulb' sign (the humeral head normally looks asymmetrical because the greater and lesser tuberosities are visible on AP views. In posterior dislocation rotation of the humerus obscures these from the X-ray shadow and the head looks symmetrical.) There may also be increased distance between the anterior rim of the glenoid and the humeral head (the 'rim' sign). On the second view (either lateral or transaxillary) the humeral head is seen to be lying behind the glenoid.

3. ***Management.*** Like anterior dislocation a posterior dislocation may be reduced in the A&E department under sedation or with analgesia. A two person technique is required. The first person extends and abducts the arm to 90° and applies traction. Whilsttraction is maintained by the first person, the second person pushes the back of the humeral head forward. Failure to achieve reduction using this technique mandates reduction under general anaesthesia. If reduction is successful the arm is strapped to the patient's side and a check X-ray obtained. The function of the axillary nerve is checked and documented and the patient referred to the next fracture clinic.

4. ***Complications***

- Recurrent dislocation.
- Humeral head (reverse Hills–Sachs lesion) or neck fracture.
- Neurovascular injury.

Inferior dislocation (luxatio erecta)

This is rare. The humeral head lies below the glenoid in the virtual space of the axilla occupied by the brachial plexus and axillary artery. The injury is obvious on inspection. The arm isfixed in the overhead position. Reduction should be achieved as a matter of urgency after X-rays have been obtained. Traction is applied to the abducted arm. The arm is them swung into adduction. Reduction may not be sucessful due to button-holing of the humeral head through a capsular tear. Open reduction will then be required. Following successful reduction the arm is strapped to the chest. An X-ray is taken to confirm reduction and the integrity of the brachial plexus is tested and documented. The patient is referred to the next fracture clinic.

1. ***Complications***

- Neurovascular injury (common, usually neuropraxia of the brachialplexus).
- Rotator cuff tear.

Further reading

McRae R. *Practical Fracture Management*. 3rd edn. Edinburgh, Churchill Livingstone, 1994.

Nicholson DA, Lang I, Hughes P, Driscoll PA. ABC of Emergency Radiology: The Shoulder. *British Medical Journal*, 1993; **307**(6912): 1129–34.

Related topic of interest

Shoulder problems – soft tissue (p. 299)

SHOULDER PROBLEMS – SOFT TISSUE

In addition to fractures there is a range of soft tissue problems that may present acutely to the A&E department. Most, but not all, are associated with an acute injury. Reaching a diagnosis in such cases rests upon a detailed history and clinical examination. These conditions may be classified into two broad groups, those affecting the rotator cuff and those affecting the tendon of the long head of biceps.

The rotator cuff

The rotator cuff comprises the four muscles running directly across the shoulder joint, supraspinatus, infraspinatus, subscapularis and teres minor. They run under the coracoacromial arch separated from it by the subacromial bursa. Several characteristic conditions can arise due to injury to or inflammation of the tendons or muscles of the cuff.

1. Supraspinatus tendinitis (chronic tendinitis). This condition is caused by degeneration of the supraspinatus tendon. The condition usually occurs in middle age and follows an intermittent course. It presents with tenderness over the point of the shoulder and pain on moving. Shoulder X-ray may show subacromial calcification of the tendon. Treatment is rest and analgesia followed by gentle mobilization. Local steroid injection may be of benefit in intractable cases.

2. Acute calcific supraspinatus tendinitis. This condition is due to deposition of hydroxyapatite in a small area of degeneration of the supraspinatus tendon. Clinically it is characterized by rapid onset of pain at rest causing severe restriction of shoulder movements. The rest pain is due to swelling within the tendon secondary to inflammation. Shoulder X-ray will demonstrate the calcific deposit within the tendon. The condition usually resolves spontaneously. In early cases the condition may be treated by aspirating the hydroxyapatite under local anaesthetic and injecting steroid. A large-bore needle is required for this procedure as the material to be aspirated has the consistency of toothpaste.

3. Acute tendinitis (painful arc syndrome). This usually occurs in younger active patients days or weeks after a bout of vigorous activity. The pain characteristically occurs between 60° and 120° of abduction (hence the term painful arc). The underlying cause is inflammation and swelling of the proximal part of the supraspinatus tendon. During abduction the tendon passes beneath the acromion (separated from it by the subacromial bursa) and above the humeral head. When the inflamed proximal portion of the tendon passes through this area it is squeezed (impingement), resulting in pain. Treatment is rest and analgesia followed by gentle mobilization. In refractory cases steroid injection into the subacromial space may help.

4. Rotator cuff tear. Partial rotator cuff tears may be difficult to distinguish from acute tendinitis. The initial management is the same, rest and analgesia followed by gentle mobilization. Complete rotator cuff tears are characterized by inability to abduct the shoulder. They may be missed initially as the inability to abduct the shoulder may be attributed to the pain of associated injuries. Complete tears may require surgical repair.

5. Frozen shoulder. This condition is characterized by pain and varying degrees of restriction of movement in the shoulder. It is often preceded by trauma, but is also associated with non-traumatic conditions such as myocardial infarction and cerebrovascular accident. The condition resolves spontaneously over a period of 12–18 months. Physiotherapy is often recommended. In severe cases manipulation under general anaesthetic may be of help.

The tendon of the long head of biceps

The tendon of the long head of biceps runs in the bicipital groove over the head of the humerus to insert into the superior part of the glenoid. There are two conditions associated with the upper part of the tendon.

1. Bicipital tendinitis. This is characterized by pain over the upper part of the humerus associated with localized tenderness over the bicipital groove. It usually follows an injury. Treatment is rest, analgesia and gentle mobilization.

2. Rupture of the long head of biceps. This occurs most commonly in the elderly. It is caused by flexing the elbow against resistance (e.g. lifting or pulling on a weight). This causes rupture of the degenerate tendon. A sensation of 'something giving' is felt. Pain is minimal. It comes to attention when the patient notices the bulge of the muscle belly in the front of the arm. This bulge may be emphasized by flexing the elbow against resistance. There is minimal functional impairment in most cases and treatment is usually conservative.

Further reading

Binder A. Management of common shoulder injuries. *British Journal of Hospital Medicine*, 1996; **56**(2–3): 66–72.

Cyriax JH, Cyriax PJ. *Cyriax's Illustrated Manual of Orthopaedic Medicine.* Oxford, Butterworth-Heinemann, 1996.

Related topics of interest

Myocardial infarction (p. 246); Shoulder dislocation (p. 295)

SICKLE CELL DISEASE

Sickle cell disease is a haemoglobin disorder in which the sickle beta globin gene (β^s) is inherited. This is most commonly manifested as homozygous sickle cell anaemia (haemoglobin SS), sickle cell trait or β thalassaemia. Sickle cell disease is commonly found in patients with an ethnic background from Africa, West Indies, India, the Mediterranean and Middle East. The frequency of sickle cell carriers is 1 in 4 in West Africans and 1 in 10 in Afro-Caribbeans. It is estimated that the number of patients with sickle cell disease in the UK is around 10 000.

Clinically patients with sickle cell disease have problems related to vaso-occlusion, caused by polymerization of deoxygenated haemoglobin S. This results in sickling of erythrocytes which can adhere to the vascular endothelium. The most common clinical problem is painful vaso-occlusive crisis resulting from a blockage of small vessels. Large vessel disease also occurs resulting in thrombotic cerebrovascular accidents, the acute sickle chest syndrome and placental infarction.

Although life expectancy of sickle cell disease continues to improve the mean for men and women with sickle cell disease is 42 and 48 years respectively and for men and women with sickle cell trait is 60 and 68 years, respectively. The most common cause of death is related to pulmonary complications, cerebrovascular accidents, infection, acute splenic sequestration and chronic organ damage/failure.

Triage

The following aims are recommended by the British Association of Accident & Emergency Medicine:

On arrival check the oxygen saturation, give oxygen and keep the patient warm. Check the Sickle Cell Disease Register if available.

Triage to the resuscitation room if:

- SaO_2 <85%.
- Neurological deficit.
- Haemoglobin <5.
- Shock.
- Organ involvement.
- Priapism.
- Obtain expert haematological advice early and/or contact the patient's base hospital if any of the following is present:
  (a) Shock.
  (b) Pregnancy >12 weeks.
  (c) Dyspnoea.
  (d) Silent abdomen.
  (e) Organ involvement.
  (f) Vomiting/dehydration >10%.
  (g) Abdominal pain/distension.
  (h) You are inexperienced in the management of this condition.

Clinical complications

The manifestations are variable and alter with age. The following complications may occur:

- Pain (dactylitis, long bones, trunk).
- Sequestration (splenic, hepatic, chest syndrome, mesenteric syndrome).
- Infection (pneumococcal, parvovirus B19, salmonella, haemophilus).
- Priapism.
- Upper airway obstruction.
- Cerebrovascular accident.
- Subarachnoid haemorrhage.
- Retinopathy.
- Gallstones.
- Avascular necrosis.
- Delayed growth and development.
- Leg ulcers.
- Chronic renal failure.
- Chronic sickle lung.

Ninety per cent of hospital admissions are for a painful crisis. Pain is as a result of oxygen deprivation of tissues and avascular necrosis of the bone marrow secondary to a vaso-occlusive crisis. Most cases of pain are treated in the community using a simple analgesic ladder, that is starting with Paracetamol then adding a non-steroidal anti-inflammatory drug, followed by codeine phosphate. If pain is uncontrolled this will then require in-patient treatment. A fast track admission policy has been shown to be effective.

Patients who develop systemic signs, tachypnoea, signs of lung involvement, neurological signs, abdominal distension and pain, splenic or hepatic enlargement, loin pain, severe pallor, or congestive cardiac failure require in-patient management.

Other complications requiring in-patient management include:

- Swollen painful joints.
- Central nervous system deficit.
- Acute sick chest syndrome or pneumonia.
- Mesenteric sickling and bowel ischaemia.
- Splenic or hepatic sequestration.
- Cholecystitis.
- Renal papillary necrosis resulting in colic or severe haematuria.
- Priapism.
- Hyphaema and retinal detachment.

Treatment

The patient will require multidisciplinary input. Initially treat as follows:

- Give high-flow oxygen.
- Give analgesia promptly – Do not underestimate the requirement for pain relief.

The individual's usual agent is stated on the front of their sickle cell card. Suitable dosages for adults are:

Diamorphine 5–10 mg i.v.
Morphine 10–15 mg i.v.
Pethidine 50–100 mg i.v.

and a suitable dosage for children is:

Pethidine 1 mg/kg i.v. or Diamorphine 0.05–0.1 mg/kg i.v.

Maintenance doses, usually given by continuous i.v. infusion are within the ranges:

Pethidine 0.1–0.5 mg/kg/h or Diamorphine 0.01–0.015 mg/kg/h.

Analgesia should be titrated according to the individual's response:

- Fluids – Either give orally or intravenously (1 litre 0.9% normal saline over 3 hours in an adult).
- Antihistamines may be needed for itching.

1. Acute sickle chest syndrome. The most common cause of death. The aetiology is unclear. Rare before puberty. The onset can be insidious or rapid, leading to death within hours. The following features are found:

- Dyspnoea.
- Sickle pain in the thoracic cage.
- Arterial desaturation.
- Pulmonary consolidation with radiological changes.

Treat with inspired oxygen, continuous positive airway ventilation and exchange transfusion. Seek help from anaesthetic and haematological colleagues.

2. Aplastic crisis. Characterized by high output CCF, decreased haematocrit and reticulocytes. Senior haematological opinion essential.

3. Sequestration. Present with severe anaemia, usually children with splenomegaly. If older present with hepatomegaly. May need urgent transfusion. Seek immediate advice from a consultant haematologist.

4. Infections. Septicaemia and meningitis require aggressive treatment, particularly prone in those patients who are hyposplenic. Pyrexia may be the only sign.

Do blood cultures, sputum cultures, throat swab, mid-stream urine. Discuss with consultant microbiologist and haematologist.

5. Neurological. Acute cerebrovascular accidents, fits and transient ischaemic attacks may present at all ages. Patients should have an emergency exchange transfusion and urgent referral to haematologist and neurologist.

6. Abdominal syndrome. Usually pain with no peritoneal signs and normal bowel sounds. Sometimes presents as acute abdomen. Do abdominal X-rays and serum amylase. Keep nil by mouth and monitor carefully. Check yersinia titres and treat if positive.

Further reading

British Association for Accident and Emergency Medicine. *Guidelines for the Management of Sickle Cell Crises*, 1997.

Davies SC, Oni L. Management of patients with sickle cell disease. *British Medical Journal*, 1997; **315:** 656–60.

SINGLE-DOSE ACTIVATED CHARCOAL

A position statement was produced by the American Academy of Clinical Toxicologists and the European Association of Poison Centres and Clinical Toxicologists.

Single-dose activated charcoal should not be administered routinely in the management of poisoned patients. The effectiveness of activated charcoal decreases with time; the greatest benefit is within one hour of ingestion. The administration of activated charcoal may therefore be considered if a patient has ingested a potentially toxic amount of a poison (which is known to be absorbed by charcoal) up to one hour previously; there are insufficient data to support or exclude its use after one hour of ingestion. There is no evidence that the administration of activated charcoal improves clinical outcome. Unless a patient has an intact or protected airway the administration of charcoal is contraindicated.

Pharmacology

Activated charcoal comes in direct contact with and adsorbs poisons in the gastrointestinal tract, decreasing the extent of absorption of the poison thereby reducing or preventing systemic toxicity.

Four brands of oral activated charcoal are available in the UK:

- Actidose-aqua.
- Carbomix.
- Liqui-Char.
- Medicoal.

Dosage

The optimal dose of activated charcoal for a poisoned patient is unknown, though available data implies a dose–response relationship that favours larger doses. Data derived from animal and human volunteer studies cannot be extrapolated directly to clinical situations.

The BNF recommends the following oral dosage regime:

- Children under one year – 1 g/kg.
- Children 1–12 years – 25–50 g.
- Adults 50 g.

1. Conscious patients should be able to drink charcoal. If the patient is unable to do so it can be delivered via a nasogastric tube. If the patient is vomiting consider giving Ondansetron (8 mg i.v.) – although expensive this drug may be justified in potentially serious poisoning e.g. Theophylline.

2. Unconscious patients. By nasogastric tube.

Contraindications

- Unprotected airway.
- A gastrointestinal tract not anatomically intact.
- When activated charcoal may increase the risk and severity of aspiration e.g. hydrocarbons.

Side effects

Few serious adverse effects have been described following single use of activated charcoal. All types are unpalatable and often result in soiled patients, staff and clothing.

The following have been described:

- Vomiting.
- Aspiration pneumonitis.
- Corneal abrasions.
- Carbomix causes constipation.

Substances not readily adsorbed by charcoal

- Acids and alkalis.
- Cyanide.
- Ethanol/methanol.
- Ethylene glycol.
- Ferrous salts.
- Lead.
- Lithium.
- Malathion.
- Mercury.
- Organic solvents.
- Petroleum distillants.
- Potassium salts.

Further reading

American Academy of Clinical Toxicology; European Association of Poisons Centres and Clinical Toxicologists. Position statement: single-dose activated charcoal. *Clinical Toxicology*, 1997; **35**(7): 721–41.

SPINE AND SPINAL CORD TRAUMA

The annual incidence of spinal cord injury within the UK is about 10–15 per million of the population. The cervical spine (55%) is the commonest site of injury, followed by the thoracic spine (15%), thoraco–lumbar region (15%) and the lumbo–sacral region (15%).

Approximately 10% of patients with a cervical spine fracture have a second associated non-contiguous vertebral column fracture.

The commonest causes of spinal injury include

- Road traffic accidents (50%)
- Domestic and industrial accidents (25%)
- Sporting injuries (15%)
- Self harm and assaults (5%)
- Others (5%).

In the unconscious patient after a fall or road traffic accident, 5% sustain a cervical spine injury. *A high index of suspicion* regarding spinal injury is necessary. At least 5% of patients experience the onset of neurological symptoms or worsening of pre-existing ones after reaching the A&E Department. This may be due to ischaemia or progression of spinal cord oedema.

An unstable spinal injury must be assumed to be present after trauma. Inadvertent manipulation or inadequate immobilization must not jeopardize the patient's spinal cord. Early consultation with a neurosurgeon and/or orthopaedic surgeon is essetial.

Examination

1. General – total spinal immobilization. This is best achieved with a stiffneck collar, securing the head to a spine board and bolster splinting the neck or with sandbags and tape. The chest, pelvis and lower extremities must also be securely immobilized to protect the thoracic and lumbar spine. Log-rolling with the help of assistants is essential when moving the patient.

Clinical finding suggesting a cervical cord injury in the unconscious patient includes:

- Flaccid areflexia, including a flaccid rectal sphincter.
- Diaphragmatic breathing – abdominal breathing and use of accessory muscles.
- Ability to flex, but not extend at the elbow.
- Grimaces to pain above, but not below the clavicle.
- Hypotension with bradycardia, especially without hypovolaemia.
- Priapism.

2. Vertebral assessment. Pain, tenderness, posterior 'step-off' deformity, prominence of spinous processes, pain with movement, oedema, bruising, visible deformity and muscle spasms may help identify and localize the site of injury.

To visualize the entire spine, the patient may be *log-rolled*, but only to the minimum degree necessary to allow the examination.

3. Neurological assessment

- Motor

 (a) *Corticospinal tract* controls ipsilateral motor power and is tested by voluntary muscle contractions or involuntary response to painful stimulation.
 (b) Certain muscles or muscle groups are identified as representing a single spinal nerve segment. The key muscles are:

 1. C5 – Deltoid;
 2. C6 – Wrist extensors;
 3. C7 – Elbow extensors (triceps);
 4. C8 – Finger flexors;
 5. T1 – Small finger abductors (abductor digiti minimi);
 6. L2 – Hip flexors (iliopsoas);
 7. L3 – Knee extensors (quadriceps);
 8. L4 – Ankle dorsiflexors (tibialis anterior);
 9. L5 – Long toe extensors (extensor hallucis longus);
 10. S1 – Ankle plantar flexors (gastrocnemius-soleus).

- Sensory

 The key sensory dermatomes are as follows:
 1. C5 – Area over the deltoid;
 2. C6 – Thumb;
 3. C7 – Middle finger;
 4. C8 – Little finger;
 5. T4 – Nipple;
 6. T8 – Xiphisternum;
 7. T10 – Umbilicus;
 8. T12 – Symphysis;
 9. L4 – Medial aspect of the leg;
 10. L5 – Space between the first and second toes;
 11. S1 – Lateral border of the foot;
 12. S3 – Ischial tuberosity area;
 13. S4 and S5 – Perianal region.

 (a) *Spinothalamic tract* controls contralateral pain and temperature sensation. It is tested by pin prick and light touch.
 (b) *Posterior columns* control ipsilateral proprioception and are tested by position sense or vibration sense.

- Reflex changes
- Autonomic

 1. Loss of bladder control.
 2. Loss of anal tone.
 3. Priapism.

Severity of the neurological injury

A complete spinal cord injury reveals no sensory or motor function below a certain level and indicates poor recovery.

An *incomplete spinal cord lesion* may be followed by recovery. *Sacral sparing* i.e. perianal sensation, voluntary anal sphincter contraction, all voluntary toe flexion and any sensation (including position sense), or voluntary movement in the lower extremities are signs of an incomplete injury and must be noted.

4. *Neurogenic and spinal shock*

- *Neurogenic shock* refers to the hypotension associated with cervical or high thoracic spinal cord injury. This is due to damage to the descending sympathetic pathways, with loss of vasomotor tone, and loss of sympathetic tone of the heart. The resultant vasodilatation, hypotension and bradycardia may be improved by increasing venous return, atropine (to overcome the bradycardia) and occasionally vasopressors.
- *Spinal shock* is the neurologic condition after spinal cord trauma. Flaccidity and loss of reflexes are present but in days to weeks this either disappears to return to normal or is replaced by spasticity.

5. *Other effects*

- *Hypoventilation* – due to paralysis of the intercostal muscles after injury to the lower cervical or upper thoracic spinal cord.
- *Diaphragmatic paralysis* – due to C-3 to C-5 damage (phrenic nerve).
- *Masking of other injuries* – due to inability to feel pain such as an acute abdominal injury.

6. *X-rays*

- *Cervical spine* – Patients who are awake, alert, not under the influence of drugs/alcohol, without neurological symptoms or signs, no neck pain and no cervical tenderness are asked to move their neck gently from side to side and if normal flex and extend. If this does not induce pain cervical spine films are not required.

  Lateral cervical spine X-rays should be obtained after life-threatening conditions are corrected. All seven cervical vertebrae and the C7/T1 junction must be visualized. The patient's shoulders are best pulled down to aid visualization. If inadequate, a *Swimmer's view* is the preferred method to visualize C7/T1. This combination of films has been reported to have an 85% sensitivity for fractures.

  After completion of the primary survey and resuscitation phases further cervical spine views are taken. These include an open-mouth odontoid and anteroposterior views. This combination of lateral, AP and open-mouth X-rays increases the sensitivity for identification of fractures to 92%. Oblique views are taken if required. Further investigations such as CT, MRI and screened lateral flexion and extension views may be required.
- *Thoracolumbar* – anteroposterior and lateral thoracic films are obtained if indicated.

  Caution: if a vertebral fracture is present it is essential to X-ray the whole of the vertebral column to exclude non-contiguous fractures.

Treatment

1. Immobilization

2. Intravenous fluids. Treatment of neurogenic shock may require additional fluids. A urinary catheter is inserted to monitor urinary output and prevent bladder distension. If the blood pressure does not improve after a fluid challenge the judicious use of vasopressors may be indicated in the presence of neurogenic shock. However, always assume hypotension is secondary to hypovolaemia in the first instance.

3. Nasogastric tube. A nasogastric tube is inserted to empty the stomach and reduce the risk of aspiration.

4. Drugs

- *Steroids.* Results from the second National Spinal Cord Injury Study showed benefit in patients with either complete or incomplete spinal cord damage if given high dose methlyprednisolone within 8 hours of injury. Complication and mortality rates were not altered.

  The effect of methylprednisolone by inhibition of lipid peroxidation is the proposed mechanism, with a secondary effect of improvement in the blood flow at the injury site. If steroids are to be given, treatment must be started within 8 hours of injury. Infuse 30 mg/kg of methlyprednisolone as soon as possible over 15 minutes. Wait for 45 minutes. Infuse 5.4 mg/kg/hour over 23 hours.

Exclusions include:

1. Greater than 8 hours since injury;
2. Age under 13 years;
3. Pregnancy;
4. Major life-threatening morbidity;
5. Injury limited to cauda equina or nerve root;
6. Abdominal trauma;
7. Systemic fungal infection.

Spinal cord injury without radiological abnormalities (SCIWORA)

SCIWORA occurs almost exclusively in children under the age of 8 years. The child's spinal column, owing to ligamentous laxity, wedge-shaped vertebrae and shallow facet joints, allows for greater flexibility. With severe trauma it may result in underlying spinal cord damage without fracture or dislocation. SCIWORA tends to occur in the cervical spine, often high up.

A high suspicion of a spinal cord lesion in the multiply injured comatose child even after normal spinal films have been obtained. Full spinal immobilization should be kept *in situ* until the child is assessed neurologically.

Further reading

ATLS. Instructor manual chapter 7 1997; 191–219.

Bracken MB *et al.* Methylprednisolone or naloxone treatment after acute spinal cord injury: 1-year follow-up data. Results of the Second National Acute Spinal Cord Injury Study. *Journal of Neurosurgery*, 1992; **72:** 23–31.

Ferguson J and Beattie T. Occult spinal cord injury in traumatised children. *Injury*, 1993; **24:** 83–84.

Related topics of interest

Abdominal trauma (p. 4); Cervical spine – acute neck sprain (p. 90); Genitourinary trauma (p. 164); Interhospital transfer (p. 194); Maxillofacial injury (p. 226); Thoracic trauma (p. 321)

SUDDEN INFANT DEATH SYNDROME

One in 450 infants die between the ages of 1 week and 1 year. Occasionally in a sudden death a cause is found, e.g. congenital heart disease, overwhelming infection, inborn errors of metabolism and very occasionally accidental or intentional suffocation. More commonly, a careful post-mortem examination reveals only evidence of minor illness, such as an URTI.

Where no cause is found, a diagnosis of *Sudden Infant Death Syndrome (SIDS)* is made and it is the commonest cause of death in this age group.

Following a cot death, parents feel a profound sense of loss, guilt and depression. For young parents, this is often the first experience of death in their family. The risk to a twin or other sibling needs consideration and the paediatrician will counsel the family and consider the use of an apnoea alarm.

Aetiology

Many theories have been put forward for a single aetiology, but it is more probably a mixture of factors.

The current hypotheses include:

- Abnormality of respiratory control.
- An abnormal response to respiratory infection.
- Hyperthermia, exacerbated by excessive warm bedding during a mild illness.
- Some association with the prone sleeping position.

Risk factors include:

- Winter months.
- Male sex.
- Premature infants.
- Twins.
- Previous apnoea attacks(s).
- Unmarried, smoking, young mothers.

Initial resuscitation

Children, who are found suddenly and unexpectedly dead are usually brought to the Accident and Emergency department. All such children should be admitted to the resuscitation room and unless rigor mortis or post-mortem lividity are present, resuscitation should be initiated. A paediatric cardiac arrest team should be in attendance.

Roles of medical staff

- To confirm the death of the infant and gather preliminary information on the cause of death (history and examination).
- To offer practical advice and support to parents.
- To inform other agencies involved.

- To ensure that the appropriate approval is obtained for the moving of the dead baby.
- To act as advocate for the parents, if they are unable to communicate clearly.

Checklist for medical staff

- Call Senior Paediatric and Senior Anaesthetic staff prior to the arrival of the baby.
- Take the baby to the resuscitation room for assessment.
- The parents are taken to a quiet room where they can stay as long as necessary.
- Examine the baby and conduct resuscitation according to European Resuscitation Council guidelines.
- Confirm death.
- Sympathetically interview the parents about their baby's health. Use the baby's first name when talking to the parents. Use present tense before death is certified.
- Record details of history, examination and resuscitation of the child.
- Ensure that all investigation procedures are carried out in accordance with the local protocol.
- After death is confirmed, remove drips, endotracheal tube etc.
- Clothe and wrap the baby and take him/her to the parents to see and hold as long as they desire.
- Explain to the parents what you think is the cause of death.
- Explain to the parents that the police and coroner have a duty to investigate all sudden and unexpected deaths, and that they will have to make a statement to the police, who may want to examine the baby's room and bedding.
- Offer support and practical advice about the post-mortem examination, funeral arrangements, cremations, registration of death etc. will be needed. It is important this information is given in written form.
- Ensure that a suitable person is looking after dependent relatives or other children at home.
- Ask whether parents would like to see a chaplain/minister, or have their baby blessed.
- If the mother is breast feeding, offer advice on suppression of lactation/expression of milk.
- Take photograph of baby for parents, offer a lock of hair or a hand/foot print, if facilities are available.
- Arrange transport to the mortuary.
- Ensure that parents have safe transport home.
- Give parents copies of 'Information for Parents' leaflet and local support contact telephone number(s).
- Explain that a paediatrician or General Practitioner will contact them in the next few days with the preliminary results of the post-mortem.
- Inform the Consultant Paediatrician.
- Inform the General Practitioner.
- Inform the Community Child Health Department or equivalent to cancel surveillance and immunization appointments.

- Inform Medical Records and cancel outpatient appointments.
- Inform Paediatric Social Work Department (if offering support in this situation).
- Inform the coroner of the death.

Further reading

Finlay FO, Rudd PT. Current concepts of the aetiology of SIDS. *British Journal of Hospital Medicine*, 1993; **49:** 727–32.

Brooks JG. Unraveling the mysteries of sudden infant death syndrome. *Current Opinion in Pediatrics*, 1993; **5:** 266–72.

SYNCOPE

Syncope is sudden, brief loss of consciousness due to transient impairment of cerebral circulation, from whatever cause, usually occurring in the absence of organic brain disease or cerebrovascular disease. Typically the onset is sudden or develops over a few seconds with blurred vision, dizziness, cold extremities and sweating. If aware of the symptoms the patient may take evasive action and sit or lie down. If however, venous return remains impaired, muscle twitching and convulsions (*convulsive syncope*) may occur.

Syncope accounts for 1–3% of A&E attendances and 3–6% of hospital attendances. In 30–50% of cases no cause is found despite extensive investigations. Subsequent case–fatality is low but morbidity remains high with about half having one or more recurrence.

Causes

The causes of syncope include:

1. Inappropriate vasodilatation

- *Vasovagal syncope* – the name given by Sir Thomas Lewis to the common type of fainting and results from vagal slowing of the heart and decreased vasomotor tone. It is usually triggered by pain or emotion.
- *Carotid sinus syncope* – the hypersensitive carotid sinus baroceptors cause vagal stimulation from either neck movement or mild pressure which may cause cardiac arrest and syncope.
- *Micturition syncope.*
- *Orthostatic hypotension* – may occur with sympathetic degeneration associated with *diabetic neuropathy, Parkinson's disease, Addison's disease* and *Shy–Drager syndrome.* A degree of postural hypotension occurs with advancing age and is exacerbated by *drugs* (hypotensives, diuretics, phenothiazines, benzodiazepines).

2. Hypovolaemia. It is vital to exclude acute blood loss as a cause of syncope. Sources of haemorrhage to be considered include the gastrointestinal tract, ruptured ectopic pregnancy, a leaking aortic aneurysm, or aortic dissection.

3. Cardiac syncope.

- *Arrhythmias* – such as bradycardias associated with heart block (Stokes Adams attacks) or sick sinus syndrome or tachycardias.
- *Myocardial ischaemia* or myocardial infarct may present with syncope.

4. Obstruction to ventricular emptying. Causes such as aortic stenosis and hypertrophic cardiomyopathy may be responsible.

5. Reduced ventricular filling occurs in cough syncope (seen in the chronic chest patient with the raised intrathoracic pressure during violent coughs), atrial myxoma and pulmonary embolism.

The differential diagnosis of syncope includes:

- Epilepsy.
- Hypoglycaemia.
- Transient ischaemic attacks.
- Labyrinthine disorders.

History and examination

The most important factor is determining the cause of syncope. In the younger patient with a history suggestive of a simple faint no further investigation is warranted. In the older patient the diagnosis should be made with caution as cardiac causes are more likely. In the elderly drugs are commonly behind the cause.

- The *lying and standing blood pressures* should be taken. Postural hypotension is shown by a significant fall in blood pressure or rise in pulse rate as the patient moves from lying to sitting (≥10 mmHg or ≥20 beats/min) or standing (≥15 mmHg or ≥ 30 beats/min).
- In all cases, except the simple faint an *ECG* is mandatory. This may reveal myocardial ischaemia, infarction, pulmonary embolism or arrhythymia, or alternatively an underlying conduction defect such as short PR interval (pre-excitation syndromes) or a long QT interval (familial syndromes).

  During ECG monitoring carotid sinus massage may reveal carotid sinus hypersensitivity. This is best done with the patient lying at 45° for 5 seconds, on one side only, and with resuscitation facilities available.

- *Full blood count* to exclude anaemia or blood loss.
- *Serum electrolytes* may indicate dehydration or Addison's disease.
- *CXR* might show evidence of cardiac disease or pulmonary embolism.
- *Further investigations* – a useful test is a *24-hour continuous ambulatory electrocardiograph* since in patients with cardiac syncope, sudden death occurs within one year in approximately 20% of cases.

Further reading

Gilliatt RW. Syncope. In: The Oxford Textbook of Medicine. Second Edition. Pp. 21.51–21.53.

Related topics of interest

Cerebrovascular syndrome – acute (p. 85); Diabetic emergencies (p. 117)

TETANUS

R J Evans

Tetanus is characterized by muscular rigidity and spasms and is induced by the exotoxin, *tetanosplasmin*, released by the bacterium that grows anaerobically at the site of injury. Between 1984 and 1995 there were 145 cases of tetanus in England and Wales. The highest risk groups are the elderly (53% aged over 65 years) and women.

Clostridium tetani is a motile, Gram-positive, spore-forming bacillus which thrives within the bowel of herbivores and humans, and the tetanus spores are located within contaminated soil. The organism is non-invasive and spores of *C. tetani* are introduced into a wound, such as a puncture wound, burn, ulcer, umbilical stump (results in neonatal tetanus) or even an unnoticed trivial wound.

The incubation period (4–21 days) is followed by a prodrome of fever, malaise and headache followed by non-specific stiffness, dysphagia. The patient classically develops *trismus* (the patient cannot close his mouth), *risus sardonicus* (grin-like position of hypertonic facial muscles), and *opisothotonus* (arched body, with hyperextended neck). *Spasms* may be initially induced by movement, noise etc. but later are spontaneous.

Routine tetanus immunization began in 1961, thus individuals born before that year will not have been immunized in infancy. After a tetanus-prone injury such individuals will therefore require a full course of immunization unless it has previously been given, as for instance in the armed services.

Immunized individuals respond rapidly to a subsequent single injection of adsorbed tetanus vaccine, even after an interval of years.

For wounds not in the above categories, such as clean cuts, antitetanus immunoglobulin should *not* be given.

Patients with impaired immunity who suffer a tetanus-prone wound may not respond to vaccine and may therefore require antitetanus immunoglobulin in addition. HIV positive individuals *should* be immunized against tetanus in the absence of contraindications.

Prognosis

- With full ITU support mortality is 11%.
- The main causes of death are *respiratory failure, pneumonia, septicaemia, cardiovascular instability* and *pulmonary embolism.*
- Other complications include *autonomic dysfunction* and *fractures/dislocations* (secondary to muscle spasms).

Treatment

1. ***Specific***
   - Wound debridement.
   - Intravenous human tetanus immunoglobulin (150 IU/kg at multiple sites).
   - Intravenous benzylpenicillin.
2. ***General***
   - Drug treatment alone with diazepam, phenobarbitone or chlorpromazine.
   - Total paralysis regime.

3. ***Vaccination.*** An attack of tetanus does not provide immunity and thus vaccination is required.

Prevention

1. ***Tetanus vaccine and adsorbed tetanus vaccine.*** Immunization is provided by *active immunization* and protects by stimulating the production of antitoxin that provided immunity against the effects of the toxin.

- *Tetanus toxoid* is prepared by treating a cell-free preparation of the toxin with formaldehyde. When used as a vaccine it is usually adsorbed onto an adjuvant, either aluminium phosphate or aluminium hydroxide.
- Plain vaccines are no longer supplied as they are less immunogenic and have no advantage in terms of reaction rates.
- Vaccines should be stored at 2 8° C. Protect from light. Do not freeze.
- The *dose* is 0.5 ml given by intramuscular or deep subcutaneous injection.
- The *immunization schedule* of infants includes primary immunization which consists of three doses starting at two months with an interval of one month between each dose, followed by a booster dose given prior to school entry and for those aged 15–19 years or before leaving school.

2. ***Treatment of a tetanus prone wound.*** The following are considered tetanus-prone wounds:

- Any wound or burn sustained more than 6 hours before surgical treatment of the wound or burn.
- Any wound or burn at any interval after injury that shows one or more of the following characteristics:
  (a) A significant degree of devitalized tissue.
  (b) Puncture-type wound.
  (c) Contact with soil or manure likely to harbour tetanus organisms.
  (d) Clinical evidence of sepsis.

- Thorough surgical toilet of all wounds is essential. The aim is to remove all contaminants that could contain tetanus spores and all dead or badly damaged tissue that could provide an anaerobic environment.

Specific anti-tetanus prophylaxis

Immunization status	*Type of wound (clean)*	*Type of wound (tetanus prone)*
Last of 3 dose course, or reinforcing dose within last 10 years	Nil	Nil – A dose of human tetanus immunoglobulin may be given if risk of infection is considered especially high, e.g. contamination with stable manure
Last of 3 dose course or reinforcing dose more than 10 years previously	A reinforcing dose of adsorbed vaccine	A reinforcing dose of adsorbed vaccine plus a dose of human tetanus immunoglobulin
Not immunized or immunization status not known with certainty	A full 3 dose course of adsorbed vaccine	A full 3 dose course of vaccine, plus a dose of tetanus immunoglobulin in a different site

3. *Adverse reactions*

- *Local reactions*, such as pain, redness and swelling at the injection site, commonly occur and persist for several days. They are more common if booster injections are given too frequently.
- *General reactions* which are uncommon include headache, lethargy, malaise, myalgia and pyrexia.
- *Acute anaphylaxis* and *urticaria* occasionally occur.
- *Peripheral neuropathy is rare.*
- *Persistent nodules* have been reported if the injection is not given deeply enough.

4. *Contraindications*

- Tetanus vaccine should not be given to an individual suffering from an *acute febrile illness* except in the presence of a tetanus-prone wound. Minor infections without fever or systemic upset are not reasons to postpone immunization.
- Immunization should not proceed in individuals who have had an *anaphylactic reaction* to a previous dose.
- *Pregnancy* is not a contraindication.

5. *Human tetanus immunoglogulin*

- *Prevention.* Intramuscular injection of 250 or 500 iu, if more than 24 hours have elapsed since injury, or there is risk of heavy contamination or following burns. Available in 1 ml ampoules containing 250 iu.

- *Treatment.* 150 iu/kg given in multiple sites.

Further reading

Department of Health, Welsh Office, Scottish Office Department of Health, DHSS (Northern Ireland). Immunisation against Infectious Disease. HMSO, London, 1996.

Related topic of interest

Anaphylaxis (p. 38)

THORACIC TRAUMA

Chest injuries cause 25% of trauma deaths. *Hypoxia* is the main complication of chest injury and may result from reduced blood volume, failure to ventilate the lungs, a ventilation/perfusion mismatch or mechanical obstruction to the lung/chest wall. Occult *haemorrhage*, which may be massive, can occur within the thoracic cavity.

The treatment of chest injuries follows the ABCs and in particular includes needle thoracentesis, tube thoracostomy, and controlled ventilation. Only 10% of blunt chest injuries require definitive surgery, and 15–30% of penetrating chest injuries require open thoracotomy.

Life-threatening injuries detectable in the primary survey

1. Airway obstruction

2. Tension pneumothorax. Air accumulates progressively when a 'one-way-valve' air leak occurs within the pleural space and collapses the lung compressing the mediastinum and thus compromises venous return and cardiac output.

The most common cause of a tension pneumothorax is mechanical ventilation with positive pressure ventilation in a patient with a pleural injury.

Patients with a pneumothorax undergoing positive-pressure ventilation are particularly at risk of developing a tension pneumothorax.

Tension pneumothorax is a clinical diagnosis and treatment should not be delayed awaiting radiological confirmation.

Signs of hypoxia and shock will be present. Specific findings include:

- Ipsilateral decreased air entry and hyperresonance;
- tracheal deviation away from the side of the pneumothorax;
- cardiovascular collapse with distended neck veins;
- cyanosis (late).

Treatment. Immediate needle *thoracocentesis* by inserting a large bore needle into the second intercostal space in the mid-clavicular line of the affected haemothorax. This converts it into a simple pneumothorax and is then followed by definitive treatment with the insertion of a chest tube into the fifth intercostal space (nipple level) between the anterior and mid-axillary line.

3. Open pneumothorax ('Sucking chest wound'). Large defects of the chest wall which remain open. If the opening is larger than approximately two thirds of the diameter of the trachea air passes preferentially through this opening as it follows the path of least resistance. Effective ventilation is therefore impaired.

Treatment. Close defect with a sterile occlusive dressing that is taped on three sides. This provides a flutter-type valve effect. A chest tube should be placed remote from the wound as soon as is practical. Definitive surgical closure of the defect is usually necessary.

4. *Massive haemothorax.* Accumulation of massive amount of blood (more than 1500 ml) in the haemothorax, more commonly associated with penetrating trauma. Will result in hypoxia and hypovolaemia. Ipsilateral absent breath sounds and dullness to percussion in association with shock are the physical findings.

Treatment

- Rapid volume resuscitation.
- Chest tube insertion.

If initial haemorrhage of 1500 ml is immediately evacuated, or continued rate of blood loss of 200 ml/hour for 2–4 hours, or patient's physiological status then consideration for thoracotomy.

5. *Flail chest.* Paradoxical movement of the flail segment occurs which may be masked by splinting, secondary to muscle spasm. Hypoventilation, hypoxia, pulmonary shunting and restricted chest wall movement all contribute to the patient's altered physiological status. Arterial blood gases need to be repeated.

Treatment. High flow oxygen, analgesia (including thoracic epidural), and consider for ventilation.

6. *Cardiac tamponade.* Commonly due to penetrating trauma. Beck's triad of hypotension, distended neck veins, and muffled heart sounds are rarely seen.

Other signs include tachycardia, pulsus paradoxus, electrical alternans (on the ECG). Kussmaul's signs (a rise in venous pressure with inspiration when breathing spontaneously) is associated with tamponade.

Cardiac tamponade should be considered in the differential diagnosis of pulseless electrical activity.

A high index of clinical suspicion is required. *Echocardiography* will provide rapid confirmation of fluid within the pericardium.

Treatment

- *Pericardiocentesis* with ECG monitoring and a subxyphoid approach will temporarily decompress the tamponade. This should only be considered in patients unresponsive to resuscitative efforts.
- A subxyphoid pericardial window or emergency thoracotomy and pericardiotomy can be performed only by an appropriate surgeon.

  A resuscitative thoracotomy may be indicated in patients with penetrating thoracic injuries who arrive pulseless but with myocardial electrical activity. Patients with blunt injuries who arrive with pulseless electrical activity are not candidates for resuscitative thoracotomy.

Potentially life threatening injuries detectable in the secondary survey

A further detailed chest examination is undertaken, an *erect chest X-ray* if possible, *arterial blood gases*, and an *ECG*.

1. *Pulmonary contusion.* Commonly seen after chest trauma and manifests as hypoxia, which worsens with time. Maintain oxygenation, and monitor respiratory function. If the patient is unable to maintain adequate ventilation then intubation and mechanical ventilation is necessary. Associated withflail chest.

2. ***Myocardial contusion.*** Underdiagnosed after blunt trauma. ECG (sinus tachycardia, ST segment changes, bundle branch block and arrhythmias), echocardiogram and myocardial enzyme changes should be sought. Arrhythmias may be found. May have associated valve damage and cardiac chamber rupture.

3. ***Aortic rupture.*** Complete ruptures are a cause of early death. Partial tears tend to occur at the level of the ligamentum arteriosum, and initial survival is dependent on a contained haematoma or a false aneurysm.

Features of CXR which suggest an aortic rupture include:

- Widened mediastinum;
- fractures of first and second ribs or scapula;
- deviation of trachea to the right;
- pleural cap or apical cap;
- obliteration of the aortic knob;
- deviation of oesophagus (nasogastric tube) to the right;
- left haemothorax.

Angiography, trans-oesophageal echocardiography or CT may further image the lesion.

Early surgery is warranted. The treatment is either primary repair or resection of the injured area and grafting.

4. ***Traumatic diaphragmatic rupture.*** More common the left side, often missed.

A CXR may reveal an elevated hemidiaphragm, or gastric contents in the chest, confirmation by the nasogastric tube in the thoracic cavity or peritoneal lavage fluid exiting from a chest tube or by contrast studies.

Undiagnosed diaphragmatic injuries can result in pulmonary compromise or entrapment and strangulation of peritoneal contents. If missed a diaphragmatic hernia will remain. Blunt trauma is associated with large tears, penetrating trauma with small tears.

Treatment is surgical repair.

5. ***Larynx, trachea, or bronchus disruption.*** Frequently fatal. Rigid bronchoscopy isthe definitive investigation.

6. ***Oesophageal trauma.*** Usually as a result of penetrating trauma. Surgical repair is essential, otherwise mediastinitis will result.

7. ***Subcutaneous emphysema.*** May result from airway injury, lung injury, or blast injury.

8. ***Traumatic asphyxia.*** Associated with facial and upper chest plethora with petechial haemorrhages. May result in cerebral oedema.

9. ***Simple pneumothorax.*** Requires treatment with a chest drain. Must be decompressed prior to positive pressure ventilation or air travel as otherwise at risk of developing a tension pneumothorax.

10. Haemothorax. Owing to haemorrhage from a lung laceration, intercostal or internal mammary vessel. Requires drainage via a large bore chest drain and will require no further intervention. If more than 1l drains or persistent drainage of more than 200 ml per hour for 4 hours then surgical intervention may prove necessary.

11. Rib fractures

- *Upper ribs (1–3)* associated with a 35% mortality and require surgical consultation as high risk of associated injury.
- *Middle ribs (4–9)* most likely to result in haemothorax and/or pneumothorax.
- *Lower ribs (10–12)* at high of hepatic and splenic injury.

Treatment consists of pain relief (intercostal block, epidural anaesthesia or systemic analgesics) to allow adequate ventilation and prevent complications of atelectasis and pneumonia.

Further reading

American College of Surgeons. *ATLS Manual.* Chapter 4, Thoracic Trauma, 1997, p. 125–156.

Related topics of interest

Abdominal trauma (p. 4); Genitourinary trauma (p. 164); Interhospital transfer (p. 194); Maxillofacial injury (p. 226); Spine and spinal cord trauma (p. 307)

TRANSFUSION REACTIONS

A confidential reporting system for major transfusion events – serious hazards of transfusion (SHOT) – was launched in 1996. Although blood transfusion is generally extremely safe it does have several potentially fatal hazards. All staff handling blood should be aware of the importance of correct identity of sample patient and blood bag at all stages.

The SHOT report revealed 366 cases over a 24-month period:

- 52% of these were related to incorrect blood/component transfused.
- 15% related to acute transfusion reactions.
- 14% delayed transfusion reaction.
- 8% acute lung injury.
- 6% post-transfusion purpura.
- 3% transfusion transmitted infections.
- 2% graft v. host disease.

There were 22 deaths from all causes and 81 cases of major morbidity.

Acute haemolytic or bacterial transfusion reactions

1. Clinical characteristics. Reactions with high morbidity may occur after only a small volume of blood has been transfused. They may result from acute haemolysis (e.g. from ABO mismatch) or, more rarely, bacterial contamination. It can be difficult to tell these apart immediately. In an unconscious patient hypotension, bleeding due to DIC and oliguria may be the only signs. ABO mismatched transfusions are usually due to human error – either at removal of the sample from the patient, in the lab, or when the blood is given.

- Usually occur soon after transfusion started.
- Patient feels unwell, agitated.
- Pain at infusion site, back pain.
- Shortness of breath.
- Fever, rigors.
- Hypotension.
- Bleeding from wounds or venepuncture sites.
- Haemoglobinuria.

2. Action

- Discontinue transfusion immediately, and remove the giving set. Leave the Iv. cannula in and attach a bag of saline.
- Check blood unit number and patient's ID against blood issue sheet.
- Take blood for:

FBC, plasma haemoglobin	(1 × EDTA tube)
Repeat grouping, DCT	(1 × Xmatch tube)
Clotting screen (including fibrinogen)	(1 × citrated tube)
U&Es, LFTs	(1 × clotted tube)
Blood cultures.	

- Resuscitate patient promptly – include broad-spectrum antibiotics. Consider immediate transfer to ITU.
- Notify blood bank and on-call haematologist immediately.
- Forward blood bags and giving set to microbiology initially for investigation.
- Monitor urine output and ECG (NB hyperkalaemia). Repeat FBC, clotting and U&Es 2–4 hourly until stable.

Anaphylaxis

1. ***Clinical characteristics.*** Bronchospasm and circulatory collapse, which may occur soon after trans-fusion commences. May be seen in IgA deficient patients reacting to transfused IgA.

2. ***Action***

- Discontinue transfusion immediately and remove the giving set. Leave the Iv. cannula in, and attach a bag of saline.
- Maintain airway and give oxygen.
- Give:
  Epinephrine (Adrenaline) 0.5 i.m. repeated every 15 min as necessary.
  Chlorpheniramine 10–20 mg slow i.v.
  Salbutamol by nebulizer.
- Notify blood bank and contact the haematology team.
- If the patient is IgA deficient any further transfusion must be planned carefully.

Non-haemolytic febrile transfusion reactions (NHFTR)

1. ***Clinical characteristics***

- Usually occur >30 min after starting transfusion.
- Patient feels fairly well, may be shivering.
- Temperature usually <38.5°C.
- BP normal.

2. ***Action***

- Stop transfusion and assess the possibility that this may be a more serious reaction.
- If no features of a more serious reaction restart transfusion at a slower rate.
- Consider the use of Paracetamol.

Minor febrile reactions are common, and can usually be dealt with by attending medical staff. Haematology advice should be sought if the reactions are recurrent, or if a more severe reaction is suspected. Hydrocortisone should not be given routinely before transfusions.

Allergic reactions

Allergic reactions are also common, and usually consist of urticaria and itch, which may begin shortly after the transfusion starts. They usually resolve if the transfusion is slowed and oral chlorpheniramine is given. No further action is indicated if there are no features of a more serious reaction.

Fluid overload

May occur, particularly in elderly patients or those with poor cardiac function, if too much fluid is given too quickly. Usually presents as respiratory distress secondary to pulmonary oedema. Treatment usually includes i.v. frusemide and oxygen. Oral frusemide (e.g. 20 mg) can be given with alternate bags of blood to elderly patients as prophylaxis.

Transfusion-related acute lung injury (TRALI)

1. ***Clinical characteristics.*** Lung injury may result following the infusion of plasma or plasma-containing blood components, due to the interaction of donor antibodies with recipient white cells (reactions between recipient plasma and donor white cells may also occur). They may resemble ARDS and may occur from 30 min to 4 days post-transfusion.

- Fever.
- Cough.
- Shortness of breath.
- CXR shows perihilar nodules and lower lung field shadows.

2. ***Action.*** Treat as for ARDS, with respiratory support as appropriate.

- Notify blood bank and contact haematology team to plan investigation and management.

Delayed haemolytic transfusion reactions (DHTR)

1. ***Clinical characteristics***

- Usually occur 5–10 days after transfusion.
- Patient may be febrile.
- Unexplained drop in haemoglobin.
- Jaundice, urobilinogenuria.

2. ***Action***

- Request FBC, U&Es, LFTs, DCT, red cell antibody screen.
- Notify blood bank and contact haematology team to plan management.

Transfusion associated graft-versus-host-disease (TA-GvHD)

1. ***Clinical characteristics.*** Transfusion of unirradiated blood or platelets to patients who are either immunocompromised or have a similar HLA type to the donor can cause a severe form of graft-versus-host disease with high mortality. This usually occurs 1–6 weeks after transfusion.

- Unexplained fever.
- Rash.
- Abnormal liver function.
- Diarrhoea.
- Pancytopenia.

2. ***Action.*** Notify blood bank and contact haematology team to plan management.

Post-transfusion purpura (PTP)

1. Clinical characteristics. Immune-mediated fall in platelet count precipitated by transfusion. Usually occurs 5–10 days post-transfusion.

2. Action. Notify blood bank and contact haematology team to plan management.

Transfusion-transmitted virus infections

1. Clinical characteristics. Now rare, but notification is important if this occurs to trace the donor. Symptoms depend on the virus, and may include jaundice, malaise, rash. Usually occurs weeks or months post transfusion.

2. Action.

- Notify blood bank immediately.
- Refer as appropriate for management of viral infection.

Iron overload

Patients on chronic transfusion regimes are prone to iron accumulation. Chelation therapy with desferrioxamine may be necessary.

TRAUMA SCORING AND INJURY SCALING

Reliable, validated methods to measure the severity of injury allow physicians to:

1. Quantify the extent of the damage.
2. Aid triage.
3. Predict outcome.
4. Audit care for quality assurance and research.

Scoring methods measure anatomical and/or physiological parameters.

Physiological scoring

Glasgow Coma Scale (GCS) is a widely accepted measure of assessing the severity of brain damage after head injury.

It correlates well with the *Glasgow Outcome Scale*, and forms part of the *Revised Trauma Score*. The GCS has been widely accepted as a reliable scale yet inexperienced or untrained users still make errors when using it. Its use in children under 4 years of age requires modification.

Glasgow Coma Scale

Eye opening	
Spontaneous	4
To speech stimulus	3
To pain stimulus	2
None	1
Best motor response	
Obeys	6
Localizes	5
Withdraws	4
Abnormal flexion*	3
Extensor response	2
No response	1
Best verbal response	
Orientated	5
Confused conversations	4
Inappropriate words	3
Incomprehensible sounds	2
No response	1
Glasgow coma score (total)	3–15

* abnormal elbow and wrist posturing without extension of the elbow.

The Children's Coma Scale (<4 years)

Eyes		
Open spontaneously		4
React to speech		3
React to pain		2
No response		1
Best motor response		
Spontaneous or obeys verbal command		6
Localizes pain		5
Withdraws to pain		4
Abnormal flexion to pain (decorticate)		3
Abnormal extension to pain (decerebrate)		2
No response		1
Best verbal response		
Smiles, orientated to sounds, follows objects, interacts		5
Crying	*Interacts*	
Consolable	Inappropriate	4
Inconsistently consolable	Moaning	3
Inconsolable	Irritable	2
No response	No response	1

Trauma score

The Trauma Score (TS) is based on five parameters:

- Glasgow Coma Scale.
- Respiratory rate.
- Respiratory expansion.
- Systolic blood pressure.
- Capillary refill.

The variables are assigned weighted points that are summed to give the TS. This has a range from 1 (worse) to 16 (normal). The TS is used as a triage tool and accurately predicts the outcome from severe injuries. Patients with a TS of less than or equal to 12 are recommended for transfer to a trauma centre as this level carries an average mortality of 10%.

A TS of 3 or less is valuable in identifying patients for who prolonged resuscitation is futile.

Revised trauma score

The Revised Trauma Score includes GCS, systolic blood pressure and respiratory rate. Two versions exist:

1. Triage Revised Trauma Score (T-RTS). Useful for the rapid identification of severely injured patients on arrival to hospital.

2. Revised Trauma Score (RTS). The RTS is a weighted sum of coded variable values and yields a more accurate outcome prediction for patients with serious head injuries than the TS.

Revised Trauma Score

	Coded × weight value	= score
Respiratory rate (breaths/min):		
10–29	4	
>29	3	
6–9	2	0.2908 ×----------
1–5	1	
0	0	
Systolic blood pressure (mmHg):		
>89	4	
76–89	3	
50–75	2	0.7326 ×----------
1–49	1	
0	0	
Glasgow Coma Scale:		
13–15	4	
9–12	3	
6–8	2	0.9368 ×----------
4–5	1	
3	0	
Total = revised trauma score:		----------

Anatomical scoring

This information is available from clinical signs, investigations, operative findings and in fatalities, the post-mortem examination.

1. Abbreviated Injury Scale (AIS). The Abbreviated Injury Scale (AIS) was developed and published in 1971 and undergoes regular revision. Every injury is assigned a code based on its anatomical site, nature and severity. Injuries are grouped by body region.

AIS code	*Description*
1	Minor.
2	Moderate.
3	Serious (non-life threatening).
4	Severe (life-threatening–survival probable).
5	Critical (survival uncertain).
6	Unsurvivable (with current treatment).

The AIS enables ranking of injury severity and correlates with patient outcome but a major disadvantage is that because it codes individual injuries, it cannot be adjusted for multiple injuries.

2. Injury Severity Score (ISS). The AIS can be used to derive the Injury Severity Score (ISS). The ISS provides a valid numerical measure of the overall severity of injury in patients with multiple injuries and correlates with mortality, morbidity and other measures such as length of hospital stay. The ISS has been validated for use with blunt and penetrating injuries in adults and also for use in children over the age of 12 years.

Every injury is given an AIS code and classified into one of the six body regions.

Body regions used in ISS:

- Head and neck.
- Face.
- Chest.
- Abdominal/pelvic contents.
- Extremities/pelvic girdle.
- External, i.e. skin and burns.

The ISS is calculated by summation of the squares of the highest AIS codes in each of the three most severely injured body regions. The maximum ISS is 75 [(5 × 5) + (5 × 5) + (5 × 5)]. Any injury coded AIS = 6 automatically converts the ISS to 75.

The ISS correlates closely with mortality and is the 'gold standard' for anatomical coding of injury severity. An ISS of 16 or more signifies major trauma with an average predicted mortality of more than 10%.

The effect of age on the outcome of injury has been incorporated into the ISS by Bull using probit analysis to derive LD_{50} values for different age-groups.

TRISS methodology

1. Trauma Score Injury Severity Score. Trauma audit using TRISS has been undertaken prospectively in the UK to show that specialized units can improve outcome.

The TRISS method estimates *the probability of patient survival based on the regression equation* and takes into account:

- Patient age.
- The severity of anatomical injury as measured by the ISS.
- The physiological status of the patient on admission based on the Revised Trauma Score.
- The type of injury (blunt or penetrating).

2. Preliminary method. Unexpected deaths or survivors can be identified by plotting the RTS and ISS for patients on a *PRE-chart.*

The *Ps 50 isobar* represents the 50% probability of survival of the baseline normal population, whilst the patients are represented by a symbol depicting outcome: L for live, D for dead.

Unexpected survivors with a Ps less than 50% (L symbols above the isobar) and *unexpected deaths* with a Ps greater than 50% (D symbols below the isobar) are identified for further study.

Definitive method – this compares outcome and the patient mix regarding severity of injury in different hospitals with the MTOS 'norm' data.

The Z statistic is a measure that can be used to test whether the observed number of survivors in a specific trauma population is significantly different from what would be expected based on the Major Trauma Outcome Study norms. Values greater than +1.96 or less than −1.96 indicate a significant difference ($P < 0.05$) from predicted, with greater or fewer survivors respectively.

The W statistic provides perspective on the clinical relevance of the Z score. A positive W value is the number of survivors more than expected from the norm predictions per 100 patients analysed.

The M statistic evaluates the match of injury severity between the study group and the MTOS baseline group. Values range from 0 to 1 and the closer to 1 the better the match of injury severity.

Further reading

Spence MT *et al.*. Trauma audit – the use of TRISS. *Health Trends*, 1988; **20:** 94–7.

Yates DW *et al.*. Preliminary analysis of the care of injured patients in 33 British hospitals: first report of the United Kingdom major trauma outcome study. *British Medical Journal*, 1992; **305:** 737–40.

Related topics of interest

Baby check (p. 60); Head injury (p. 173)

UROLOGICAL CONDITIONS

The cardinal symptoms of acute urological conditions are pain, haematuria, retention of urine and rarely priapism. The common conditions accounting for these symptoms are stone, urinary tract infection, testicular torsion, prostatic obstruction and malignancy.

Pain

Pain is generally located in the loin or testicle (or groin). Loin pain is usually due to infection (pyelonephritis) or stone. Other causes of loin pain, e.g. aneurysm, testicular torsion or ovarian pathology should be excluded by examination and where necessary ultrasound examination.

Haematuria

Haematuria may be painful or painless. As a rule any adult presenting with haematuria where a benign cause cannot be excluded should be referred to the urology clinic for investigation to excluded malignancy. Such investigation will usually require imaging of the renal tract (IVU or renal ultrasound and plain X-ray) and cystoscopy. Similarly all children presenting with haematuria required follow up. Haematuria is often classified into initial stream, whole stream or terminal. In practice this classification does little to aid diagnosis or management. It should be remembered that haematuria may be the presenting complaint in medical as well as surgical conditions (e.g. nephritis).

Retention of urine

In men this is commonly caused by prostatic outflow obstruction. There is usually a long preceding history of progressive difficulty in passing urine.

Retention of urine is uncommon in women and never due to urethral obstruction. Causes include faecal impaction and pelvic tumours (including the pregnant uterus).

In children urinary retention may be secondary to faecal impaction or in boys to phimosis (either secondary to trauma from forced retraction of the prepuce or balanitis xerotica obliterans). Catheterization is rarely required. The child may require admission for management of the underlying cause. The temptation to manage this condition in the A&E department should be avoided as it will usually result in unnecessary upset to the child.

In all cases of urinary retention a neurological cause should be considered and actively excluded by detailed neurological examination including rectal examination.

Priapism

This is persistent erection of the penis. Causes include:

- Intracorporeal injection of papaverine.
- Malignancy (usually leukaemia).

- Sickle cell disease.
- Spinal cord trauma.

It is essential to refer cases of priapism early to a urologist as intracorporeal thrombosis leading to fibrosis may occur within 12 hours. Treatment options include decompression of the corpora cavernosa either with a biopsy needle or surgically.

Stone

Renal tract stone usually presents with severe loin pain radiating down to the groin. It may be associated with haematuria. Initial management in the A&E department should be centred round the exclusion of other causes including testicular torsion, ovarian pathology and aortic aneurysm. An ultrasound examination of the abdomen may be required to exclude aneurysm as not all are palpable.

Pain should be treatment with parenteral or rectal diclofenac (or in patients in whom NSAIDs are contraindicated parenteral opiates).

The diagnosis is best made by performing an immediate IVU. This will confirm the diagnosis and show the level of the stone. If an IVU cannot be performed immediately then a KUB should be done. In a proportion of patients referred for elective IVU the stone will have passed before the IVU is done. The baseline KUB may well help to establish the diagnosis in such cases.

If diclofenac controls the pain and there are no other reasons for admission (e.g. obstruction) then the patient can be discharged with an out-patient appointment.

Urinary tract infection

Urinary tract infections (UTI) are common in women. This is attributed to the short length of the urethra. In women it is recommended that if more than three UTIs occur in any one year investigation is warranted. In men and children it is recommended that any episode of proven UTI should be investigated. Urine should be taken for stick analysis and culture to establish the organism and sensitivities. Once urine has been taken an appropriate antibiotic is prescribed and follow up arranged as appropriate.

In children if a UTI is suspected anti-microbial therapy should not be commenced until adequate cultures have been obtained to establish the diagnosis and causative organism. All children with UTI required follow up investigations looking for underlying structural causes of the infection and for the presence of renal scarring.

The majority of patients with UTI can be managed without admission. Exceptions include the very young (generally children under one year are admitted as the organism is likely to have spread via the bloodstream), the elderly where the infection has precipitated an acute confusional state and those who are otherwise compromised (e.g. diabetics).

Testicular torsion

This is most common in teenagers around the time of puberty and young adults. Torsion presents as pain localized to the testicle associated with swelling of the affected testicle. The pain may be accompanied by nausea or vomiting. There may be a history of preceding episodes of pain which have resolved spontaneously. The testicle has a horizontal lie and may be red. Urine examination is usually normal. The differential diagnosis includes torsion of an appendix, testis or epididymitis. In practice it can be difficult to differentiate these conditions clinically. Doppler ultrasound may demonstrate the absence of blood flow in the testis, but may delay surgery. Because of the risk of testicular infarction (which may occur within 6–12 hours of onset of symptoms) it is recommended that any male under the age of 35 years with testicular pain undergoes exploration of the scrotum to exclude torsion. It is usual to fix the normal side at operation as the incidence of subsequent torsion in this is 10%.

Prostatic obstruction

The patient usually presents because of pain. In chronic cases there may be little pain, inability to void being the presenting complaint. Having excluded a neurological cause the obstruction is relieved by inserting a urinary catheter aseptically using local anaesthetic gel. In chronic cases catheterization can lead to haematuria, post-obstruction diuresis or renal failure. All patients catheterized for obstruction require admission for monitoring. If there is any difficulty in passing the catheter force should not be used as this may lead to stricture formation or the creation of a false passage. The patient should be referred to the urology team.

Malignancy

Prostatic cancer commonly presents as outflow obstruction and may be an incidental finding on histology of prostatic chippings following transurethral resection. It may present as a result of lumbar spine pain because of secondary deposits.

Bladder tumours commonly present as an episode of haematuria. Patients may recall only a single episode of haematuria, hence the importance of considering referral of all patients with haematuria for investigation.

Further reading

Blandy J. Urology (5th edn). Oxford, Blackwell Science Ltd, 1998.

Related topics of interest

Genitourinary trauma (p. 164); Gynaecology (p. 168)

WRIST INJURY

Wrist fractures occur at all ages. Frequently the result of a fall onto the outstretched hand, the pattern of injury varies with age. Wrist fractures usually present as an isolated injury. On occasion however they occur in association with a second upper limb fracture. The whole of the upper limb must therefore be examined lest a more serious injury be missed.

Colles' fracture

In 1814 Abraham Colles' described a fracture involving the distal radius within an inch of the wrist joint which is dorsally angulated. It most commonly occurs in elderly women, particularly those with coexisting osteoporosis.

1. Classification. Frykman described an eight stage classification in 1967. This classification is based upon the severity of the fracture and is of some value in predicting outcome. The following summarizes the classification. Odd-numbered types indicate no fracture of the ulna. Even-numbered types indicate an associated distal ulna fracture. Prognosis for functional recovery is worse the higher the number.

- *Type 1 and 2*
  Extra-articular fracture.
- *Type 3 and 4*
  Intra-articular fracture involving the radio-carpal joint.
- *Type 5 and 6*
  Intra-articular fracture involving the distal radio-ulnar joint.
- *Type 7 and 8*
  Intra-articular fracture involving both radio-carpal and distal radio-ulnar joints.

2. Clinical features. The wrist is swollen, painful and tender. In all but the least severe cases there is a classical 'dinner fork' deformity of the dorsum of the wrist due to dorsal angulation of the distal fragment. Bruising may be present.

3. Pathology. The constant feature is a fracture of the distal radius within one inch of the wrist joint. This may be associated with some or all of the following:

- Displacement: radially and/or dorsally of the distal fragment.
- Impaction of the distal fragment.
- Avulsion of the ulna styloid (due to avulsion of the insertion of the triangular ligament of the distal radio-ulnar joint).
- Angulation: ulnar and/or anterior of the distal fragment.
- Torsional deformity of the distal fragment.

4. Diagnosis. The history and examination suggests that a fracture may be present. If a scaphoid fracture is not suspected simple AP and lateral views will allow the diagnosis to be made. In examining the X-rays two features of the normal wrist X-ray should be kept in mind. On the lateral view the articular surface of the radius has a 5–10° forward tilt. In the AP view the radius extends further forward than the ulna.

5. ***Management.*** Most undisplaced or minimally displaced fractures can be managed conservatively in a Colles' plaster. The decision as to whether a fracture required reduction rests as much on the patient's age, and expectations of function as on the radiological appearances. The following factors should suggest the need for reduction:

- Shortening of the radius (seen on the AP view).
- A loss of the normal 5–10° anterior tilt of the articular surface of the radius.
- Significant dorsal or radial displacement.
- There are various means of effecting adequate analgesia for reduction varying from a full general anaesthetic to regional block, local haematoma block and sedation. Local protocols vary.
- The fracture should be immobilized in a Colles' backslab with the wrist flexed and with ulnar deviation. The patient should be referred to the next fracture clinic.

6. ***Complications.*** Swelling. This is most likely to occur in the first 24–48 hours. This is why a backslab is applied for the first day or two. The patient should be advised to return immediately if swelling occurs, particularly if it is associated with pain or numbness. The plaster should be split to the skin and opened out. In severe cases the plaster should be totally removed and reduction repeated at a later stage.

- Mal-union.
- Non-union.
- Stiffness after removal of the plaster. This may persist for some time. The patient is encouraged to mobilize as soon as possible after plaster removal.
- Carpal tunnel syndrome. This may present up to several weeks or months after the injury. Once the diagnosis is confirmed by nerve conduction studies surgical decompression may be required.
- Extensor pollicis longus rupture. This is often delayed. It is thought to be due to compromise to the vascular supply of the tendon at the level of the tuber cle of Lister and results in loss of thumb extension at the interphalangeal joint. It may be treated by tendon transfer if it is causing significant functional impairment.
- Reflex sympathetic dystrophy (Sudek's atrophy). This is said to be due to autonomic dysfunction. It presents in its most extreme form with a painful, stiff, swollen hand. This skin is shiny and dystrophic. X-ray reveals generalized osteoporosis of the bones of the hand. Treatment is often unsatisfactory and includes physiotherapy to encourage mobilization and Guanethidine block or surgical sympathectomy.
- Shoulder hand syndrome.

Smith's fracture

In 1847 Robert Smith described an extra-articular fracture of the distal radius with anterior displacement. The fracture follows a fall onto the flexed wrist and is also known as the reverse Colles' fracture.

1. ***Clinical features.*** This fracture is much less common than the Colles' fracture but the clinical features are similar. Definitive diagnosis is made after careful examination of the standard AP and lateral wrist X-rays.

2. ***Diagnosis.*** Although the characteristic deformity (anterior displacement) is visible on the lateral wrist view, the fracture is often misdiagnosed initially as the far more common Colles' fracture. The most important consideration in looking at the lateral view is to correctly orientate oneself. The volar surface of the wrist is identified by the position of the thumb. The distal fragment of the radius will be seen to be anteriorly displaced as opposed to the posterior displacement of the distal fragment in a Colles' fracture.

3. ***Management.*** These fractures are inherently unstable. If satisfactory closed reduction can be obtained the fracture may be immobilized in an above arm plaster with the forearm in full supination and the wrist extended. Often, however, the fracture slips into an unsatisfactory position and open reduction and internal fixation is required.

4. ***Complications.*** These are similar to those seen in Colles' fracture.

Barton's fracture

In 1838, John Barton described an intra-articular fracture of the distal radius through the anterior portion of the radius, often with displacement of the fragment anteriorly. This fracture is unstable and usually requires open reduction and internal fixation. The complications are as for Colles' fracture.

Scaphoid fracture

See chapter on scaphoid fracture.

Radial styloid fracture

This fracture is intra-articular, but usually minimally displaced. It is generally treated conservatively in a Colles' plaster. If significantly displaced it may require open reduction and internal fixation.

Galeazzi fracture-dislocation

This is a fracture of the radius associated with distal radio-ulnar dislocation. Normally the distal end of the ulna (excluding the ulna styloid) lies just proximal to the radial articular surface. If this normal arrangement is disturbed an associated radial fracture should be considered. X-ray of the entire forearm including wrist and elbow joint should be requested. This fracture requires open reduction and internal fixation.

Carpal fractures and/or dislocations

There are various injuries within this group. They are easy to miss unless the wrist X-ray is carefully examined, paying particular attention to the relationship between the lunate and the radius and other carpal bones on standard wrist views. There are three common patterns:

1. ***Isolated lunate dislocation.*** The lunate is dislocated anteriorly into the carpal tunnel with consequent compression of the median nerve. The dislocation is best seen on the lateral wrist view when the anteriorly displaced lunate can be seen as a crescent moon-shaped body. On the AP view the normal quadrilateral shape of the lunate is triangular. Urgent referral for reduction is required in order to decompress the median nerve.

2. ***Perilunar dislocations.*** The lunate remains in its normal position with respect to the radius. The entirety of the remaining carpus is dislocated posteriorly. Again urgent referral for reduction is required.

3. ***Trans-scaphoid perilunar dislocation.*** This is similar to a perilunar dislocation with the addition of a scaphoid fracture. The lunate and proximal pole of the scaphoid retain their normal relationship with the radius. The remainder of the carpal bones along with the distal fragment of the scaphoid is displaced posteriorly. On the AP view this injury is characterized by widening of the gap between the scaphoid and lunate (the 'missing tooth' or 'Terry Thomas' sign).

Wrist sprain

The diagnosis of wrist sprain is a diagnosis of exclusion. It probably should not be made in the absence of appropriate radiographic exclusion of fracture (but note that scaphoid fracture cannot be excluded on initial X-ray). If there is no suspicion of a scaphoid fracture clinically and standard wrist views are normal, it is appropriate to treat the sprain conservatively for a week. If symptoms persist beyond this period the patient should be reviewed.

Carpal instability

This is ligamentous instability to the carpus following an injury. It is rarely diagnosed on first visit, the pain being attributed to a 'sprain'. On review following conservative management for the sprain the patient will complain of persisting pain, weakness and poor function. Standard AP and lateral views are normal. A lateral view of the wrist with the fist clenched may show the instability. There is no consensus on the best form of treatment. Many less severe cases probably settle with time. Persistent cases, particularly if they are affecting the ability to work should be referred for expert advice.

Further reading

McRae R. *Practical Fracture Management*, 3rd edn. Edinburgh, Churchill Livingstone, 1994.

Related topic of interest

Scaphoid fracture (p. 283)

INDEX